Malignant Lymphoma

Modern Surgical Monographs

Series Consultant
Richard H. Egdahl, M.D.
Professor and Chairman, Department of Survey,
Boston University School of Medicine

Malignant Lymphoma:

NODAL AND EXTRANODAL DISEASES

Yeu-Tsu N. Lee, M.D., F.A.C.S.

*Associate Professor of Surgery, University of Southern California
School of Medicine, Los Angeles, California;
Head Physician, Tumor Surgery Service, L.A. County–U.S.C.
Medical Center, Los Angeles, California;
Formerly Assistant Professor, University of Missouri
School of Medicine, Columbia, Missouri;
Formerly Assistant Scientist and Surgeon, Cancer Research Center and
Ellis Fischel State Cancer Hospital, Columbia, Missouri*

John S. Spratt, Jr., M.S.P.H., M.D., F.A.C.S.

*Chief Surgeon, Ellis Fischel State Cancer Hospital,
Columbia, Missouri;
Director, Cancer Research Center, Columbia, Missouri;
Professor of Surgery, University of Missouri School of Medicine,
Columbia, Missouri;
Lecturer in Surgery, Washington University School of Medicine,
St. Louis, Missouri;
Coordinator for Cancer Control, State of Missouri*

B. Komen, M.D.

GRUNE & STRATTON

A Subsidiary of Harcourt Brace Jovanovich, Publishers

New York and London

Library of Congress Cataloging in Publication Data

Lee, Yeu-Tsu N   1936-
    Malignant lymphoma: nodal and extranodal diseases.

    (Modern surgical monographs)
    Bibliography: p.
    1. Lymphoma. I. Spratt, John S., 1929-   joint
author. II. Title. III. Series.
[DNLM: 1. Lymphoma. WH525 L482m 1974]
RC280.L9L43   616.4'2   73-19919
ISBN 0-8089-0824-3

Grune & Stratton, Inc.
111 Fifth Avenue
New York, New York 10003

Library of Congress Catalog Card Number 73-19919
International Standard Book Number 0-8089-0824-3
Printed in the United States of America

Contents

Preface

In the past decade, great progress has been made in our knowledge of the natural history and treatment of malignant lymphoma, especially Hodgkin's disease. Supravoltage radiotherapy is curative for patients with local and regional lesions and combination chemotherapy has greatly improved the outlook for those with advanced disease. Under these circumstances, why should two surgeons write a book about malignant lymphoma?

Statistically, malignant lymphoma accounted for less than 5 percent of all the cancers in this country. Histologically, Hodgkin's disease can be classified into four subtypes; and non-Hodgkin's lymphoma, more than six. Each subtype has its own pattern of involvement and natural history. Extranodal malignant lymphoma can present as lesions of a great variety of unusual sites, each with its unique clinical manifestations. Such cases offer special challenges and surgeons are more likely to be consulted.

Since the experiences of most physicians, even those who specialize in oncology, are limited to isolated cases, it is difficult for individual clinicians or even institutions to formulate a rational and standardized approach to specific problems. A good scientific guideline to follow when one does not have the answer is to read and ask others. Therefore, in addition to a detailed review of our own clinical experiences of over 30 years at the Ellis Fischel State Cancer Hospital (EFSCH) in Columbia, Missouri, we have incorporated many of the important papers published in the past 10 to 15 years. Many of the data have not been published before. Current literatures, including findings reported in 1973, are reviewed extensively.

The purposes of this book are to present broad and comprehensive views of malignant lymphoma including Hodgkin's disease and non-Hodgkin's lymphomas. Conditions affecting both nodal and extranodal tissues are covered. The contributions of radiation therapy and chemotherapy are emphasized. The changing roles of surgery are discussed in their proper perspective. The radiobiological changes in normal tissues that affect surgical evaluation, decisions and techniques are reviewed in detail. The clinical and pathological aspects of malignant lymphomas involving different organs and systems are presented. The pertinent diagnostic and therapeutic approaches are discussed. It is hoped that the information and references will be of value for students of neoplastic disease in all medical and surgical specialties, but the orientation is primarily toward surgeons.

Since case material presented here are taken from the record of Ellis Fischel State Cancer Hospital, the contribution of all the professional staff members and residents who participated in patient care are gratefully acknowledged. Particular appreciation is expressed to Dr. Jose M. Hori who reviewed all the pathological slides and to Dr. Carlos Say who assisted in abstracting the patients' records. The cooperation of the Social Service Department under the direction of Mrs. Miriam G. Hoag and Record Room personnel under the direction of Mrs. Freda Tarr was vital in gathering follow-up information and making all charts readily available. Mr. Robert Hahn, the Cancer Research Center librarian, provided invaluable service in gathering necessary references and in checking the bibliography lists. Mrs. Linda Wilson contributed to the graphic illustrations and photography. The computer programs for life tables were developed by the Biomathematics unit of the Cancer Research Center under Dr. Francis R. Watson. Mr. Richard Le Duc, chief programmer under Dr. Watson, provided valuable consultations. Many of the statistical tables were compiled by Dr. Jean E. Holt. Mrs. Mary Lou Kaltenbach completed proofreading and final editing. Many secretaries, all hereby acknowledged collectively, contributed to the typing.

During the final stage of preparation of this book, one of the authors (Y.N.L.) spent a year of her sabbatical leave at the Division of Oncology, Department of Surgery, University of California at Los Angeles. The kindness of Dr. William P. Longmire and Dr. Donald L. Morton is much appreciated. We are indebted to the editors and publisher of the American Journal of Roentgenology, Radium Therapy and Nuclear Medicine for their permission to reprint many of the figures used in Chapter 1. Finally, Miss Janet Feller and the staff of Grune & Stratton deserve all the credit for making the final product a reality.

Yeu-Tsu N. Lee
John S. Spratt, Jr.

This investigation was supported in part by Public Health Service Research Grants No. CA-08023 and CA-08018 from the National Cancer Institute and by General Research Support Grant No. FR-05618 from the National Institutes of Health.

Malignant Lymphoma

1

Clinical and Pathological Aspects

INTRODUCTION

The term "malignant lymphoma" is used in this book to cover essentially only two conditions: Hodgkin's disease and other non-Hodgkin's lymphomas. Non-Hodgkin's lymphomas, as used here, include all the diseases formerly called reticulum cell sarcoma, lymphosarcoma, giant follicular lymphoma, lymphoblastoma, and lymphoma, unspecified. Many of these terms are still in common use. The term lymphosarcoma has often been used in a general sense to cover all of the non-Hodgkin's lymphomas. Other conditions specifically excluded here are the leukemias, histiocytosis, multiple myeloma, mycosis fungoides, myeloid metaplasia, polycythemia, and reticuloendotheliosis.

Table 1-1 gives the relative distribution of Hodgkin's disease and non-Hodgkin's lymphoma as reported in the literature. Hodgkin's disease accounted for about 40 percent of the malignant lymphomas. In the past 10 to 15 years, great progress has been made in the diagnosis and treatment of malignant lymphoma, especially Hodgkin's disease (Table 1-2). The End Result Group of the National Cancer Institute has collected information on approximately 18,000 patients with diagnosed lymphoma from 1940 to 1968. The overall 5-year survival rate for Hodgkin's disease has risen from 23 percent for the period 1940–1949 to about 40 percent for 1964–1968 (Shimkin 1973).

Similar to many other diseases, improvement in clinical management and prognosis came only after the basic pathological characteristics had been well defined and important clinicopathological correlations delineated. The Luke's classification and its modifications recommended at the Rye

1

Table 1-1
Relative Incidence of Various Subtypes of Malignant Lymphomas

Year	Authors	Patient No.	HD* (%)	LS* (%)	RCS* (%)	GFL* (%)
1942	Gall and Mallory	618	37.0	35.6	20.4	7.0
1947	Jackson and Parker	847	32.6	43.3	19.6	4.6
1947	Hellwig	127	20.5	61.4	16.6	1.5
1956	Hall and Olson	116	56.0	34.4	3.4	6.2
1961	Rosenberg et al	2,600†	51.2	32.0	10.2	6.6
1963	Molander and Pack	883	35.0	30.5	22.5	12.0
1966	Catlin	249	22.0	30.0	48.0	
1968	Peters et al	1,406	35.9	44.9	19.2	
1969	Lennert	218	66.5	17.4	16.1	
1972	EFSCH	527	30.9	39.8	24.7	4.6
	Total	7,591	40.9	36.3	17.6	5.2

*HD = Hodgkin's disease; LS = lymphosarcoma; RCS = reticulum cell sarcoma; GFL = giant follicular lymphoma.

†Estimated from figures given by Rosenberg et al (1961) and Molander and Pack (1963).

Conference have fulfilled this expectation for Hodgkin's disease. For non-Hodgkin's lymphomas, the terminology and descriptions of Rappaport appear to be more useful than the old classifications. Presently in our own hospital and in almost all of the cooperative oncological protocol studies involving multiple medical institutions, all the malignant lymphomas are classified according to these two new systems. Since the names lymphosarcoma and reticulum cell sarcoma are still being used quite frequently in the literature, out of necessity and for convenience, we have quoted them directly without modification in this book.

Pathologically, malignant lymphomas are tumors of the reticular tissues. Clinically, in contrast to histiocytosis and leukemias which are invariably disseminated by the time they are diagnosed, malignant lymphomas often initially affect only one lymph node group or one extranodal site. The diagnosis of malignant lymphoma can only be made by histological examination of tissue biopsies. In addition, there are many unique aspects in the clinical management of these conditions that require, and are benefited by the participation of surgeons.

In the United States for the year of 1972, there were 25,100 new cases of malignant lymphoma, and 19,800 patients died of it (Silverberg and Holleb 1972). But malignant lymphoma as defined here accounted for less than 5 percent of all the cancer cases in this country. Different subtypes of lymphoma have different natural courses, and each mode of presentation may reflect a certain pattern of involvement. And malignant lymphoma of extranodal sites includes widely scattered and heterogenous lesions, each with its unique clinical problems. It is not commonly known that extranodal

Table 1-2
History of Hodgkin's Disease

1832 Hodgkin:	Described 7 cases of lymph node disease (3 cases qualified as Hodgkin's disease today)
1898 Sternberg; 1902 Reed	Characterized the diagnostic multinucleated giant cells; correlated the pathological features with clinical findings
1902 Pusey:	First report of radiotherapeutic management
1917 Yates and Bunting:	Championed surgical removal of localized Hodgkin's disease
1946 Goodman et al:	First successful treatment with nitrogen mustard
1947 Jackson and Parker:	First histological classification: paragranuloma, granuloma, sarcoma
1950 Peters:	Devised three clinical stages according to the number of nodal regions involved (I, II, III), and separated those with or without symptoms
1962 Kaplan:	Gave high-dose prophylactic radiotherapy to all the main lymphatics using "mantle" and "inverted Y" fields; separated stage IV from old stage III for disease involving extranodal tissues
1963 Easson and Russell:	Showed that patients with localized disease could be cured by radiotherapy, because their survival curve paralleled normal population 10 years after diagnosis
1963 Lukes:	Proposed 6 histological classifications
1966 Rye Conference:	Defined 4 clinical stages (I, II, III, IV), each divided into A or B, according to the absence or presence of fever, night sweat, or pruritis; modified Luke's histological types into 4 (lymphocyte predominance, nodular sclerosis, mixed cellularity, lymphocyte depletion)
1969 Glatstein et al:	Reported on the use of laparotomy and splenectomy for more accurate staging
1969 De Vita et al:	Tried combination chemotherapy (MOPP) in the treatment of advance Hodgkin's disease
1971 Ann Arbor Conference:	Proposed changes of Rye's clinical staging system: Combine stage I$_2$ into Stage II, delete pruritus from substage B, add weight loss as one of the 3 significant symptoms, classify extranodal disease similar to nodal disease

lymphoma is the first recognized site(s) of involvement in nearly half of the patients with non-Hodgkin's lymphoma (Peters et al 1968).

Thus it is difficult for individual clinicians or even institutions to accumulate enough clinical experience to formulate a rational and standardized approach to specific problems. Therefore, in addition to a review of the experience at our own hospital for the past 30 years, we have incorporated all the important reports published in the literature, concentrating on findings of the last 10 to 15 years.

Within each major topic, and whenever possible, the information is presented in chronological order to provide an historical background. Obviously there are areas of controversy, and no simple hard and fast rules can be given. Whenever pertinent, we present the exact number of patients and the results reported, in order to give the reader a greater appreciation of the "state of the art" so that he may evaluate his own opinions more intelligently.

CLINICAL MANIFESTATIONS

The most common early manifestation of malignant lymphoma of any type is a progressive, usually painless, enlargement of a single superficial lymph node or lymph node group in an otherwise asymptomatic patient. Since no physical finding nor any clinical history is characteristically reliable, biopsy is the only means of establishing a diagnosis. In some instances, especially for non-Hodgkin's lymphoma, the involvement of extranodal sites occurs early in the disease; such sites include the skin, nasopharynx, tonsil, thyroid, lung, breast, gastrointestinal tract, gonad, and bone. Whether the early involvement of any one of these organs indicates that it is a primary site for the tumor or is merely an early clinical manifestation of an already disseminated disease is often difficult to determine (Rappaport 1966). Symptoms and physical signs that are indicative of systemic malignant lymphoma, such as fever, night sweat, weight loss, weakness, anemia, enlargements of the spleen and liver, and generalized enlargement of the lymph nodes, usually appear as the disease progresses, although they may occur as early clinical manifestations of the disease.

In order to better understand the similarities and differences of the clinical courses of Hodgkin's disease and other malignant lymphomas, we have conducted a detailed retrospective and comprehensive review of 527 patients with histologically confirmed diagnosis seen at the Ellis Fischel State Cancer Hospital (EFSCH) from 1940 to 1971. The institution is a referral center and has admitted 40,610 patients during the same period, although about one-third of the patients had nonmalignant diseases. Very few pediatric cases are admitted and about six to eight percent of the new cancer cases in the state of Missouri are seen at this hospital.

There were 163 patients with Hodgkin's disease and 364 with other malignant lymphomas. More than 200 clinicopathological factors were abstracted from patient records, including details of radiotherapy and chemotherapy. Survival data presented are adjusted for age, sex, and decade of admission and are calculated from the time of tissue diagnosis by the life-table method. All patients who had major surgical procedures or required surgical consultation were studied in detail and are discussed under appropriate topics in this book. Whenever applicable, data from this EFSCH series will be used to illustrate the clinical manifestations, pathological variations and factors important for prognosis (Lee et al 1973). Pertinent and current reports in the literature will be included in the discussion to supplement our data.

Age and Sex

In the EFSCH series, there were 99 males and 64 females with Hodgkin's disease (M : F = 1.5 : 1). The age range was 4 to 81 years (median = 40, mean = 43.3). There were 220 males and 144 females with other lymphomas. The male-to-female sex ratio is also 1.5. The age range was 4 to 88 years (median = 62, mean = 58.5). Figure 1-1 shows the age distributions. In our series, as in others, the non-Hodgkin's lymphomas appeared mainly in older patients.

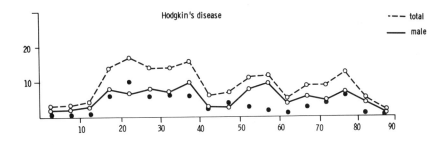

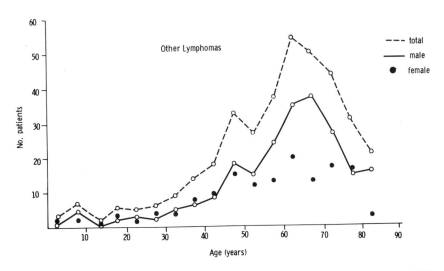

Fig. 1-1. Age and sex distribution of 163 cases of Hodgkin's disease and 364 cases of other lymphomas (EFSCH series).

In the EFSCH series, our overall survival rates were similar for the patients with Hodgkin's disease and those with other lymphomas (adjusted 5-year survival rate = 24 percent, 10-year = 16 percent; Fig. 1-2). Similar to numerous other reports, females had a better survival curve in both groups, but statistically it was not significant (p > 0.05).* Patients who belong to the age group of 21 to 40 years had the best survival rate (Fig. 1-3), and the difference was significant (p < 0.05). Within each age decade, females fared better than males, especially those who were younger than 40 years old. Within each sex group, the age factor holds equally true. Jelliffe and Thompson (1955) also found that the outlook was best in the third and fourth decades, and this was particularly marked among the female cases. Lampe and Fayos (1968) found a 5-year survival rate of 27.7 percent in males and 41.0 percent in females. Within each stage, the 5-year survival was found to decrease with increasing age.

MacMahon (1957) found that the age-incidence curve of Hodgkin's disease was distinctly bimodal, with one peak in the age group 25–29 and a second in the 70–74 group, whereas the curve for non-Hodgkin's lymphoma increased approximately linearly through life to age 75. Later, three age groups were described: 0–14, 15–34, and 50 years and over (MacMahon 1966). This suggested that Hodgkin's disease might include the clinical and pathological end results of at least two distinct etiological processes: disease in young adults behaves more like a chronic granulomatous inflammation, whereas that occurring in persons over 50 is a neoplasm.

Hodgkin's disease in children occurs most frequently in boys. For patients from 5 through 11 years old, Miller (1966) reported a male to female sex ratio of 3 : 1, and MacMahon (1966) found that in children younger than 10 years of age, the sex ratio was almost 6 : 1. Butler (1969) reported that the prognosis was better for children, especially girls, who were 10 years old or older and those with early unifocal disease.

In this country, many reports showed that less than 10 percent of Hodgkin's disease occurred in children below 15 years of age (Shimkin 1955; MacMahon 1957; Razis et al 1959). Azzam (1966) found that more than 20 percent of the cases of Hodgkin's disease in Lebanon occurred in children below 15 years of age, and Solidoro et al (1966) and Albujar (1973), reported the comparable figure in Peru was 40 percent. Correa and O'Connor (1971) confirmed the finding that there is a higher frequency of Hodgkin's disease in male children in poverty-stricken communities. Compared to European countries, cases in Africa and South America had more mixed cellularity and lymphocyte depletion subtypes. By contrast, in wealthy communities the disease affects young adults more frequently, and also the favorable

---

*P value of 0.05 means that the probability that the observed difference was due to change alone was one in 20. Conventionally when p value is less than 0.05, the difference seen are considered as statistically significant.

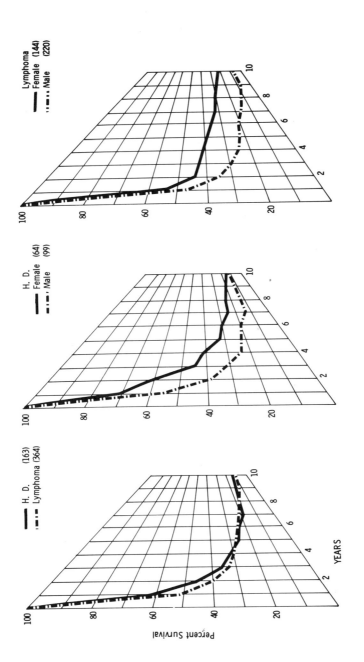

Fig. 1-2. Survival curves according to diagnosis and sex (EFSCH series).

7

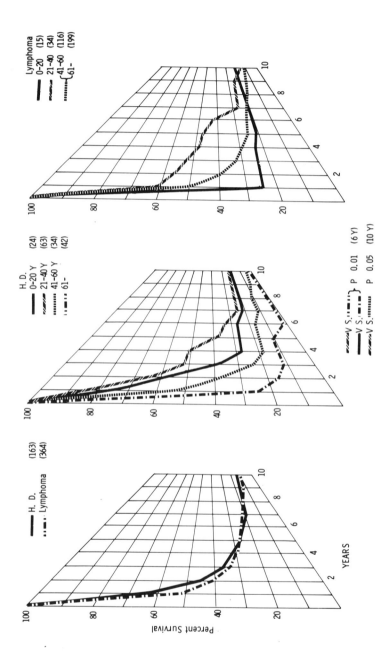

Fig. 1-3. Survival curves according to diagnosis and age (EFSCH series).

8

form of nodular sclerosis predominates. MacMahon (1971) has summarized many distinct clinical and pathological differences among patients of different age groups with Hodgkin's disease.

In the United States, most of the patients with Hodgkin's disease come from the higher economic groups. And high mortality ratios in the upper social classes are characteristics of the lymphomas as a group, except multiple myeloma which is more common in nonwhites. However, "it remains to be seen, which of the several closely related variables—socioeconomic status, duration of education, intelligence, and occupational class—is most closely related to Hodgkin's disease's risk" (MacMahon 1966).

Many epidemiological aspects of Hodgkin's disease are interesting, but have not shed any light regarding its etiology (Cole 1972, Kaplan 1972, Lee 1973). Vianna et al (1972) reported an unusual cluster of cases of malignant lymphoma in a group of high school students, their relatives, and friends. There were 34 interlinked cases, 31 of Hodgkin's disease and 3 of other lymphomas, diagnosed from 1948 to 1971. Their findings suggest that Hodgkin's disease could be similar to an infectious condition, transmitted either from patient to patient or through some healthy carrier, with a long incubation period. Heath (1972) commented that many other epidemiological studies did not show very strong nor consistent evidence of such spread.

Clinical Staging

Studies on large series of patients with malignant lymphoma have shown that the important prognostic factors included age, sex, presence or absence of symptoms, histological types and clinical stages. However, Keller et al (1968) found that age and sex contributed little additional prognostic information beyond that determined by histological type and clinical stages, and Patchefsky et al (1973) showed that age, sex, and systemic symptoms were weaker prognostic variables. Thus, in talking about the natural course of patients with malignant lymphomas, we will concentrate on these two latter distinct but interrelated factors.

Clinical staging of malignant disease, in general, reflects the extent of involvement based on physical findings supplemented by standard diagnostic procedures. Progressively more advanced stages have progressively shorter median survivals. The objectives of clinical staging as stated by the International Union Against Cancer (1966) included: (1) aiding the clinician in planning treatment; (2) aiding the clinician in estimating the prognosis; (3) assisting in the evaluation of the results of treatment; (4) facilitating the exchange of information between treatment centers; and (5) assisting in the continuing investigation of human cancer.

As early as 1920, Longcope and McAlpin described seven clinical subtypes of Hodgkin's disease: (1) localized, (2) mediastinal, (3) generalized, (4) acute, (5) concealed, (6) splenomegalic, and (7) osteoperiosteal. Later

Craver (1948) used three subtypes: localized, regional, and generalized. Peters (1950) devised three stages (I, II, III) according to the number of nodal regions involved and further subdivided the stages according to those patients with and without systemic symptoms. Kaplan (1962) added a stage IV, separate from the previous stage III, to include patients who had visceral disease such as lesions of the bone marrow, bone, lungs, skin, subcutaneous area, gastrointestinal tract, or kidney.

In the 1965 Rye Conference, the Committee on Staging of Hodgkin's Disease recommended a clinical staging system which found wide acceptance (Rosenberg 1966). The criterion for involvement of the spleen was either palpable enlargement or abnormal radioisotopic scan. Liver involvement was defined as hepatomegaly and elevated alkaline phosphatase, or two abnormal liver function tests, or an abnormal liver scan and one abnormal liver function test.

Subsequently, several drawbacks of the Rye Classification were found, especially regarding the group with stage IV diseases. Excluding patients with lesions of the liver, lung, and bone marrow, Peters et al (1968) showed that patients with localized extranodal presentations fared as well as the patients whose diseases were limited to the nodal presentations. Musshoff et al (1970) suggested that survival rates of patients with organ involvement from local invasion from a node, especially those of lung, pleura, bone, and soft tissues were much better than those with visceral lesions secondary to generalized disease. Rosenberg and Kaplan (1970) also found that many localized extralymphatic foci were amenable to treatment with tumoricidal doses of radiotherapy. Thus, a new staging system applicable to extralymphatic and non-Hodgkin's lymphoma was proposed and recommended for use by the 1971 Ann Arbor Conference (Carbone et al 1971).

Table 1-3 summarizes these clinical staging systems. In order to have meaningful staging designations, the methods used to define the extent of the disease need to be standardized. The staging procedures recommended by the Committee on Hodgkin's Disease Staging Procedure are listed in Table 1-4 (Rosenberg et al 1971). They are divided into four groups: required procedures for all untreated patients; those procedures necessary under certain conditions; useful auxiliary procedures; and those promising experimental procedures to be done at selected centers. Although these procedures are recommended for the staging of Hodgkin's disease only, many of them have also been found useful in cases of non-Hodgkin's lymphomas. Details and pertinent discussions of many of the tests and procedures are given elsewhere in this book.

In the EFSCH study of 527 patients with histologically proven Hodgkin's disease and other lymphomas, we have used the Rye staging system, with the exception that hepatomegaly and splenomegaly as such were considered as involvement of the liver and spleen, respectively. The modern techniques of lymphangiogram and staging laparotomy were used rarely in the EFSCH series. The basic work-up consisted of complete blood counts,

Table 1-3
Clinical Staging of Malignant Lymphoma

A. Rye Conference (1966)
    1. 4 stages:
        Stage I. Disease limited to one anatomic region (Stage I_1) or two contiguous anatomic regions (stage I_2) on the same side of the diaphragm.
        Stage II. Disease in more than 2 anatomic regions or in 2 noncontiguous regions on the same side of the diaphragm.
        Stage III. Disease on both sides of the diaphragm but not extending beyond the involvement of lymph nodes, spleen, and/or Waldeyer's ring.
        Stage IV. Involvement of the bone marrow, lung parenchyma, pleura, liver, bone, skin, kidneys, gastrointestinal tract, or any tissue or organ in addition to lymph nodes, spleen, or Waldeyer's ring.
    2. All stages are subclassified as A or B to indicate absence or presence of the following systemic symptoms: fever; night sweats; pruritus.
    3. Anatomically, the lymphoid regions are defined as follows:
        Above diaphragm: Waldeyer's ring; neck; mediastinal or hilar; infraclavicular; axillary and pectoral; epitrochlear and brachial.
        Below diaphragm: Spleen; para-aortic; mesentery; iliac; inguinal and femoral; popliteal.
B. EFSCH Study (1940–1971)
        Same as above, except hepatomegaly or splenomegaly were considered involvement of liver and spleen, respectively.
C. Ann Arbor Conference (1971)
    1. Clinical stages same as those proposed at Rye Conference except:
        Delete symptom of pruritis from subclass B; replace with "unexplained weight loss of more than 10% of body weight in the 6 months prior to admission."
        Combining previous stage I_2 into stage II.
        Add appendix and Peyer's patches to the list of lymphoid tissues.
        Staging lesions originated from extralymphatic organ or site in the same way as lesions of lymphoid tissue, but add subscript E, e.g., stage III_E= localized lesion of extralymphatic site and involvement of lymph node regions on both sides of diaphragm.
    2. Add pathological stages to incorporate the results of histopathological findings of tissues biopsied at staging laparotomy or other procedures. Abbreviations used:
        D = skin
        H = liver
        L = lung
        M = marrow
        N = abdominal node
        O = bone
        P = pleura
        S = spleen

urinalysis, blood typing, chest x-ray, and electrocardiogram. As listed in Table 1-5, lymphangiogram and radioisotope liver scans were used in less than 10 percent of the patients. Thirty to 50 percent of the patients had gastrointestinal x-rays and about 70 percent had intravenous pyelograms. Bone marrow biopsy—the majority done by needle aspiration—was obtained for approximately 50 percent of the patients.

Table 1-4.

Staging Procedures Recommended for Hodgkin's Disease [Committee on Hodgkin's Disease Staging Procedures, Ann Arbor Conference, Rosenberg et al (1971)]

A. Required Evaluation Procedures
  1. Surgical biopsy
  2. Detailed history, specifically:
     a. fever and duration
     b. night sweat and severity
     c. pruritus, extent and severity
     d. weight loss, amount and duration
     e. other desirable facts:
        1. family history
        2. history of infectious mononucleosis
        3. history of tonsillectomy
        4. drug usage, especially anticonvulsant
        5. alcohol-induced pain
  3. Complete physical examination, specifically:
     a. peripheral lymph nodes
     b. Waldeyer's ring
     c. liver and spleen
     d. bone tenderness
  4. Necessary laboratory tests:
     a. CBC, platelet count, sedimentation rate
     b. serum alkaline phosphatase
     c. renal function test
     d. liver function test
  5. Radiological studies:
     a. chest x-ray, PA, and lateral views
     b. intravenous pyelogram
     c. lower extremity lymphangiogram
     d. bone x-ray of vertebra, pelvis, proximal extremities, and sites with symptoms

B. Required Procedures under Certain Conditions
  1. Whole chest tomography
  2. Inferior cavography
  3. Bone-marrow biopsy
  4. Exploratory laparotomy and splenectomy

C. Useful Ancillary Procedures
  1. Skeletal scintigrams
  2. Liver and spleen scintigrams
  3. Serum calcium and uric acid
  4. Skin test for delayed hypersensitivity

D. Experimental Procedures for Study at Selected Centers
  1. Whole-body gallium and selenium scintigrams
  2. Special tests:
     a. serum iron and iron-binding capacity
     b. Serum copper and ceruloplasm
     c. serum zinc
     d. serum haptoglobin
     e. serum fibrinogen
     f. serum gamma-2-globulin
     g. urinary hydroxproline
     h. leukocyte alkaline phosphatase
     i. absolute lymphocyte count
     j. antibodies to Epstein-Barr virus
     k. human lymphocyte antibody typing

Table 1-5
Additional Pretherapy Special Procedures (EFSCH series)

	Hodgkin's disease		Other lymphomas	
	No.	*%*	*No.*	*%*
Lymphangiogram	16 (6)*	10	22(13)*	6
(since 1962)				
Liver scan	10	6	11	3
(since 1965)				
IVP x-ray	107(21)	66	251(56)	69
GI x-ray	51 (2)	31	188(41)	52
Bone marrow Bx	78 (2)	49	182(37)	50
Operation for staging	12	7	3	1
(since 1969)				
Operation for diagnosis	7	4	82	23
Celiotomy	3		55	
Radical mastectomy	1		3	
Node dissection	2		8	
Wide excision			8	
Other	1		8	
Total patients	163		364	

*Parentheses indicate numbers of patients with abnormal tests.

Even though our staging designation is not as precise as it should be according to present-day standards, our data show that clinical staging does haveimportant prognostic values. In both Hodgkin's disease and non-Hodgkin's lymphoma, patients with stage I or II disease have better survival curves than those with stage III or IV (Fig. 1-4). The latter two groups had very similar prognoses, especially those with Hodgkin's disease. We found that the survival curves of stage I_2 (disease limited to two adjacent lymph nodal groups) and II (disease involving two nonadjacent, or more than two nodal groups) were very close. This agrees with the recommendation of Carbone et al (1971) that the old Rye stage I_2 should be combined with stage II. Figure 1-5 demonstrates the distribution of age and sex versus clinical stage, and shows that the clinical pattern appears to be different between those with Hodgkin's disease and those with other lymphomas. Male and female patients had similar age distribution curves except those with stage III Hodgkin's disease and those with stage II malignant lymphomas. In patients with Hodgkin's disease, females fared better within each of the clinical stages (Fig. 1-6). For patients with non-Hodgkin's diseases, females had better survival only in stage II (Fig. 1-7).

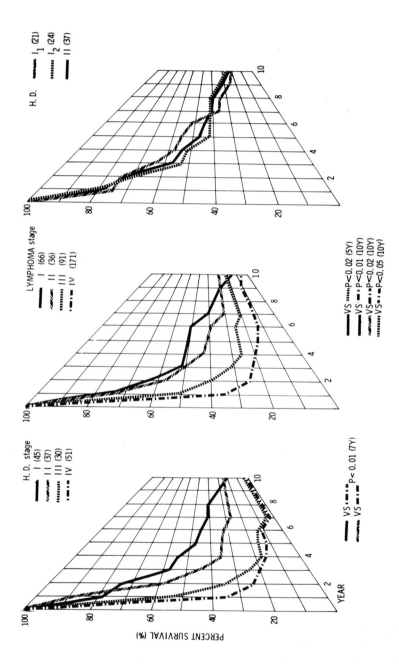

Fig. 1-4. Survival curves according to clinical stage (EFSCH series).

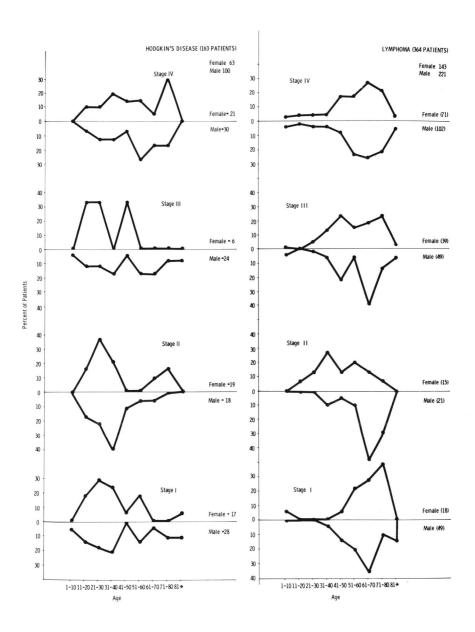

Fig. 1-5. Distribution of clinical stages according to age and sex (EFSCH series).

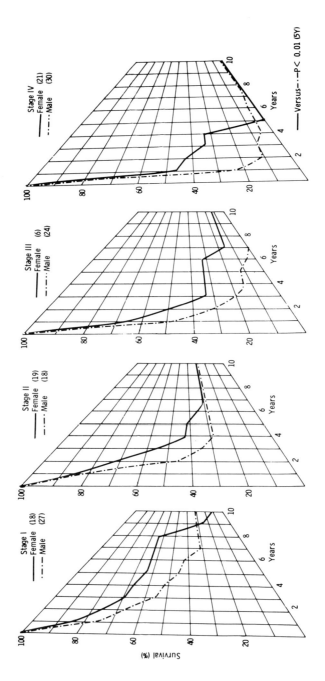

Fig. 1-6. Survival curves of patients with Hodgkin's disease according to clinical stage and sex (EFSCH series).

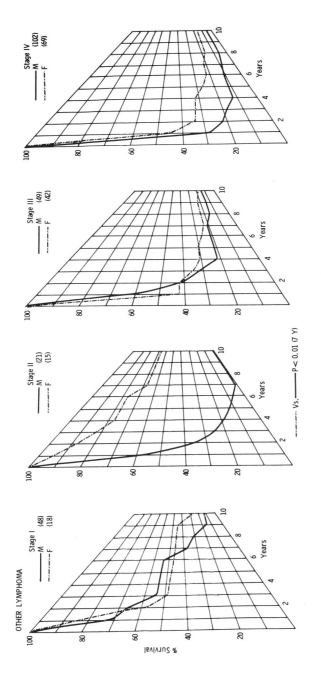

Fig. 1-7. Survival curves of patients with other lymphomas according to clinical stage and sex (EFSCH series).

Constitutional Symptoms

In the clinical staging system proposed at the Rye Conference, fever, night sweats, and pruritus were accepted as important and significant symptoms. Other symptoms and signs which also should be documented included weight loss, malaise, weakness, fatigue, anemia, leukocytosis, leukopenia, lymphopenia, elevated sedimentation rate, cutaneous anergy, or alcohol pain. Subsequently, the prognostic significance of pruritus, which occurred only in about 10 percent of the patients anyway, was questioned, because there was no correlation between survival and the symptom of pruritus, whether localized or generalized. Thus, pruritus was deleted from subclass B at the Ann Arbor Conference, and, instead, weight loss of more than 10 percent in the 6 months prior to admission was added.

In the present EFSCH study of 163 patients with Hodgkin's disease and 364 patients with non-Hodgkin's lymphoma, the presence of any systemic symptoms, such as fever, pruritus, weight loss, or weakness decreased the survival rates (Figs. 1-8 and 1-9). For patients with Hodgkin's disease, we have compared the subclassification of A and B according to the criteria suggested at the Rye and Ann Arbor Conferences. It is interesting to note that they both separated the prognosis of patients in the early stages (I and II) nicely, but did not show any difference in survival in patients with advanced diseases (III and IV). In our EFSCH series, the differences are not statistically significant and we cannot tell whether deletion of pruritis and addition of weight loss will improve the prognostic value of the new system or not.

Constitutional symptoms appeared to correlate with the extent of the disease. Hilton and Sutton (1962) showed none of those patients with the disease localized to one site (stage I) had severe symptoms; conversely, almost all the patients with the generalized disease did. Cohen et al (1964), studied 14 interrelated signs and symptoms in 388 patients with Hodgkin's disease. In the order of decreasing frequency, these were weakness, fever, weight loss, fatigue, cough, pain in the affected area, anorexia, evidence of anemia, dyspnea, neuralgia, splenomegaly, pruritus, hepatomegaly, and other neurological symptoms. The number of signs at diagnosis were associated with the histological types, the number of sites of adenopathy, and the extent of deep organ involvement. Thus, they showed that the survival curve of patients with no or one symptom was much better than those with two or three symptoms, and the prognosis of those with more than 7 symptoms was the worst.

Peters (1950) showed that 85 percent of Hodgkin's patients without constitutional symptoms (i.e., weight loss, lack of energy, fluctuating fever, or pruritus) survived 5 years in contrast with less than 36 percent of those who had such symptoms. Keller et al (1968) showed that the presence or absence of constitutional symptoms not only correlated with clinical stages,

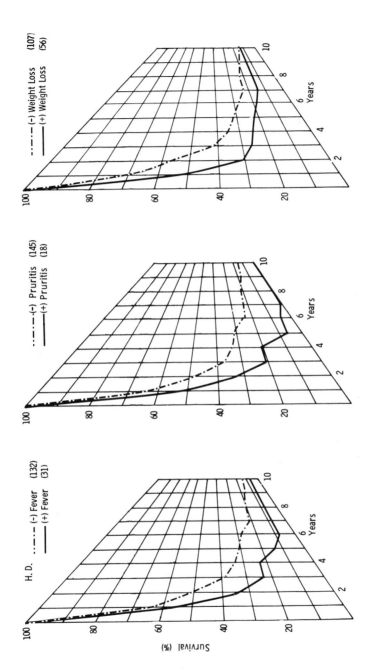

Fig. 1-8. Survival curves of patients with Hodgkin's disease according to presence or absence of systemic symptoms (EFSCH series).

19

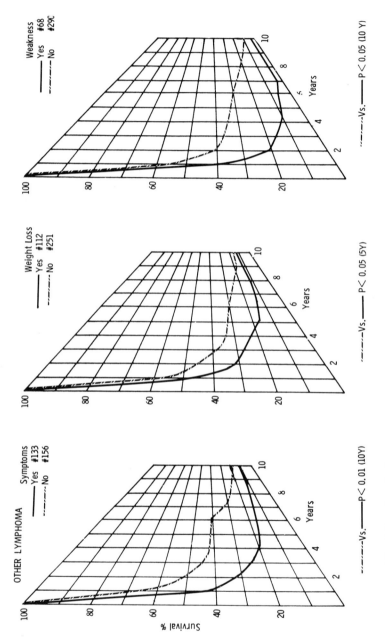

Fig. 1-9. Survival curves of patients with other lymphomas according to presence or absence of systemic symptoms (EFSCH series).

but also with histological subtypes of Hodgkin's disease. Patients with lymphocyte predominance had mostly stage I and II lesions on presentation, and very few had systemic symptoms, whereas most of those patients with lymphocyte depletion belonged to stage III and IV, and the majority had symptoms.

Lacher (1969) pointed out that, although patients with stage IA and IIA disease had the best survival rate, patients with extensive disease (IIB and IIIB) also could achieve survivals of 10 years or more and should not be considered hopeless. In 402 patients with Hodgkin's disease, he reported a 10-year survival rate of 22 percent; specifically, the figure was 13 percent for those with symptoms and 35 percent for those without.

Cross and Dixon (1971) showed that in the Hodgkin's patient who had no constitutional symptoms, there was little difference in survival time between those in whom glands were initially involved in a single region and those in whom glands were involved in many regions. They felt that clinical staging was not as valuable in prognosis as the combined assessment of the degree of differentiation of the lesion histologically and the presence or absence of constitutional symptoms. In patients with reticulum cell sarcoma, Reilly et al (1972) found that an overall rating of disease activity based upon general performance status and rate of progression of the disease was more important than anatomical staging in the predication of either tumor response to radiotherapy or survival.

Aisenberg (1973) described a group of newly uncovered expressions of Hodgkin's disease that are associated with such phenomena as fever, itching, leucocytosis, thrombocytosis, eosinophilia, seizures and depressed cellular immunity as systemic manifestations that are not clearly linked to hematogenous dissemination. The newly described phenomena include abnormal liver chemical findings that are seen with nonspecific liver-biopsy changes, enlarged spleens that are free of lymphoma, abdominal node hyperplasia without biopsy evidence of Hodgkin's disease that accounts for many equivocal lymphangiograms, nephrotic syndromes associated with active Hodgkin's disease, and the disseminated granulomas seen in some 12 percent of patients without other evidence of spread of Hodgkin's disease.

An interesting symptom associated with Hodgkin's disease is that of alcohol-induced pain, which was first mentioned by Hoster (1950). James (1960) reviewed 58 cases with this sign reported in the literature and studied 13 such cases himself. His finding suggested that Hodgkin's disease with alcohol-induced pain might be a separate entity. The sex incidence favored women; clinically, more of the patients had mediastinal involvement, and histological sections of the lesions showed more eosinophils and fibrosis. Brewin (1966 a,b) studied 155 patients with various neoplasms who had documented alcohol intolerance (84 of these had malignant lymphomas). He showed that such intolerance might appear as a very early symptom of localized neoplastic change and that there might be different ways of intolerance to alcohol; i.e., alcohol pain of the lesion itself is only one of the most common signs. When the focus of disease is treated with radiotherapy or surgery, the form of alcohol intolerance may shift from one site to another. Brewin (1967) also showed that a higher proportion of patients with adenocarcinoma of the uterus and ovary gave a history of alcohol intolerance than those with breast cancers. Kaplan (1972) commented that, although this alcoholic pain appeared to have some degree of specificity for Hodgkin's disease, the fact that it occurred in only 1.6 percent of his patients severely limited its prognostic value. The pathophysiologic mechanisms of alcohol intolerance in Hodgkin's disease is unknown. Lockwood (1973) mentioned 2 patients with Hodgkin's disease and alcohol intolerance who had identical symptoms after the use of marihuana.

Site of Nodal Presentations

Ultmann and Moran (1973) found that in 90 to 93 percent of the cases, Hodgkin's disease is manifested by superficial lymph node involvement: 60 to 80 percent in the cervical, 6 to 20 percent in the axillary, and 6 to 12 percent in the inguinal areas. Primary mediastinal involvement is seen in 6 to 11 percent, and retroperitoneal disease in 25 percent of the cases.

In the EFSCH series, as noted in Table 1-6, at the time of diagnosis about 75 percent of the patients with Hodgkin's disease showed nodal involvement and 25 percent had both nodal and extranodal lesions. The comparable figures for patients with non-Hodgkin's lymphomas were 51 percent and 49 percent. About 8 to 10 percent of all the patients apparently showed involvement of a single nodal region. In both Hodgkin's disease and other lymphomas, cervical nodes were the most common site of involvement. However, Hodgkin's disease had a higher predilection for developing mediastinal adenopathy, whereas non-Hodgkin's lymphomas had a higher involvement rate of the mesenteric and groin nodes. The distribution of nodal involvement according to clinical stages is presented in Figure 1-10.

In the EFSCH series, the spleen was enlarged in about 18 percent of the patients. Comparing 58 patients with Hodgkin's disease who survived for 10 years or more with 465 patients who had shorter survivals, Chawla et al (1970) found that splenomegaly and/or retroperitoneal adenopathy carried bad prognosis: the median survival after either of these findings was 4 years. However, one-fourth of the patients with splenomegaly did live 10 years or more after these abnormalities were demonstrated.

Since the ultilization of exploratory laparotomy and splenectomy for staging Hodgkin's disease (Glatstein et al 1969), it was found that approximately half of the patients with clinically enlarged spleens did not have histologic involvement of that organ; conversely, approximately one in three

Table 1-6
Distribution of Lymphadenopathy at the Time of Diagnosis (EFSCH series)

	Hodgkin's disease			Other lymphomas		
		Combination			Combination	
	Single No.	No.	Percent (of 163)	Single No.	No.	Percent (of 364)
Neck						
Upper-R	2	38	23	7	113	39
Upper-L	2	58	36	4	121	42
Lower-R	2	71	43	1	81	28
Lower-L	6	97	59	1	92	32
Mediastinum		60	37		57	20
Axilla-R	2	51	31	2	120	41
Axilla-L		60	39	5	124	43
Groin-R	2	33	20	2	122	42
Groin-L		34	21	4	118	41
Spleen		31	18		52	18
Other nodes						
Epitrochlear		2	1		15	5
Infraclavicular		4	0.2		13	4
Mesentery		1	0.6		49	43.5
Retroperitoneum		8	5	1	17	6
Tonsil		1	0.6		13	4
Nasopharynx				1	4	1
Subtotal:						
Single node	16		10	28		8
Single organ	1*			29*		8
Multiple nodes		107	65		156	43
Nodes and organ		39	25		151	41

*Sites in 30 patients with single-organ involvements:

Stomach	(12 patients)	Soft Tissue	(3 patients; 1 with Hodgkin's disease)
Ileum/cecum	(8 patients)	Skin	(2 patients)
Spinal cord	(4 patients)	Bone	(1 patient)

spleens, which were normal in size, contained demonstrable foci of Hodgkin's disease. However, histological involvement of the spleen carried more serious implications than if it were a lymph node because splenic disease usually preceded hepatic involvement and reflected a poorer prognostic consequence. (For a more detailed discussion, see pp. 203–205.)

Since Lukes (1963) and Hanson (1964) described the histological subtype of nodular sclerosis, it became known that this lesion had a remarkably high incidence of mediastinal involvement. Keller et al (1968) documented that nodular sclerosis in stages I and II involved the mediastinal and cervical nodes more often than did other types. In fact, every case of this type involved, in part, either the mediastinum or the cervical nodes, and none had lesions below the diaphragm.

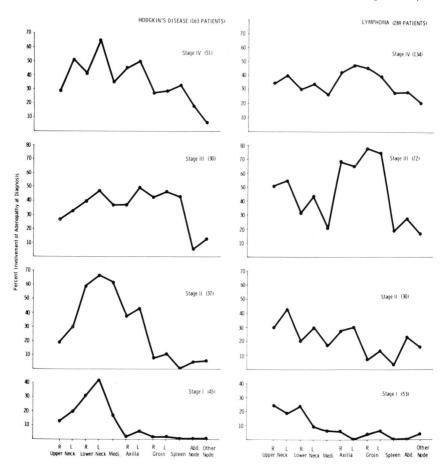

Fig. 1-10.   Distribution of lymphadenopathy at time of diagnosis according to clinical stage (EFSCH series).

Hutchison (1971) reported that mixed cellularity types were more concentrated in cases with involvement of one nodal region (47 percent) but had smaller proportions with two, three, four, or five regions involved. Nodular sclerosis was relatively unlikely to present with one site involved (22 percent) and was substantially more likely to have two or three regions involved. Later, Hutchison (1972) showed that nodular sclerosis commonly first involved mediastinum, then spread by contiguity to the neck, either left or right. In contrast, mixed cellularity types had significantly more (noncontiguous) lesions involving both axillae than were expected to occur on a random basis.

In patients with stage I Hodgkin's disease, Peters (1971) found no difference in survival between those who presented with cervical adenopathy and those with all other presentations. In those with two or more nodal regions affected and all remaining above the diaphragm (stage II), mediastinal involvement had better prognosis. In patients with stage III disease, the survival rates were distinctly better in the group without mediastinal involvement.

In the present EFSCH series, the clinical stage designation was similar to Peters' 1971 series in the sense that lymphangiogram was rarely used. We have found that all Hodgkin's patients with mediastinal involvement had better survivals, especially those with stage II disease (Fig. 1-11); whereas in patients with non-Hodgkin's lymphomas, those who had mediastinal adenopathy had a poorer prognosis in all stages (Fig. 1-12). Jones et al (1973) also found that mediastinal involvement in non-Hodgkin's patients with stage II and III disease had a poorer survival curve than those without mediastinal involvement, although the difference was statistically significant only in patients who had nodular mixed cell and nodular poorly differentiated lymphocytic types.

In Hodgkin's disease, Teillet et al (1971) described four major forms in relation to the site of disease onset: (1) high cervical forms, without mediastinal involvement; (2) mediastinal forms, with dissemination to supraclavicular and/or axillary areas; (3) retroperitoneal forms with frequent supraclavicular disease (especially on the left side) but without mediastinal disease; (4) axillary forms. Histologically, lymphocyte predominance is frequent in high cervical forms; it and mixed cellularity are also more frequent in retroperitoneal forms. In addition, high cervical adenopathy is more frequent in males and children; the mediastinal form is more frequent in females; and retroperitoneal forms are seen most often in older patients.

Fuller et al (1970) found that the occurrence of Hodgkin's disease on one side of the upper neck was limited almost exclusively to young males, the specific histology being mixed cellularity. Only 2 of 15 patients with Hodgkin's disease involving one side of the upper neck developed new disease after radiotherapy; whereas over 50 percent of those with initial disease of the lower neck did so. Axillary adenopathy reflected a poor prognosis, suggesting that this was merely a manifestation of a more generalized disease process which probably included involvement of the upper abdomen. In patients with localized Hodgkin's disease treated with regional radiation, Fuller et al (1971) found the 5-year survival rate of patients with disease presented at the neck, mediastinum, axilla, and lower torso was 71, 74, 44, and 56 percent, respectively. The difference in survivals between lesions of the mediastinum and axilla or lower torso was statistically significant (p < 0.05). In addition, the prognosis of patients with disease limited to one side of the upper neck was much better than that of the lower neck (5-year survival = 93 percent versus 65 percent).

Peters et al (1973), pointed out that in Hodgkin's disease, and probably also in non-Hodgkin's lymphomas, the supraclavicular area should not be

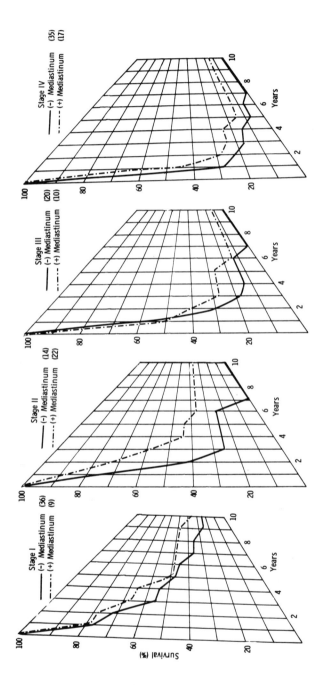

Fig. 1-11. Survival curves of patients with Hodgkin's disease according to presence or absence of mediastinal involvement (EFSCH series).

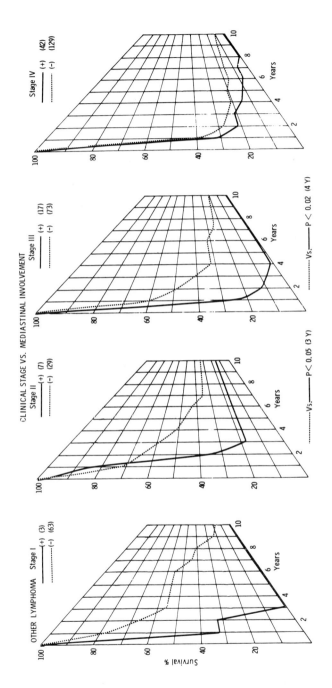

Fig. 1-12. Survival curves of patients with other lymphomas according to presence or absence of mediastinal involvement (EFSCH series).

considered a peripheral lymphoid region since medial supraclavicular disease alone is almost always associated with upper anterior mediastinal disease and lateral supraclavicular involvement is often associated with intraabdominal disease. Stage I disease in the neck seems to be confined to the upper, midcervical, or submandibular chains. The size and distribution of lymphadenopathy also had clinical significance. In general, if lymph nodes are small and numerous within one or more regions, especially distributed in a noncontiguous fashion, the patient is very likely to have generalized disease, possibly stage IV. If most of the individual nodes are large, i.e., more than 2 cm, the diagnosis is more likely to be limited to the major lymphatic system and could even be stage I. In 64 patients who had staging laparotomy, 37 of the 40 patients with negative findings had large lymph nodes, whereas most of the 24 patients who had positive biopsies had small peripheral nodes, either widely spread or noncontiguous.

Extranodal Involvement

Primary extranodal lesions in Hodgkin's disease are rare. Most such lesions occur as direct extensions from adjacent involved lymphoid tissues. For example, involvement of the lung presumably arises from mediastinal or hilar lymph nodes. Less frequently, the sternum, clavicle, vertebra, pericardium, pleura, and adjacent subcutaneous tissue and skin could be invaded subsequent to disease of the regional lymph nodes. All such lesions, if limited in extent, may still allow aggressive radiotherapy to be delivered and are associated with a good prognosis (Rosenberg 1970).

Comparing 58 Hodgkin's patients who survived 10 or more years with 465 patients who survived less than 10 years, Chawla et al (1970) found that during the course of the disease there was a significantly higher frequency of bone, skin, and subcutaneous lesions among long-term survivors (p >0.05 and 0.01, respectively). The most unfavorable manifestations were involvement of liver or lung; median survival after either of these was only 2 years. Medina et al (1971) studied the instances of extranodal Hodgkin's disease occurring in 4 selected sites in 150 patients. There was involvement of epidura in 13, skin in 12, lung in 10 and bone in 9. The corresponding lymph nodes were involved before the appearance of extranodal disease in 75 percent of the cases, suggesting retrograde lymphatic embolization of Hodgkin's cells as the mechanism of extranodal spread.

Wood and Coltman (1973) reviewed the world literature for well-documented cases of localized, primary extranodal Hodgkin's disease. They estimated the incidence of this unusual form of Hodgkin's disease to be one-fourth of 1 percent of the overall incidence of Hodgkin's disease. Localized primary extranodal Hodgkin's disease seems to have an excellent prognosis in some cases, including skin, tongue, lung, stomach, small bowel, and thyroid. Thus, it appears that Hodgkin's disease can arise and may be localized in surprisingly diverse sites and may well be related to small foci of lymphatic tissue within these extralymphatic organs that undergo malignant transformation.

Many reports have emphasized the fact that non-Hodgkin's lymphoma frequently presents, or is associated with, extranodal involvement early in the course of the disease. Peters et al (1968) reported that the first sites of involvement in patients with Hodgkin's disease were 91 percent nodal and 9 percent extranodal. The comparable figures for reticulum cell sarcoma were 39 percent and 61 percent, and lymphosarcoma, 60 percent and 40 percent (Table 1-7). The gastrointestinal tract was the most common extranodal site; it accounted for 2 percent in Hodgkin's disease and 13–25 percent in non-Hodgkin's lymphoma. Banfi et al (1968) showed that extranodal disease was more common in children with malignant lymphomas. Jenkin et al (1969) reported that about one-third of children with non-Hodgkin's lymphomas had primary lesions of the gastrointestinal tract.

Freeman et al (1972), from the End Results Study Group of the National Cancer Institute, studied 12,947 cases recorded in the years 1950–1964 and noted 2,194 in whom a lymphoma was said to have arisen at some site other than the lymph nodes. Approximately 24 percent of reticulum cell sarcomas, 15 percent of lymphosarcomas, 5 percent of giant follicular lymphomas, and perhaps 5 percent of Hodgkin's disease arose extranodally in their series. The most common sites in children were the large and small intestines and bone; in young adults, the adenoid and skin. Males were affected more often than females, but the latter was especially prone to disease at certain sites: 94 percent of thyroid and breast lymphomas and 55 percent of salivary gland lymphomas were seen in females.

Histologically, bone, testis, and thyroid lymphomas are predominantly reticulum cell sarcomas, which are unusual in skin and lung lymphomas. Lung, breast, and small intestine lymphomas are usually lymphosarcomas, which are seen infrequently in bone. The specific organ distribution of extranodal lymphomas and survival rates are given in more detail on page 170.

Aisenberg (1973) pointed out that the prognosis seen in many non-Hodgkin's lymphomas of extranodal sites is rather favorable as contrasted with the poor prognosis of nodal non-Hodgkin's lymphomas. For example, the typical 5-year survival figures for the following sites are: primary reticulum cell sarcoma of bone, 58 percent; primary lymphoma of the Waldeyer's ring, 50 percent; primary lymphoma of the thyroid, 44 percent; and primary lymphoma of the stomach and small intestine, 34 percent, and colon, 55 percent.

At the time of diagnosis in the EFSCH series (Table 1-7), 25 percent of the patients with Hodgkin's disease had extranodal involvement, and 49 percent of those with non-Hodgkin's had such lesions—in 8 percent, the disease appeared to be localized to single extranodal sites (Table 1-6).

Table 1-7
Distribution of Extranodal Involvement in Malignant Lymphoma

Extranodal type	RCS Patient No.	RCS %	LS Patient No.	LS %	RCS & LS Patient No.	RCS & LS %	HD Patient No.	HD %	HD Patient No.	HD %	Non-HD Patient No.	Non-HD %
Gastrointestinal	67	25	78	13	145	17	12	2			31	10
Liver			2		2				1*			
Pancreas	1		3		4						7*	
Head and neck												
Pharynx	33	14	60	13	93	13	9	3				
Parotid	1		12		13		3					
Orbit	1		7		8							
Thyroid	2		4		6		3					
Skin/soft tissue	20	16	30	8	50	10	2	1	5		29	12
Breast	1		4		5							
Bone	21	16	17	8	38	10	3		7	8	15	
Genital tract											5	1
Testis	3	3	6	2	9	2	1					
Ovary	2		5		7		1					
Uterus/Vagina	3		2		5							
CNS												
Extradural	7	3	10	2	17	2					6	2
Brain	1		3		4		3					
Urinary												
Bladder			1		1							
Kidney	1		1		2				5	3	4	1

As first recognized sites (Peters et al 1968)

As recognized sites at time of diagnosis (EFSCH series)

Site													
Chest													
Lung	2		6	1	8	1	6	2	8	12	13		13
Pleura				1		1				25	33		33
Thymus			1		1		3		2				
Bone marrow									2		37	12	10
Total extranodal	166	61	252	40	418	46	43	9	40	100	180	25	49
Grand total	270	100	631	100	901	100	505	100	163		364		100

*Only patients with positive liver biopsies are included here.

Our classification system was modified from the old Rye system; thus, patients with hepatomegaly and/or extranodal lesions were classified as stage IV. Specific problems in management and the different natural history of malignant lymphomas at specific extranodal sites will be discussed in Chapters 7 to 10. Certain aspects will be mentioned in general terms here.

Our patients with stage IV disease had the lowest survival rate among the four stages (Figure 1-4). Within stage IV, hepatomegaly detected only by physical examination without reference to laboratory findings or biopsy specimen had a negative effect on survival (Fig. 1-13). Ultmann, et al (1966) also showed that Hodgkin's patients with hepatomegaly had a survival rate much lower than other patients with pruritis and/or fever but without hepatomegaly. In the EFSCH series, among patients with stage IV disease, those who had involvement of skin and/or soft tissue, pleura and/or lung, or bone marrow, showed no significant difference in survival from those who had no such lesions. But patients with lesions of the gastrointestinal tract appeared to have better survival rates than those without (Fig. 1-13). Most of these had surgical resection supplemented with radiotherapy (pp. 252–254).

Since the Committee on Hodgkin's Disease Staging Classification at the Ann Arbor Conference specifically stated that appendix and Peyer's patch should be considered as lymphatic structures (Carbone et al 1971), many of the presently so-called "extranodal" lesions, e.g., primary malignant lymphoma of the gastrointestinal tract, currently classified as stage IV, will be reclassified as "nodal" lesions and stage I in the future. It is hoped that this revision in classification will better define the prognosis and improve our understanding of the natural history of malignant lymphoma. However, it appears that neoplasms of lymphoid tissues of the viscera do behave somewhat differently than peripheral lymph nodes. We must await the results of clinical studies which correlate this revised staging system and histopathologic classifications before having confidence in the proposed new system.

One interesting physical finding associated with extranodal malignant lymphoma is digital clubbing. Apparently, Hippocrates described this first, and his name was associated with this sign (Henderson 1963). Clubbing of the fingers occurred in about 10 percent of patients with primary intestinal lymphomas and malabsorption syndromes (Eidelmen et al 1966; al-Bahrani and Bakir 1971). Novis et al (1971) reported 23 cases of abdominal lymphomas presented with malabsorption syndrome. Finger clubbing, peripheral edema and intermittent abdominal pain were present in 50 percent of the cases.

Mullins and Lenhard (1971) also described digital clubbing in 3 patients with Hodgkin's disease. However, only mediastinal involvement was present in each case; and in one patient, the nail changes disappeared after mediastinal irradiation.

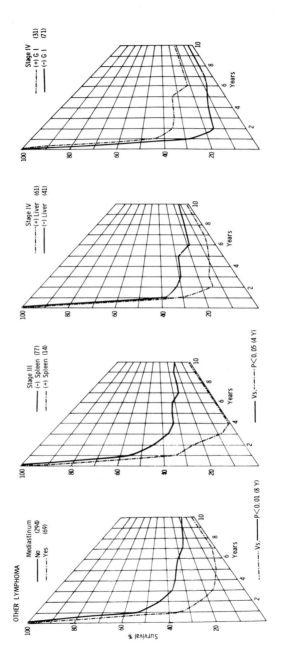

Fig. 1-13. Survival curves of patients with non-Hodgkin's lymphomas according to specific sites of involvement (EFSCH series).

33

HISTOPATHOLOGICAL CLASSIFICATION

Pathologically, malignant lymphomas are characterized by tumors of reticular tissue that are composed of primitive reticular cells, their histiocytic or lymphocytic derivations, or combinations of these cell types. Hodgkin's disease is diagnosed by the presence of the characteristic malignant de-differentiated histiocyte of the Reed-Sternberg, or Sternberg-Reed, type. Rather (1972) has reviewed the moot but interesting question: Who discovered the pathognomonic giant cell of Hodgkin's disease? His conclusion was that many investigators in Germany, France, England, and elsewhere, beginning in the 1860s, recognized and described one and sometimes two varieties of large cells in clinical patients with this disease. Who had priority in discovering these characteristic cells cannot be known with certainty. Non-Hodgkin's lymphoma in this book covers all the conditions commonly and formerly called reticulum cell sarcoma, lymphosarcoma, giant follicular lymphoma, and unspecified lymphoma. In the EFSCH study, the subgroups of Hodgkin's disease were classified according to Lukes' proposal, modified and recommended at the 1965 Rye Conference (Lukes et al 1966b). The non-Hodgkin's lymphomas were classified according to the terminology of Rappaport (1966). A review of the historical evolution of these new classifications and their clinical and prognostic importance is given below.

Hodgkin's Disease

Jackson and Parker (1944) showed that the histological classification of lesions into paragranuloma and sarcoma could be correlated with the very good and bad prognoses of the disease. However, their class of granuloma was rather heterogeneous and covered 80 to 90 percent of the cases reported.

Lukes (1963) proposed six new histologic types and showed that, when used in conjunction with clinical stages, they provided an effective basis for prognosis. The six types were: (1) lymphocytic and/or histocytic, nodular; (2) lymphocytic and/or histocytic, diffuse; (3) nodular sclerosis; (4) mixed; (5) diffuse fibrosis; and (6) reticular. In particular, the nodular sclerosis subtype was associated with a remarkably high incidence of mediastinal involvement (59 percent versus 24 percent of other types). In his series, it was the most common type observed in patients with stage I disease, and had a median survival of 11 years.

In subsequent papers, Lukes (1964, 1968), Lukes et al (1966a), and Lukes and Butler (1966) further documented the definite relationship between the six new histologic types, the clinical stages, and survival. The lymphocytic and histiocytic types represented essentially a predominance of lymphocytic proliferation, while diffuse fibrosis and reticular were associated with lymphocytic depletion; the former types correspond with quiescence of the disease, and the latter, with more malignant or progressive disease. Nodular sclerosis appeared to be a regional expression of Hodgkin's disease in the mediastinum. The mixed type appeared to reflect a changing disease state. Thus, the Committee on Nomenclature at the Rye Conference decided to adopt Lukes' histological system, but consolidated it into four readily usable groups, reflecting the dynamic state of the host response (Lukes et al 1966b). The histological terms recommended were: (1) lymphocyte predominance, (2) nodular sclerosis, (3) mixed cellularity, and (4) lymphocyte depletion. A description of each is given in Table 1-8. Lukes (1972) felt that the histological components associated with Reed-Sternberg cells were a reflection of the host and related to many of the immunologic abnormalities described in Hodgkin's disease. Lymphocyte depletion in Hodgkin's disease, although very rare, is a distinctive clinicopathologic entity of rapidly fatal disease with fever, pancytopenia, lymphocytopenia, and abnormalities of hepatic function, frequently without peripheral lymphadenopathy (Neiman et al 1973).

Table 1-8
Histological Classification of Hodgkin's Disease
[Nomenclature Committee, Rye Conference (Lukes et al 1966b)]

LP:	Lymphocyte predominance. Prominently composed of well-differentiated lymphocytes or histiocytes or any degree of combination of the two cell types. Eosinophils and plasma cells are rare or absent. There are no fibrosis and necrosis. The diagnostic Reed-Sternberg and mononuclear cells were rare and difficult to find. The histologic pattern may be nodular (LPN) or diffuse (LPD).
NS:	Nodular sclerosis. Bands of collagenous connective tissue that partially or entirely subdivide the abnormal lymphoid tissue into isolated nodules. The Reed-Sternberg cells are found in apparent lacunae or in clusters. The rest of the cells, within and outside the nodules, may be prominently lymphocytic or of a mixed composition, with eosinophils or mature granulocytes being numerous and prominent. Total sclerosis appears to be the end result of this type.
MC:	Mixed cellularity. It shows a variable composition. Histiocytes of the reactive type, mature neutrophils, eosinophils, plasma cells, and a variable number of lymphocytes with a slight-to-moderate degree of disorderly fibrosis without collagen formation are observed in variable numbers. The diagnostic cells are usually numerous. Small foci of necrosis may be present but usually are not prominent.
LD:	Lymphocyte depletion. It shows a general cellular depletion with small cellular areas with predominantly Reed-Sternberg cells. The lymph node may show diffuse fibrosis with small areas of predominantly Reed-Sternberg proliferation. Focal necrosis is commonly found.
UC:	Unclassified. Lesions diagnosed as Hodgkin's disease but which could not be classified into any of the above four subgroups.

Between the different pathological subtypes of Hodgkin's disease, there is a definite pattern of progression. Andersen et al (1970) studied 91 cases who had repeated biopsies taken later in the course or at autopsy. Lymphocyte depletion was present in 54 out of the 58 patients who died. In only 4 cases were the changes in the subsequent histological preparations less "advanced" than in the primary biopsies; while in 54 the histologic type was more "advanced." Strum and Rappaport (1971) studied sequential biopsy materials of 81 patients. In over 75 percent of the cases, they found that the four subtypes remained constant over long periods of observation. The highest degree of persistence was observed in that of the nodular sclerosis type (91.7 percent), and the least, in lymphocytic predominance (38.5 percent). When progression did occur, it usually occurred toward a histologically more malignant form.

It needs to be pointed out that the diagnosis of Hodgkin's disease and its subgroups can be a difficult problem at times. On assigning lesions to any one of the four subgroups by three different pathologists, Keller et al (1968) reported that unanimous agreement was seen in only two-thirds of the cases. Coppleson et al (1970) studied observer disagreement by giving each slide to three different pathologists. They found that when individual pathologists examined the same material in two separate occasions, the mean disagreement was about 28 out of 100 cases. The amount of complete agreement between observers ranged between 25.8 percent and 66.7 percent. Thus, they recommended the use of a panel of three pathologists working together since the consensus of three observers increased the accuracy of classifying individual cases beyond that which could be achieved by even the most experienced pathologists working alone.

Strum and Rappaport (1970b) showed that there was an early "cellular" phase of nodular sclerosis in which lacunar cells were conspicuous but bands of collagen could not be demonstrated. This suggested that the lacunar cells were probably the most significant feature of this subtype. Lukes (1971) further described the progressive variants of nodular sclerosis as focal cellular, early cellular, early sclerosis, and advanced sclerosis. He commented that the principal problem in histological classification, in general, was the separation of nodular sclerosis and its varied expressions from the remaining histologic types, and the acquisition of extensive experience with the essential criteria that permitted critical differentiation between the closely related remaining subtypes.

In the present EFSCH series, about 18 percent of the slides were not available or technically insufficient for subclassification. The distribution of the Rye histological subtypes according to sex and age is presented in Figure 1-14, according to clinical stages in Table 1-9. Similar to many other reports, patients with nodular sclerosis belonged to the younger age groups, were more frequently female than male, and had better survival rates than those with other histological types (Fig. 1-15). It is obvious also that the majority of patients with nodular sclerosis belonged to the early stages, whereas the reverse is true for those with lymphocyte depletion lesions (Table 1-9).

Butler (1971) summarized the relationship of histological subtypes and

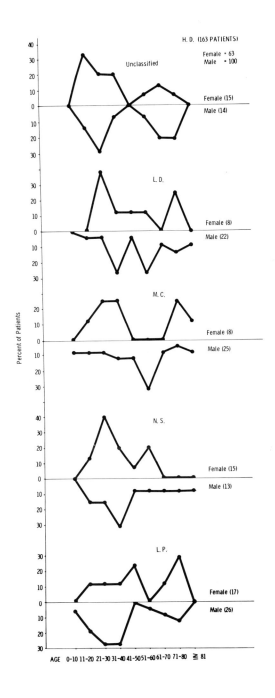

Fig. 1-14. Distribution of histological subtypes of Hodgkin's disease according to age and sex (EFSCH series).

Table 1-9
Sex and Clinical Stages versus Pathological Subtypes of Malignant Lymphoma (EFSCH series)

	I		II		III		IV		All Stages			
	M/F Ratio	Patient No.	M/F Ratio	Patient No.	M/F Ratio	Patient No.	M/F Ratio	Patient No.	M/F Ratio	Patient No.	% of 163	% of 134
I. Hodgkin's Disease												
LP	2.3	10	2.0	12	4.0	10	3.8	11	1.5	43	26	32
NS	0.4	11	1.3	7	*	2	1	8	0.9	28	18	21
MC	5.5	13	1.5	5	*	5	1.5	10	3.1	33	20	24
LD	2.0	3	0.4	7	2.5	7	*	13	2.8	30	18	13
Unclass.	1.7	8	0.2	6	2.0	6	0.8	9	0.9	29	18	0
Subtotal	1.6	45	1.0	37	4.0	30	1.4	51	1.5	163	100	100
									M/F Ratio	Patient No.	% of 364	% of 323
II. Non-Hodgkin's Disease												
LW	1.6	18	1.5	10	0.8	31	1.3	37	1.2	96	26	30
LP	1.7	8	1.3	7	1.5	20	1.0	44	1.2	79	22	24
Hist.	2.1	22	1.0	8	1.0	12	2.7	33	1.9	75	21	23
Pleo-Mixed	9.0	10	1.0	6	3.3	17	1.2	40	1.9	73	20	23
Unclass.	*	9	4.0	5	1.0	8	2.2	19	2.7	41	11	0
Subtotal	2.7	67	1.4	36	1.3	88	1.4	173	1.5	364	100	100

*All male patients.

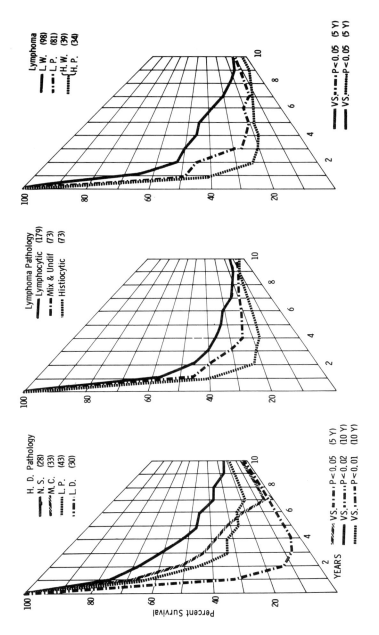

Fig. 1-15. Survival curves according to pathologic classifications (EFSCH series).

39

survivals in a total of 1220 patients with Hodgkin's disease collected from eight separate series (Franssila et al 1967; Fuller et al 1971; Gough 1970; Hamann et al 1970; Keller et al 1968; Landberg and Larsson 1969; Lukes and Butler 1966; and one of Lukes' personal series). In all eight studies, there was a clearcut difference in the survival rates between the nodular sclerosis and mixed cellularity groups. In five of the eight series, patients with the lymphocyte predominance type had the best prognosis; those with the nodular sclerosis type, the second best; those with mixed cellularity, the third; and those with the lymphocyte depletion type, the poorest prognosis. In two of the series, the survival was the same for the mixed cellularity and lymphocyte depletion groups. In another series (Landberg and Larsson 1969) patients with nodular sclerosis had a slightly better survival rate than those with the lymphocyte predominance type. Otherwise, the ranking of these three series was the same as the other five.

We have combined Butler's information and three other reports not summarized by him (Anderson et al 1970; Berard et al 1971; Selzer et al 1972), together with the data of the present EFSCH series in Table 1-10. Our results are comparable to others except for the subtype of lymphocyte predominance, although Anderson et al (1970) and Berard et al (1971) showed the survival of lymphocyte predominance was lower than that of nodular sclerosis; and Selzer et al (1972) showed that lymphocyte predominance and nodular sclerosis were very similar.

One explanation for the poor results of patients with this diagnosis in the EFSCH series could be that the majority (76 percent) of patients with lymphocyte predominance was admitted before 1960, as contrasted with only 46 percent of those with nodular sclerosis (p < 0.02). Also there has been a higher proportion of Hodgkin's disease patients who received combined radiotherapy and chemotherapy since 1960 (Fig. 1-16). We have data that show the prognosis of patients with Hodgkin's disease admitted after 1960 was much better than those admitted before, and the prognosis of patients who received both radiotherapy and chemotherapy was better than either treatment alone (Fig. 1-17). Presently, we cannot separate these interrelated factors in our small series of patients treated over the past 30 years by various different programs. Another explanation of our results could be difficulty in assigning certain lesions to one of the four particular types since all of the slides were reviewed and classified by only one pathologist in the present series. Our precentage of lesions of the lymphocyte predominance subtype was unusually high (26 percent versus 10–17 percent as reported by others, Table 1-10).

Many studies have demonstrated that the different histological subtypes also have distinct clinical manifestations, modes of spread, responses to therapy, and prognosis. Nodular sclerosis appears to be the most unique lesion. Such cases were appreciably younger than the other groups and had a high female to male ratio of 1.5 : 1 (Hanson 1964). Enlarged cervical

Table 1-10
Distribution and Survival Rates of Hodgkin's Disease versus Pathology Subtypes

		LP	NS	MC	LD	UC	Total
Patient Number							
Butler (1971)*	1942–1966	9–63	14–149	28–97	5–68		1220
Andersen et al (1970)	1955–1964	24	46	48	24		142
Berard et al (1971)	1953–1968	45	96	92	37	7	277
Selzer et al (1972)	1952–1967	17	32	43	30		122
EFSCH	1940–1971	43	28	33	30	29	163
Percent							
Butler (1971)*		10–17	40–53	26–33	4–18		100
Andersen et al (1970)		17	32	34	17		100
Berard et al (1971)		16	35	33	13	3	100
Selzer et al (1972)		14	26	35	25		100
EFSCH		26	18	20	18	18	100
5-Year Survival %							
Butler (1971)*		50–88	44–72	3–58	0–38		26–57
Andersen et al (1970)		27	44	15	24		33
Berard et al (1971)		51	61	33			43
Selzer et al (1972)		57	66	30	4		37
EFSCH		26	46	34	5		28
10-Year Survival %							
Butler (1971)*		44–69	25–53	14–37	4–20		22–51
Selzer et al (1972)		30	30	13	4		16
EFSCH		20	20	7	5		16

*Butler's summarization of eight reported series.

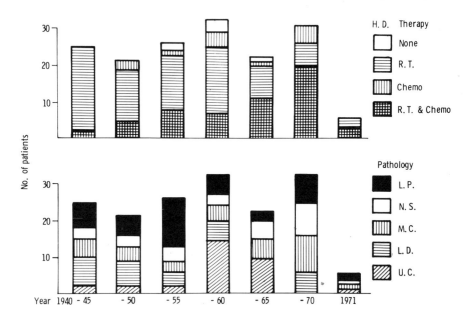

Fig. 1-16. Distribution of types of therapy, pathological subtypes, and years of admission (EFSCH series).

nodes were present in 97 percent of the patients at onset, and mediastinal mass was present in 87 percent. Berard et al (1971) found that about 80 percent of their patients with nodular sclerosis were between 15 and 34 years of age, and this particular subtype was infrequent in patients over 50 years old. Keller et al (1968) showed that the usual manner of spread in Hodgkin's disease was to adjacent lymph node groups. Noncontiguous dissemination, when it occurred, was more than twice as frequent in the mixed cellularity and lymphocyte depletion types, as compared to nodular sclerosis; and nodular sclerosis involving the lung has shown a favorable prognosis, unlike mixed cellularity. They found this histological classification system effective in predicting different prognosis even within similar clinical staging groups.

Strangly, Franssila et al (1967) found that 22 percent of the patients with nodular sclerosis had evidence of bony metastasis by x-ray, whereas there was not a single case in the other groups. Similar to the findings in adults, Butler (1969) reported that children with lymphocyte predominance lesions had the best prognosis. Next were those with the nodular sclerosis, which were also the only ones who exhibited involvement of the lungs, soft tissues of the chest wall, extremity and spinal cord compression.

Strum and Rappaport (1970a) studied 35 children with Hodgkin's disease. In 30 of 31 classified cases, the histologic sections showed either nodular sclerosis or lymphocyte predominance. Regardless of classification,

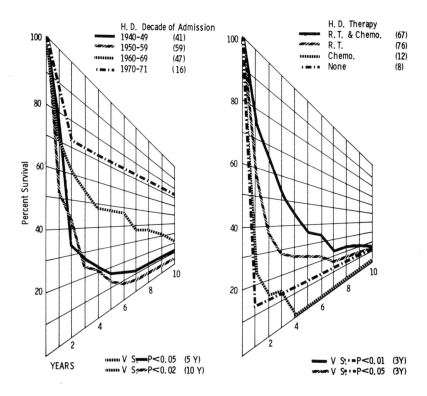

Fig. 1-17. Survival curves of patients with Hodgkin's disease according to decade of admission and type of therapy (EFSCH series).

most of the cases exhibited a striking predominance of mature lymphocytes in tissue sections, suggesting a particular host response characterizing the disease in the young. Schnitzer et al (1973) found nodular sclerosis was the most frequent histologic type seen in children aged 11 through 15, whereas no preponderant histologic type was seen in those in their first decade of life. Prognosis of patients with nodular sclerosis was considerably worse than that of children with lymphocytic predominance.

Peters (1970) reported a series of 150 new patients, two-thirds of whom had lymphangiographic studies as part of the initial assessment (only 6 had lymphocytic depletion). The author said that histological subtypes appeared to have the most important prognostic meanings because they governed the chronicity and the pattern of the natural course of Hodgkin's disease. Only 22 percent of those with nodular sclerosis and lymphocyte predominance presented with stages IIIB and IV disease, whereas 43 percent of those with mixed cellularity presented with similar stages. Berard et al (1971) also found that lymphocyte predominance was associated strongly with clinical stages I and II, while lymphocyte depletion was seen primarily with clinical stages III and IV. Mixed cellularity occurred in all clinical stages without any strong associations. Nodular sclerosis was associated predominantly with clinical stage II and was the only histological subtype with an apparently distinctive pattern of anatomic distribution, namely a strong propensity to involve the lower cervical lymph nodes, mediastinum, and contiguous structures. The other three histological groups exhibited variable degrees of association with clinical stages, but within clinical stages, they did not appear to have different sites of predilection. With regard to survival, the prognostic advantage of nodular sclerosis was largely restricted to patients in clinical stages I and II. There was no significant evidence of survival advantage in stage III or IV. In particular, in patients with stage I disease, only lymphocyte depletion had a poor survival; the other three subtypes had superimposable survival curves for the first 5 years. For patients with stage IV disease, lymphocyte predominance had the best prognosis; survival rates for the other three types were equally bad.

In patients with localized diseases (stage I and II), Gough (1970) showed that those having nodular sclerosis lesions had similar survival rates as those with mixed cellularity for the first 5 years. However, Fuller et al (1971) reported that the 5-year survival rates were 72 percent for those with nodular sclerosis and 58 percent for those with mixed cellularity. Furthermore, a breakdown of the nodular sclerosis group by stages (IA, IIA, IIB) or site of presentation (head and neck, or mediastinum) failed to demonstrate any statistically significant difference. In patients with mixed cellularity, a highly significant difference was noted in the 5-year survival figures for stages IA and IIA (72 percent versus 27 percent). Of the patients with stage IA disease of the upper neck, which was composed almost entirely of mixed cellularity cases, the 5-year survival rate was 93 percent. In contrast, patients in the stage IIA mixed cellularity group were almost totally ones with axillary or lower torso adenopathies.

Frei and Gehan (1971) presented the data of Fuller et al (1971) in a different way, showing that the different prognoses of different histopathological groups could be correlated with the individual propensity of postradiotherapeutic recurrence: (1) All patients with lymphocyte depletion had a very short relapse-free interval. (2) Patients with nodular sclerosis and mixed cellularity had a gradual decrease in the risk of recurrence during the first 4 years and, after that, the risk of recurrence was minimal (approximately 5 percent). (3) For patients with lymphocyte predominance, the risk of recurrence per year remained constant after the fourth up through the eighth year, suggesting this disease would be more indolent. Selzer et al (1972) found that the duration of remission following the initial therapy had important prognostic values. Those patients who had at least a 2-year remission had a much better survival rate than those who had shorter periods of remission. In particular, 2-year remissions were most frequent in patients with lesions of lymphocyte predominance with stage I disease (47 percent);

and there was a progressively diminishing frequency of such occurrence in the nodular sclerosis and mixed cellularity types at the advanced stages.

Many other histologic features of prognostic importance in Hodgkin's disease have also been described. Strum and Rappaport (1970b) reported 6 cases in which lymph node biopsy sections demonstrated only minute foci of Hodgkin's disease. They commented that such focal involvement of abdominal lymph nodes was much more likely to occur in cases which appeared clinically to be stage I or II. Henry (1970) studied 27 patients who survived for 10 years or longer. He confirmed the favorable outcome of the lymphocyte predominance and nodular sclerosis varieties. Other features indicating a good prognosis included a pseudofollicular pattern, incomplete involvement of the lymph node architecture, and the presence of lymphoid follicles within the tumor. Later, he (Henry 1971) showed that such favorable effect could be demonstrated in the mixed type and in the long-term survival of the nodular sclerosis variety, but not in the lymphocyte predominance or lymphocyte depletion forms.

Cross and Dixon (1971) divided Hodgkin's disease into three groups: reticular (paragranuloma), histiocytic, and nodular sclerosis. Each group was subclassified into well or poorly differentiated types. He indicated that patients with histologically well differentiated lesions showed a significantly higher survival rate than those with the poorly differentiated tumors. Patchefsky et al (1973) felt that the nodular sclerosis histological group could be further subdivided into subgroups by cellular composition and degree of fibrosis. Patients whose lesions composed predominately of mature lymphocytes, few Reed-Sternberg cells and minimal fibrosis had the best survival rates, especially at 6th year. Thus it appears that it may be possible to pick out those patients having the most and least favorable prognosis, based on quantitative and qualitative assessment of these histologic features.

Vascular invasion in Hodgkin's disease was first reported by Rappaport and Strum (1970), who found this most frequent in lesions of the lymphocyte depletion type. About 80 percent of the patients with vascular invasion were stage III or IV and had relatively short survivals. Further observations showed that vascular invasion could be detected in 5.9 percent of 153 patients who had lymph node biopsy for stage I or II diseases (Strum et al 1971a). Of the 9 cases with vascular invasion, 4 occurred in lesions of the nodular sclerosis type and 4 in mixed cellularity. This finding was associated with a greater than twofold increase in extension of the disease to nonadjacent areas and with a survival at 18 months almost one-half that of cases without such invasion, suggesting the poor prognosis of this finding even though the lesion was one of the favorable types (Rappaport et al 1971a). In a later series of 29 patients who had exploratory laparotomy for staging, 20.7 percent showed vascular invasion either in sections of the nodal biopsy or in the splenectomy specimen (Strum et al 1971b). Patients with this histological feature had either stage III or IV disease, whereas only 43.5 percent of those without such finding had such extensive disease. In addition, involvement of the liver, lung, or bone marrow was found in 5 of 6 patients with vascular invasion, in contrast to only 1 patient without this finding. In 2 of the 3 patients who had vascular invasion in the spleen, there was unequivocal liver involvement, suggesting that hematogenous dissemination via the portal system might be important. Thus, the Committee on Histopathological Criteria Contributing to Staging of Hodgkin's Disease at the Ann Arbor Conference recommended the routine use of special stain for elastica on all tissue sections in order to facilitate the diagnosis of vascular invasion and to correlate this with the prevalence of extranodal and disseminated disease (Rappaport et al 1971b).

However, Lamoureux et al (1973) did not find evidence of vascular invasion in a retrospective study of 11 patients who developed extranodal dissemination of disease following radiotherapy among 136 consecutive patients who had early (stage I and II) Hodgkin's disease. Vascular invasion was also not seen in any of the disease-free patients from the same series matched for age, sex, clinical stage of disease, and histological subclassification. In their experience, a more reliable index of high risk for extranodal dissemination is provided by clinicohistologic correlation, the greatest risk is seen in patients having constitutional symptoms associated with mixed cellularity and lymphocyte depletion histology.

Non-Hodgkin's Lymphoma

Virchow distinguished lymphosarcoma from leukemia in 1867. Kundrat (1893) separated lymphosarcoma from Hodgkin's disease and "pseudo-leukemias." Brill et al (1925) and Symmers (1927) described the picture of so-called giant follicular lymphoma. Gall and Mallory (1942) divided the histology of non-Hodgkin's lymphoma into: (1) reticulum cell sarcoma, (2) lymphoblastic lymphoma, (3) lymphocytic lymphoma, and (4) follicular lymphoma. Lymphosarcoma, a general term which was used synonymously with malignant lymphoma by many authors, corresponds roughly with the two middle groups. Rappaport et al (1956) pointed out that malignant lymphoma of any cellular composition might have either a nodular (follicular) or a diffuse pattern. Patients with tumors of the follicular pattern had better survival rates, and follicular lesions had a tendency to progress into diffuse patterns. Among patients with non-Hodgkin's lymphomas, Gellhorn (1957) showed that the survival curve of patients with giant follicular lymphomas was the best (60 percent at 5 years), and those with reticulum cell sarcomas, the poorest (4 percent at 5 years).

Based on the cellular composition, cellular differentiation, and patterns of proliferation, Gall and Rappaport (1958) proposed a new classification system. Rappaport (1966) described their proposal in more detail in a monograph (Table 1-11). In the present EFSCH series, 364 patients had non-

Table 1-11
Histological Classification of Non-Hodgkin's Lymphoma* (Rappaport 1966)

LW:	Lymphocytic, well-differentiated—A malignant proliferation of lymphocytes that appear to be mature and that show moderate variations in either nuclear size or shape. Mitotic figures are usually absent. Histological separation from lymphocytic leukemias are sometimes impossible.
LP:	Lymphocytic, poorly differentiated—Malignant tumor composed of lymphocytes that show varying degrees of nuclear atypia and immaturity. The size of the cells are between a mature lymphocyte and a histiocyte. Clear evidence of mitotic activity. The chromatin structure is relatively coarse. A single, distinct nucleolus can be detected. A few malignant reticulum cells and occasional reticulum fiber formation can be found. Fibrosis is rare.
Und:	Undifferentiated—Tumor composed of primitive reticular cells showing no appreciable histiocytic or lymphocytic differentiation. The nuclei are two to four times larger than those of a normal lymphocyte. Few lymphoblasts and lymphocytes can be detected. Burkitt's tumor is included in this classification. Histiocytes containing nuclear fragments are not uncommon.
HW/HP:	Histiocytic (reticulum cell sarcoma)—Malignant tumor composed of prominently neoplastic histiocytes in various stages of maturation and differentiation: well-differentiated (HW), or poorly differentiated (HP). The more differentiated cells may resemble monocytes. There is abnormal formation of reticulum. The variant "pleomorphic cell type" of reticulum cell sarcoma shows cytological features similar to those of histiocytic lymphomas except that they contain bizarre atypical giant cells. Morphologically they are similar to Reed-Sternberg cells.
MC:	Mixed cell (histiocytic-lymphocytic)—This is a malignant tumor characterized by proliferation of neoplastic histiocytes and lymphocytes without appreciable predominance of either cell type. With time, they will progress into histiocytic or occasionally into poorly differentiated lymphocytic types. Another common feature is they tend to exhibit a nodular or follicular pattern
UC:	Unclassified—Lesion diagnosed as malignant lymphoma but could not be classified into any of the above five subgroups.

*Each subgroup can then be divided into D (diffuse) or N (nodular) subtype.

Hodgkin's lymphomas. A comparison of the distribution of histological subtypes according to the old diagnosis versus the new Rappaport classification is given in Table 1-12. There are very few reports in the literature correlating the different distributions of non-Hodgkin's lymphoma between the old histologic types and the new classifications. Talvalkar (1971) reported a series of 58 patients with giant follicular lymphomas. On reclassification, a well differentiated lymphocytic type was seen in 18; poorly differentiated, 32; mixed cell type, 6; histiocytic type, 1; and Hodgkin's disease, 1.

About 11 percent of the slides in the EFSCH series could not be reclassified. The sex and clinical stage distribution in each pathological subtype is given in Table 1-9. Figure 1-18 shows the sex and age distribution graphically. Almost all of the subtypes are more concentrated in the older age groups, and the variations between males and females are much less than that of Hodgkin's disease.

Table 1-12
Distribution and Survival Rates of Non-Hodgkin's Lymphoma versus Pathology Subtypes (EFSCH series)

Old diagnosis	Survival (%)		No. of patients	New Diagnosis						
	5 yr	10 yr		Lymphocytic		Histiocytic		Mixed cell	Undifferentiated	Cannot classify
				WD*	PD*	WD*	PD*			
Reticulum cell sarcoma	24	15	121	12	19	21	20	12	22	15
Lymphocytic lymphoma			138	54	29	12	6	11	10	16
Lymphoblastic lymphoma	31	15	61	13	23	5	4	3	7	6
Giant follicular lymphoma			23	14	4	1	1	2		1
Hodgkin's disease	59	17	21	5	.6	1	3	4	1	1
No. of patients			364	98	81	40	34	32	40	39
Total patients (%)			100	27	22	11	9	9	11	11
Survival (%)										
5 year			30	46	21	18	18	24	24	38
10 year			14	16	13	0	11	10	10	28

*WD = well-differentiated, PD = poorly differentiated

48

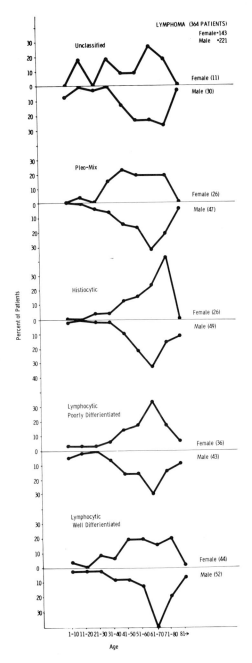

Fig. 1-18. Distribution of histological subtypes of non-Hodgkin's lymphoma according to age and sex (EFSCH series).

The survival curves according to histological subtypes in the EFSCH series are given in Figures 1-15 and 1-19. We found that patients with well differentiated lymphocytic lymphoma and those with the older diagnosis of giant follicular lymphoma had much better survival curves than all the other types. The survival curves of those with the histiocytic type were the worst; and those of the poorly differentiated lymphocytic, undif-ferentiated, or mixed cell types, intermediate (Lee et al, 1973). In all subtypes, the presence of nodular or follicular patterns reflected better prognosis (Fig. 1-19). The favorable prognostic effect of well differentiated lymphocytic histology was especially noticeable in female patients and in those in the early stages of the disease (Fig. 1-20). Among patients with well differentiated lymphocytic lesions, those who were females, of the younger age group, without symptoms, and who were treated since 1960 also fared better; although, statistically, the difference was not significant (Fig. 1-21). In early lesions (stages I and II), but not in advanced stages, those without capsular invasion meant better survival for the patients (Fig. 1-22). Hansen (1969) also found that extension outside the capsule led to a poorer prognosis.

Lukes (1967) pointed out that the new classification system of Gall and Rappaport could relate better to the histologic pattern of involvement, the clinical distribution of the process, the occurrence of leukemic manifesta-tions, and the immunologic state. The transition and progression among the various subtypes also followed certain well-defined pathways. Sheehan and Rappaport (1968) said the general tendency was for initial nodular pat-terns to become diffuse and for the mixed cell type to become histiocytic. Butler (1970) said all nodular and well differentiated lymphocytic lymphomas appeared to have stable or slowly progressive courses; histiocytic and undif-ferentiated types, rapidly progressive; and poorly differentiated lymphocytic types, moderately progressive.

Using the scheme of Rappaport, Jones et al (1972) reported that patients with histiocytic lymphomas uncommonly had initial marrow involvement, whereas patients with mixed and lymphocytic types frequently had bone marrow lesions. They commented that the older terminology of reticulum cell sarcoma, lymphosarcoma, and giant follicular lymphoma would not have shown this important clinical and pathological finding. Reviewing the results of radiotherapy in patients with localized non-Hodgkin's lymphomas, they also found that those who had *diffuse* histiocytic lesions had a short median survival of 13 months and a high risk of relapse within 1 year of treatment. In contrast, patients with *nodular* mixed cell type or lymphocytic poorly differentiated lymphomas exhibited a median survival of 80 months and a pattern of continued late relapse.

Jones et al (1973) further reported that nodular lymphoma constituted 44 percent of their 405 patients. Patients under the age of 35 years and those over 60 tended to have diffuse lymphomas. In each cellular category, patients with nodular lymphomas survived significantly longer than those

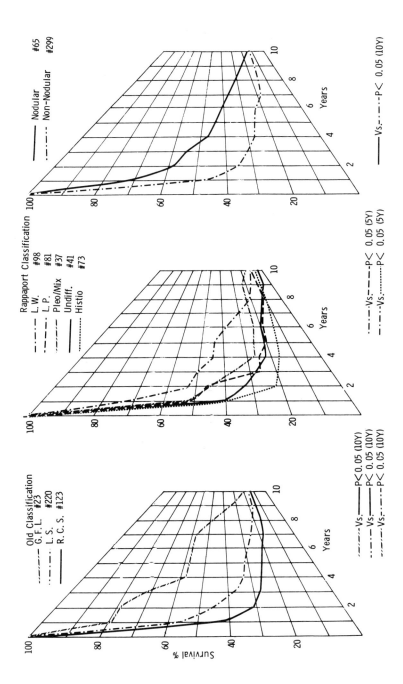

Fig. 1-19. Survival curves of patients with non-Hodgkin's lymphoma according to pathological subtypes and presence or absence of nodular pattern (EFSCH series).

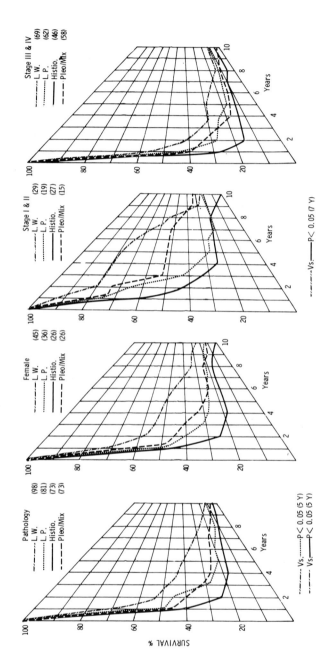

Fig. 1-20. Survival curves of patients with non-Hodgkin's lymphoma according to pathologic subtype, sex, and clinical stage (EFSCH series).

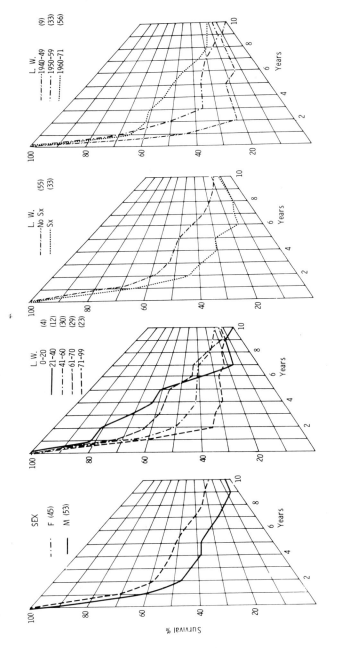

Fig. 1-21. Survival curves of 98 patients with well-differentiated lymphocytic lymphoma according to sex, age, presence or absence of systemic symptoms, and decade of admission (EFSCH series).

53

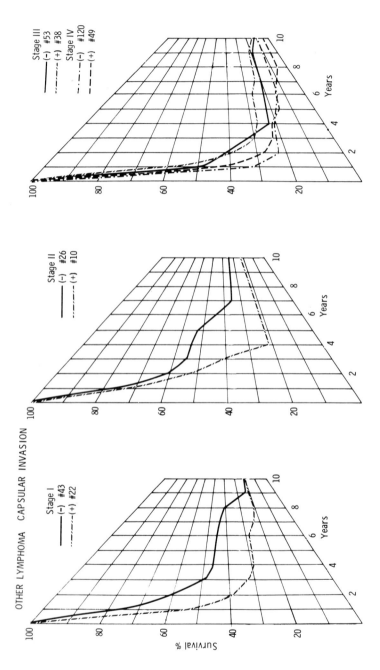

Fig. 1-22. Survival curves of patients with non-Hodgkin's lymphoma according to presence and absence of capsular invasion of lymph node lesions (EFSCH series).

with diffuse lymphomas. Localized extralymphatic involvement occurred more often in patients with diffuse than with nodular lymphomas (p < 0.001). Two frequently observed sites of initial extralymphatic involvement were bone marrow and gastrointestinal tract, each occurred in 16 percent of the patients; the former was observed more often in advanced lymphocytic lymphomas, whether nodular or diffuse, and the latter in advanced diffuse lymphomas. Patients with either initial bone marrow or gastrointestinal tract involvement survived longer if their lymphoma had a nodular pattern. They also found that 81 percent of evaluable patients with nodular lymphoma and 90 percent of those with diffuse lymphoma had contiguous sites of involvement.

Several other histiological features were shown to have prognostic significance. Oels et al (1968) reviewed the incidence of histiocytic phagocytosis ("starry-sky" appearance). They found this phenomenon was associated predominantly with lymphoblastic rather than lymphocytic lesions, and the degree of histiophagocytosis was greater in patients with more advanced disease. The life expectancy for patients with advanced and moderate phagocytosis was considerably less than that for those without phagocytosis, regardless of the clinical stage at diagnosis.

Bennett and Millett (1969) described a clinicopathological entity of "nodular sclerotic lymphosarcoma." The fibrosis was seen most commonly between the fifth and seventh decades and was not seen before the fourth decade. Women were affected more commonly, and most patients with such lesions presented with glands in the groin or retroperitoneum. This variant of lymphosarcoma appeared to be less malignant than that showing diffuse infiltration of the lymph node without fibrous banding, and the prognosis approximated that of follicular lymphoma. In a later report of 233 patients, 21 percent of all the patients with nodular lymphosarcoma had this particular histology (Millett et al 1969). The improvement in survival rates was more marked in patients presenting with generalized disease. With localized disease, the 5-year survival rate was similar in follicular lymphoma, diffuse lymphosarcoma, and nodular sclerotic lymphosarcoma, but a greater percentage of the last group continued to survive, free from clinical evidence of disease, for periods up to 19 years.

Recently, Rosas-Uribe and Rappaport (1972) also described a unique morphological pattern of "histiocytic type with sclerosis." The most striking histologic feature was pronounced fibrosis and a peculiar compartmentalization of the tumor tissue. Clinically, 4 of the 9 patients survived 5 years or longer with only local therapy (excision and/or local radiotherapy). The disease was initially localized to the axilla in 6 patients, the cervical chain in 2, and the inguinal region in one. In their series, they purposely excluded cases with sclerotic features in retroperitoneal nodes since it was felt that these might be a desmoplastic reaction to fatty acids released by tumor invasion and destruction of fatty tissue.

B. Kon

Thus, similar to the nodular sclerosis subtype of Hodgkin's disease, the presence of abundant collagen formation in non-Hodgkin's lymphoma also indicated a more favorable prognosis. It is conceivable that the pronounced fibrosis might represent a peculiar host reaction, perhaps indicative of a resistance to the spread of the disease. On the other hand, the particular malignant reticuloendothelial cell might act as a facultative fibroblast.

Rosas-Uribe et al (1973) reported a heretofore undescribed finding of proteinaceous precipitate within the neoplastic nodules of malignant lymphoma with nodular patterns. In their series of 13 patients, there was no correlation found between the amount of precipitate and the clinical course of the disease, the cytologic type of lymphoma, or its anatomical location.

SUMMARY

In the past decade, great progress has been made in the diagnosis and treatment of malignant lymphoma, especially the Hodgkin's disease which accounted for about 40 percent of the lymphoma cases. Nearly half of the patients with non-Hodgkin's lymphoma may have disease of the extranodal sites on presentation.

The important prognostic factors of malignant lymphoma included age, sex, presence or absence of systemic symptoms, clinical stages, and histological types. All these factors are interrelated and the last two, stage of the disease and histological subtype of the lesion, appeared to be most significant. Female patients and those who belong to the age group of 21 to 40 years had the best survival rate. Patients with stage I or II disease have better survival curves than those with stage III or IV. The presence of systemic symptoms, such as fever, night sweat, weight loss, etc., affected the survival adversely.

Sites of lymphadenopathy have been studied in detail in patients with Hodgkin's disease, and patterns of initial nodal involvement might have prognostic importance. Primary extranodal lesions in Hodgkin's disease are rare. But in 60 percent of the patients with reticulum cell sarcoma, and in 40 percent of those with lymphosarcoma, the first site of involvement was extranodal. Lesions of the gastrointestinal tract were most common and accounted for about half of the extranodal lymphomas.

Histopathologically, Hodgkin's disease can be classified as lymphocyte predominance (LP), nodular sclerosis (NS), mixed cellularity (MC), and lymphocyte depletion (LD). Many studies have demonstrated that the different histological subtypes also have distinct clinical manifestations, modes of spread, response to therapy, and prognoses. Nodular sclerosis appeared to be most unique in that patients who had this lesion belonged to the younger age groups, were more likely to be females, had a higher incidence of mediastinal disease and involvement of contiguous structures. Histological subtype seems to be the most important prognostic factor, because it reflects different survival rates even within the same clinical stages. Several other useful pathological features have been described; the most important one is vascular invasion, the presence of which correlated with disseminated disease and poor prognosis.

According to the Rappaport system, non-Hodgkin's lymphoma can be subdivided into lymphocytic, well and poorly differentiated (LW, LP), histiocytic, well and poorly differentiated (HW, HP), mixed cell (MC), and undifferentiated (UND) types. Each subtype can be divided into either a nodular or a diffuse pattern. Nodular lesions with well-differentiated lymphocytic types had the best prognosis. Different histological subtypes had different frequency of involvement of the bone marrow and separate patterns of relapse after radiotherapy.

REFERENCE

Aisenberg AC: Malignant lymphoma, N Engl J Med 288:883–890, 935–941, 1973

Albujar PF: Hodgkin's disease in Trujillo, Peru: Clinical and histologic presentation. Cancer 31:1520–1522, 1973

Andersen AP, Brincker H. Lass F: Prognosis in Hodgkin's disease with special reference to histologic type: Results of treatment predominantly by cytostatics. Acta Radiol [Ther] (Stockh) 9:81–101, 1970

Azzam SA: High incidence of Hodgkin's disease in children in Lebanon. Cancer Res 26:1202–1203, 1966

al-Bahrani ZR, Bakir F: Primary intestinal lymphoma: A challenging problem in abdominal pain. Ann R Coll Surg Engl 49:103–113, 1971

Banfi A, Bonadonna G, Carnevali G, et al: Preferential sites of involvement and spread in malignant lymphomas. Eur J Cancer 4:319–324, 1968

Bennett MH, Millett YL: Nodular sclerotic lymphosarcoma: A possible new clinico-pathological entity. Clin Radiol 20:339–343, 1969

Berard CW, Thomas LB, Axtell LM, et al: The relationship of histopathological subtype to clinical stage of Hodgkin's disease at diagnosis. Cancer Res 31:1776–1785, 1971

Brewin TB: Alcohol intolerance in neoplastic disease. Br Med J 2:437–441, 1966a

Brewin TB: Alcohol shift and alcohol dysphagia in Hodgkin's disease, carcinoma of cervix, and other neoplasms. Br J Cancer 20:688–702, 1966b

Brewin TB: The incidence of alcohol intolerance in women with tumours of the uterus, ovary, or breast. Proc R Soc Med 60:1308–1309, 1967

Brill NE, Baehr G, Rosenthal N: Generalized giant lymph follicle hyperplasia of lymph nodes and spleen: A hitherto undescribed type. JAMA 84:668–671, 1925

Butler JJ: Histopathology of malignant lymphomas and Hodgkin's disease. Leukemia-Lymphoma. Chicago, Year Book, 1970, pp 123–142

Butler JJ: Hodgkin's disease in children. Neoplasia in Childhood. Chicago, Year Book, 1969, pp 267–279

Butler JJ: Relationship of histological findings to survival in Hodgkin's disease. Cancer Res 31:1770–1775, 1971

Carbone PP, Kaplan HS, Musshoff K, et al: Report of the Committee on Hodgkin's Disease Staging Classification. Cancer Res 31:1860–1861, 1971

Catlin D: Surgery for head and neck lymphomas. Surgery 60:1160–1166, 1966

Chawla PL, Stutzman L, Dubois RE, et al: Long survival in Hodgkin's disease. Am J Med 48:85–95, 1970

Cohen BM, Smetana HF, Miller RW: Hodgkin's disease: Long survival in a study of 388 World War II army cases. Cancer 17:856–866, 1964

Cole P: Epidemiology of Hodgkin's disease. JAMA 222:1636–1639, 1972

Coppleson LW, Factor RM, Strum SB, et al: Observer disagreement in the classification and histology of Hodgkin's disease. J Natl Cancer Insti 45:731–740, 1970

Correa P, O'Conor GT: Epidemiological patterns of Hodgkin's disease. Int J Cancer 8:192–201, 1971

Craver LF: Recent advances in treatment of lymphomas, leukemias, and allied disorders. Bull NY Acad Med 24:3–25, 1948

Cross RM, Dixon FW: A combined clinical and histological assessment of survival of patients with Hodgkin's disease. J Clin Pathol 24:385–393, 1971

De Vita VT, Serpick A, Carbone PP: Combination chemotherapy of advanced Hodgkin's disease (HD): The NCI program, a progress report. Proc Am Assoc Cancer Res 10:19, 1969

Easson EC, Russell MH: The cure of Hodgkin's disease. Br Med J 1:1704–1707, 1963

Eidelman S, Parkins A, Rubin CE: Abdominal lymphoma presenting as malabsorption: A clinico-pathologic study of nine cases in Israel and a review of the literature. Medicine 45:111–137, 1966

Franssila KO, Kalima TV, Voutilainen A: Histologic classification of Hodgkin's disease. Cancer 20:1594–1601, 1967

Freeman C, Berg JW, Cutler SJ: Occurrence and prognosis of extranodal lymphomas. Cancer 29:252–260, 1972

Frei E III, Gehan EA: Definition of cure for Hodgkin's disease. Cancer Res 31:1828–1833, 1971

Fuller LM, Gamble JF, Butler JJ: Leukemia-Lymphoma. Chicago, Year Book, 1970, pp 241–259

Fuller LM, Gamble JF, Shullenberger CC, el al: Prognostic factors in localized Hodgkin's disease treated with regional radiation. Radiology 98:641–654, 1971

Gall EA, Mallory TB: Malignant lymphoma: Clinico-pathologic survey of 618 cases. Am J Pathol 18:381–429, 1942

Gall EA, Rappaport H: Seminar on diseases of lymph nodes and spleen. In McDonald (ed): Proceedings of the Twenty-third Seminar. New Orleans, La., Am Soc Clin Pathol, 1958, p 107

Gellhorn A: End-results in lymphosarcoma and Hodgkin's disease. Proceedings of the Third National Cancer Conference, Philadelphia, Lippincott, 1957, pp 862–869

Glatstein E, Guernsey JM, Rosenberg SA, et al: The value of laparotomy and splenectomy in the staging of Hodgkin's disease. Cancer 24:709–718, 1969

Goodman LS, Wintrobe MM, Dameshek W, et al: Nitrogen mustard therapy: Use of methyl-bis (beta-chloroethyl) amine hydrochloride and tris (beta-chloroethyl) amine hydrochloride for Hodgkin's disease, lymphosarcoma, leukemia and certain allied and miscellaneous disorders. JAMA 132:236–132, 1946

Gough J: Hodgkin's disease: A correlation of histopathology with survival. Int J Cancer 5:273–281, 1970

Hall CA, Olson KB: Prognosis of the malignant lymphomas. Ann Intern Med 44:687–706, 1956

Hamann W, Oehlert W, Musshoff K, et al: The histologic classification of Hodgkin's disease and its relevance to prognosis. Ger Med Mon 15:509–514, 1970

Hansen HS: Reticulum cell sarcoma treated by radiotherapy. Significance of clinical features upon the prognosis. Acta Radiol [Ther] (Stockh) 8:439–458, 1969

Hanson TA: Histological classification and survival in Hodgkin's disease: A study of 251 cases with special reference to nodular sclerosing Hodgkin's disease. Cancer 17:1595–1603, 1964

Heath CW Jr: The epidemiology of Hodgkin's disease. Ann Intern Med 77:313–314, 1972

Hellwig CA: Malignant lymphoma: The value of radical surgery in selected cases. Surg Gynecol Obstet 84:950–958, 1947

Henderson RD: Occult manifestations of cancer. Can Med Assoc J 88:31–36, 1963

Henry L: Long survival in Hodgkin's disease. Clin Radiol 21:203–210, 1970

Henry L: Partial involvement of the lymph node in Hodgkin's disease. Clin Radiol 22:405–410, 1971

Hilton G, Sutton PM: Malignant lymphomas: Classification, prognosis, and treatment. Lancet 1:283–287, 1962

Hodgkin T: On some morbid appearances of the absorbent glands and spleen. Medico-Chir Trans 17:68–114, 1832

Hoster HA: Hodgkin's disease. Am J Roentgenol Radium Ther Nucl Med 64:913–918, 1950

Hutchison G: Formal discussion of Brian MacMahon's paper, Epidemiological considerations of staging in Hodgkin's disease. Cancer Res 31:1858–1859, 1971

Hutchison GB: Anatomic patterns by histologic type of localized Hodgkin's disease of the upper torso. Lymphology 5:1–14, 1972

International Union Against Cancer: Clinical stage classification. Research Commission Report, 1966

Jackson H Jr, Parker F Jr: Hodgkin's disease. II. Pathology. N Engl J Med 231:35–44, 1944

Jackson H Jr, Parker F Jr: Hodgkin's Disease and Allied Disorders. New York, Oxford University Press, 1947

James AH: Hodgkin's disease with and without alcohol-induced pain: A clinical and histological comparison. Q J Med 29:47–66, 1960

Jelliffe AM, Thompson AD: The prognosis in Hodgkin's disease. Br J Cancer 9:21–36, 1955

Jenkin RD, Sonley MJ, Stephens CA, et al: Primary gastrointestinal tract lymphoma in childhood. Radiology 92:763–767, 1969

Jones SE, Fuks Z, Bull M, et al: Non-Hodgkin's lymphomas: IV. Clinicopathologic correlation in 405 cases. Cancer 31:806–823, 1973

Jones SE, Kaplan HS, Rosenberg SA: Non-Hodgkin's lymphomas: III. Preliminary results of radiotherapy and a proposal for new clinical trials. Radiology 103:657–662, 1972

Kaplan HS: Hodgkin's disease. Cambridge, Mass., Harvard University Press, 1972, p 90

Kaplan HS: The radical radiotherapy of regionally localized Hodgkin's disease. Radiology 78:553–561, 1962

Keller AR, Kaplan HS, Lukes RJ, et al: Correlation of histopathology with other prognostic indicators in Hodgkin's disease. Cancer 22:487–499, 1968

Kundrat H: Ueber Lympho-Sarkomatosis. Wien Klin Wochenscha 6:211–213, 1893

Lacher MJ: Long survival in Hodgkin's disease. Ann Intern Med 70:7–17, 1969

Lamoureux KB, Jaffe ES, Berard CW, et al: Lack of identifiable vascular invasion in patients with extranodal dissemination of Hodgkin's disease. Cancer 31:824–825, 1973

Lampe I, Fayos JV: Hodgkin's disease—radiotherapeutic experience, in Zarafonetis CJ (ed): Proceedings of the International Conference on Leukemia-Lymphoma. Philadelphia, Lea & Febiger, 1968, pp 393–401

Landberg T, Larsson L: Hodgkin's disease: Retrospective clinicopathologic study in 149 patients. Acta Radiol Ther (Stockh) 8:390–414, 1969

Lee YN: Aggregation of Hodgkin's disease. J Am Wom MA 28:529–536, 1973

Lee YN, Say C, Hori JM, et al: Clinical courses of Hodgkin's disease and other malignant lymphomas. Am J Roentgenol Radium Ther Nucl Med 117:19–29, 1973

Lee YN, Say C, Hori JM, et al: Histopathological features and survival in malignant lymphoma. Proc Amer Assoc Cancer Res 14:114, 1973

Lennert K: Pathologisch anatomische Klassification der malignen Lymphome. Strahlentherapie Sonderb 69:1–7, 1969

Longcope WT, McAlpin FR: Hodgkin's disease. Oxford Medicine, vol 4, part 1, 1920 pp 1–43

Lockwood AH: Marihuana and alcohol intolerance in Hodgkin's disease. N Engl J Med 288:526, 1973

Lukes RF: Criteria for involvement of lymph node, bone marrow, spleen, and liver in Hodgkin's disease. Cancer Res 31:1755–1767, 1971

Lukes RF: Current concepts in cancer. I. Hodgkin's disease, prognosis and relationship of histologic features to clinical stage. JAMA 190:914–915, 1964

Lukes RJ: Current concepts in cancer. 36. Updated Hodgkin,s disease, prognosis and relationship of histologic features to clinical stage. JAMA 222:1294–1296, 1972

Lukes RJ: The pathologic picture of the malignant lymphomas, in Zarafonetis (ed): Proceedings of the International Conference on Leukemia-Lymphoma. Philadelphia, Lea & Febiger, 1968, pp 333–356

Lukes RJ: Relationship of histologic features to clinical stages in Hodgkin's disease. Am J Roentgenol Radium Ther Nucl Med 90:944–955, 1963

Lukes RJ: A review of the American concept of malignant lymphoma: The evolution of a modern classification, in Ruttimann A (ed): Progress in Lymphology, vol. I. Stuttgart, Thieme, 1967, pp 109–119

Lukes RJ, Butler JJ: The pathology and nomenclature of Hodgkin's disease. Cancer Res 26:1063–1081, 1966

Lukes RJ, Butler JJ, Hicks EB: Natural history of Hodgkin's disease as related to its pathologic picture. Cancer 19:317–344, 1966a

Lukes RJ, Craver LF, Hall TC, et al: Report of the Nomenclature Committee. Cancer Res 26:1311, 1966b

MacMahon B: Epidemiological considerations in staging of Hodgkin's disease. Cancer Res 31:1854–1857, 1971

MacMahon B: Epidemiological evidence on the nature of Hodgkin's disease. Cancer 10:1045–1054, 1957

MacMahon B: Epidemiology of Hodgkin's disease. Cancer Res 26:1189–1200, 1966

Medina A, Benninghoff DL, Camiel MR: Extranodal spread of Hodgkin's disease. Am J Roentgenol Radium Ther Nucl Med 111:368–375, 1971

Miller RW: Mortality in childhood Hodgkin's disease: An etiologic clue. JAMA 198: 1216–1217, 1966

Millett YL, Bennett MH, Jelliffe AM, et al: Nodular sclerotic lymphosarcoma: A further review. Br J Cancer 23:683–692, 1969

Molànder DW, Pack GT: Lymphosarcoma: Choice of treatment and end-results in 567 patients; role of surgical treatment for cure and palliation. Rev Surg 20:3–31, 1963

Mullins GM, Lenhard RE Jr: Digital clubbing in Hodgkin's disease. Johns Hopkins Med J 128:153–157, 1971

Musshoff K, Renemann H, Boutis L, et al: Malignant lymphoma: The differentiation of two different types of Stage IV Hodgkin's disease in Viamonte M, Koehler PR, Witte M, et al (eds): Progress in Lymphology, vol 2. Stuttgart, Thieme, 1970, pp 272

Neiman RS, Rosen PJ, Lukes RJ: Lymphocyte-depletion Hodgkin's disease: A clinicopathological entity. New Engl J Med 288:751–755, 1973

Novis BH, Bank S, Marks IN, et al: Abdominal lymphoma presenting with malabsorption. Q J Med 40:521–540, 1971

Oels HC, Harrison EG Jr, Kiely JM: Lymphoblastic lymphoma with histiocytic phagocytosis ("starry-sky" appearance) in adults: Guide to prognosis. Cancer 21:368–375, 1968

Patchefsky AS, Brodovsky H, Southard M, et al: Hodgkin's disease: A clinical and pathologic study of 235 cases. Cancer 32:150–161, 1973

Peters MV: Changing concepts in radiotherapy for the Lymphomas. Leukemia-Lymphoma. Chicago, Year Book, 1970, pp 261–274

Peters MV: The need for a new clinical classification in Hodgkin's disease: Keynote address. Cancer Res 31:1713–1722, 1971

Peters MV: A study of survivals in Hodgkin's disease treated radiologically. Am J Roentgenol Radium Ther Nucl Med 63:299–311, 1950

Peters MV, Brown TC, Rideout DF: Current concepts in cancer. 39. Updated Hodgkin's Disease, prognostic influences and radiation therapy according to pattern of disease. JAMA 233:53–59, 1973

Peters MV, Hasselback R, Brown TC: The natural history of the lymphomas related to the clinical classification, in Zarafonetis CJ (ed): Proceedings of the International Conference on Leukemia-Lymphoma. Philadelphia, Lea & Febiger, 1968, pp 357–371

Pusey WA: Cases of sarcoma and of Hodgkin's disease treated by exposures to x-rays—a preliminary report. JAMA 38: 166–169, 1902

Rappaport H: Tumors of the hematopoietic system, Atlas of Tumor Pathology, Section III, Fascicle 8. Armed Forces Institute of Pathology, 1966

Rappaport H, Berard CW, Butler JJ, et al: Report of the Committee on Histopathological Criteria Contributing to Staging of Hodgkin's disease. Cancer Res 31:1864–1865, 1971b

Rappaport H, Strum SB: Vascular invasion in Hodgkin's disease: Its incidence and relationship to the spread of the disease. Cancer 25:1304–1313, 1970

Rappaport H, Strum SB, Hutchison G, et al: Clinical and biological significance of vascular invasion in Hodgkin's disease. Cancer Res 31:1794–1798, 1971a

Rappaport H, Winter WJ, Hicks EB: Follicular lymphoma: A re-evaluation of its position in the scheme of malignant lymphoma, based on a survey of 253 cases. Cancer 9:792–821, 1956

Rather LJ: Who discovered the pathognomonic giant cell of Hodgkin's disease? Bull NY Acad Med 48:943–950, 1972

Razis DV, Diamond HD, Craver LF: Familial Hodgkin's disease: Its significance and implications. Ann Intern Med 51:933–971, 1959

Reed DH: On the pathological changes in Hodgkin's disease, with especial reference to its relation to tuberculosis. Johns Hopkins Hosp Rep 10:133–196, 1902

Reilly CJ, Han T, Stutzman L, et al: Reticulum-cell sarcoma: A review of radiotherapeutic experience. Cancer 29:1314–1320, 1972

Rosas-Uribe A, Rappaport H: Malignant lymphoma, histiocytic type with sclerosis (sclerosing reticulum cell sarcoma). Cancer 29:946–953, 1972

Rosas-Uribe A, Variakojis D, Rappaport H: Proteinaceous precipitate in nodular (follicular) lymphomas. Cancer 31:534–542, 1973

Rosenberg SA: Report of the Committee on the Staging of Hodgkin's Disease. Cancer Res 26:1310, 1966

Rosenberg SA: The clinical evaluation and staging of patients with malignant lymphoma, in Clark RL, Cumley RW, McCay JE, et al (eds): Oncology 1970, vol 4. Chicago, Year Book, 1971, pp 507–518

Rosenberg SA, Boiron M, DeVita VT Jr, et al: Report of the Committee on Hodgkin's Disease Staging Procedures. Cancer Res 31:1862–1863, 1971

Rosenberg SA, Diamond HD, Jaslowitz B, et al: Lymphosarcoma: A review of 1269 cases. Medicine 40:31–84, 1961

Rosenberg SA, Kaplan HS: Hodgkin's disease and other malignant lymphomas. Calif Med 113:23–38, 1970

Schnitzer B, Nishiyama RH, Heidelberger KP, et al: Hodgkin's disease in children. Cancer 31:560–567, 1973

Selzer G, Kahn IB, Sealy R: Hodgkin's disease. A clinico-pathologic study of 122 cases. Cancer 29:1090–1100, 1972

Sheehan WW, Rappaport H: Morphological criteria in the classification of the malignant lymphomas. Proc Natl Cancer Conf 6:59–71, 1968

Shimkin MB: Current concepts in cancer. No 40. Updated Hodgkin's Disease, evaluation of recent results. JAMA 233:169–170, 1973

Shimkin MB: Hodgkin's disease: Mortality in the United States, 1921–1951; race, sex and age distribution; comparison with leukemia. Blood 10:1214–1227, 1955

Silverberg E, Holleb AI: Cancer statistics 1972. CA 22:2–20, 1972

Solidoro A, Guzman C, Chang A: Relative increased incidence of childhood Hodgkin's disease in Peru. Cancer Res 26:1204–1208, 1966

Sternberg C: Uber eine eigenartige unter dem Bilde der Pseudoleukamis verlaufende Tuberculose des lymphatischen Apparates. Ztschr Heilk 19:21–90, 1898

Strum SB, Allen LW, Rappaport H: Vascular invasion in Hodgkin's disease: Its relationship to involvement of the spleen and other extranodal sites. Cancer 28:1329–1334, 1971b

Strum SB, Hutchison GB, Park JK, et al: Further observations on the biologic significance of vascular invasion in Hodgkin's disease. Cancer 27:1–6, 1971a

Strum SB, Rappaport H: Hodgkin's disease in the first decade of life. Pediatrics 46:748–759, 1970a

Strum SB, Rappaport B: Interrelations of the histologic types of Hodgkin's disease. Arch Pathol 91:127–134, 1971

Strum SB, Rappaport H: Significance of focal involvement of lymph nodes for the diagnosis and staging of Hodgkin's disease. Cancer 25:1314–1319, 1970b

Symmers D: Certain clinical and pathologic aspects of lymphosarcoma. Am J Med Sci 174:9–29, 1927

Symposium on obstacles to the control of Hodgkin's disease. Cancer Res 26:1041–1311, 1966

Symposium on staging in Hodgkin's disease. Cancer Res 31:1707–1870, 1971

Talvalkar GV: Giant follicular lymphoma: Clinico-pathologic review of 58 cases. Indian J Cancer 8:7–20, 1971

Teillet F, Boiron M, Bernard J: A reappraisal of clinical and biological signs in staging of Hodgkin's disease. Cancer Res 31: 1723–1729, 1971

Ultmann JE, Cunningham JK, Gellhorn A: The clinical picture of Hodgkin's disease. Cancer Res 26:1047–1060, 1966

Ultmann JE, Moran EM: Clinical course and complications in Hodgkin's disease. Arch Intern Med 131:332–353, 1973

Vianna NJ, Greenwald P. Brady J, et al: Hodgkin's disease: Cases with features of a community outbreak. Ann Intern Med 77:169–180, 1972

Wood NL, Coltman CA: Localized primary extranodal Hodgkin's disease. Ann Intern Med 78:113–118, 1973

Yates JL Bunting CH: Results of treatment in Hodgkin's disease. JAMA 68:747–751, 1917

2

Special Diagnostic Tests

It is reported that even after the most careful evaluative physical examinations and tests, about one-third of the cases were assigned to the wrong clinical stages (Peters and Middlemiss 1958). Thus, special radiological studies were added in order to decrease this margin of error. Routine investigation of the stomach, small bowel, and colon is usually not worthwhile in untreated patients with Hodgkin's disease, but in the non-Hodgkin's patients, they are always important since involvement of these viscera is more frequent (Rosenberg 1971). For examination of retroperitoneal nodes, both intravenous pyelogram and inferior venacavogram were relatively ineffective because the nodes had to be grossly enlarged to displace the ureters from which they were separated by distances as great as 3 cm; and the opacified vena cava reflected changes in the right paravertebral lymphatic chain only. After conducting studies in 231 patients with various lymphomas, Lee (1967) stated that inferior venacavography demonstrated retroperitoneal disease with about 65 percent reliability and intraenous pyelography with about 30 percent reliability.

LYMPHANGIOGRAM

Lymphangiography, developed in the 1950s by Kinmonth, is the only available method of direct roentgenographic visualization of lymphatics and lymph nodes. This procedure was not used to any great extent in patients with malignant lymphomas until after 1965. Lower extremity lymphangiogram, as it is employed at the present time, is accomplished by injecting radiopaque contrast material (Ethiodol) into the subcutaneous lymphatic trunks of the feet.

In patients with Hodgkin's disease, Peters et al (1967), performed lymphangiograms first; intravenous pyelograms and inferior venacavograms were done subsequently, if disease was not apparent in the lymphangiograms. Rosenberg (1971) also used lymphangiograms in the initial evaluations of all patients with malignant lymphomas and added the venacavogram only in selected cases, especially for evaluation of the region above the second lumbar vertebra which was not usually visualized on the lymphangiogram. Peters et al (1973) estimated that about 60 percent of the cases on presentation were classed as stage I or II, and 40 percent as more advanced before 1965. Since 1965, when routine lymphangiogram and complementary tests were done, the ratio has been reversed, with 40 percent in stages I and II and 60 percent in stages III and IV.

Clinicopathological Correlations

In 110 patients with Hodgkin's disease, Lee et al (1964) found that retroperitoneal nodes were abnormal on lymphangiograms in 35 percent of those with clinical stage I disease; 51 percent, stage II; and 89 percent, stage III or above. Only 10–15 percent of stage I patients with cervical presentation had abnormal retroperitoneal nodes, whereas 6 out of 6 patients with groin presentation did so (Lee 1966). The presence of systemic symptoms correlated highly with the presence of retroperitoneal disease—one-third of those with stage IIA disease had abnormality below the diaphragm, whereas nearly 90 percent of those with symptoms did so. Of 12 patients who had stage IV disease above the diaphragm involving the lung or chest wall, abnormal lymphangiograms were seen only in those with systemic symptoms (Lee 1968).

Davidson et al (1967) reported that abnormal lymphangiograms were found in 36 percent of those Hodgkin's cases clinically diagnosed as stages I and II; whereas, if suspicious lymphangiograms were also counted as abnormal, the figure became 52 percent. More specifically, 38 percent of stage I and 43 percent of stage II cases advanced to stage III because of abnormal lymphangiograms (Davidson and Clarke 1968). Among the 12 patients with lesions of the groin, only 9 had retroperitoneal disease, in contrast with the 100 percent rate reported by Lee (1966). Among the patients with stages I and II disease, 32 percent of those with neck adenophy and 52 percent of those with axilla lesions had clinically occult abnormality in lymph nodes on the opposite side of the diaphragm.

The incidence of disease in the abdominal nodes was similar for all histological subtypes of Hodgkin's disease. However, Davidson and Clarke (1970) found that lesions of lymphocyte predominance involved mainly superficial and retroperitoneal nodes and that lesions of nodular sclerosis involved the mediastinal and adjacent lymph glands. Thus, lymphographic studies reconfirmed what was described by pathologists. It is suggested that the lymphangiogram is also useful in the diagnosis and localization of lesions in patients with obscure pruritis, autoimmune hemolytic anemia, jaundice, or back pain (Lee 1967).

Lymphangiograms showed a higher incidence of abdominal lymph node involvement in patients with reticulum cell sarcomas and lymphosarcomas. Among 76 patients, Lee et al (1964) found that over 80 percent of those with clinical stage I disease and 90 percent of those with more advanced lesions had retroperitoneal abnormality. In a series of 118 patients with Hodgkin's disease and 88 with non-Hodgkin's lymphomas, Takahashi and Abrams (1967) found that the diagnostic accuracy rate of lymphangiograms was about 80 percent. The false positive rate was 5 percent and the false negative, 15 percent. Among the false negative cases, there were relatively more cases of Hodgkin's disease and giant follicular lymphomas than reticulum cell sarcomas and lymphosarcomas. In 60 children with all types of malignant tumors, Musumeci et al (1972) found that the use of lympho-graphy was just as important as in adults. In about 27 percent of children with Hodgkin's disease and in 19 percent with lymphoreticular sarcomas clinically classified as stages I and II, lymphangiograms detected abnormal lymph nodes in the retroperitoneal space.

The variability of interpreting lymphangiograms among different observers appeared to be low. During a collaborative study of patients with Hodgkin's disease, the reading of the consultant radiologist concurred with the local radiologist in 130 negative and 10 positive reports (Viamonte 1971). There were 11 discordant reports (7 percent); of these, the report was changed to positive in 3 cases and to negative in 8 by the consultants.

The diagnosis of malignant lymphoma by lymphangiogram is based upon two criteria: nodal enlargement and abnormal contrast pattern. Viamonte (1972) emphasized that there are no adenographic patterns pathognomonic of Hodgkin's disease or other lymphomas. Fischer and Thornbury (1965) pointed out the limitations of the technique: (1) It can be applied only to a portion of the lymphatic system, i.e., inguinal, iliac, abdominoaortic, and rarely axillary node regions; (2) In cases of massive involvement, diseased nodes closest to the site of injection may take up almost all the injected contrast material, preventing visualization of nodes further away. Eichner (1971) showed that some nodes, such as obturator and deep pelvic nodes, were not seen on the usual lower extremity lymphangiograms at all. Escobar-Prieto et al (1971) emphasized that evidence of lymphatic channel obstruction and patterns of altered flow dynamics were also important abnormal findings. These were manifested by dilation of channels, stasis of lymph flow, extravasation, backflow, and collateral circulation.

In about 60 percent of the cases, it is possible to diagnose the histological subtypes of malignant lymphomas from the lymphangiographic appearances (Dolan 1964). Oh et al (1969) showed the appearance of giant follicular lymphomas was not very specific, since it was indistinguishable from other types of malignant lymphomas and granulomatous disorders. In Hodgkin's disease, Wiljasalo (1969) found that a foamy appearance was predominant in the early stages and filling defects in the later stages. But filling defects were also typical of the nodular sclerosis subtype, and an accuracy rate of 70 percent was found which distinguished this subgroup from the others. Fuchs and Härtel (1970) found that irregular and solitary filling defects were common in the initial stages of Hodgkin's disease; cystic foamy storage patterns and the rare forms of fibrosis were common mainly in the terminal stages.

Lee and Stephenson (1970) found that the results of lymphangiograms per se also had prognostic value. Patients with stages I and II disease who had negative lymphangiograms and those with stage IIIA disease did well regardless of the mode of radiation therapy. However, patients with stage IIIB disease who received extended radiotherapy to all of their node bearing areas appeared to do better than those who were treated with local ports.

Morbidity and Mortality

Minor complications of lymphangiography included fever; nausea; vomiting; pain of limb, groin, back, or intraabdominal nodes. In a series of 176 patients, Lee et al (1964) encountered 11 complications: 4 of pulmonary insufficiency; 5 of infection at the site of the cutdown; and 2 of allergic skin reaction. Thus, pulmonary parenchymal disease and history of allergy to iodine compound should be considered as contraindications to the use of lymphangiograms. Lee (1966) added that the lymphangiogram should not be used in those patients with known stage III disease, especially those with palpable nodes below the diaphragm.

Fallat et al (1970) studied the clearance of radioactive ^{131}I-labeled Ethiodol from the lungs following a lymphangiogram. Maximum deposition in the lungs occurred within the first 24 hours, and often over 40 percent of the total dose was found there. Clearance was slow and variable; the mean biological half-life in the lung was 8 days. Diffusing capacity of the lung decreased 16–34 percent below control levels and persisted even when much of the radioactive iodine had cleared.

Lee (1966) reported a patient who died after a lymphangiogram for Hodgkin's disease. The patient had stage III disease but did not have any apparent pulmonary abnormality. He knew of two other deaths attributable to lymphangiograms in patients with generalized lymphomas and radiation fibrosis of the lungs (Lee et al 1964). In retrospect, lymphangiograms were unnecessary in these patients. Another patient died of anaphylactic reaction to the patent blue dye which was used for labeling the subcutaneous lymphatics. Lee (1967) commented that the amount of dye given in this particular patient was three times the usual amount. Routinely, no more than 2 ml of patent blue dye was required in each foot, and 5–7 ml of Ethiodol on each side gave excellent films. In children, 1–3 ml in each foot is sufficient. Davidson (1971) utilized a slightly different technique by dividing the contrast material unequally so that the left side received 0.5–1 ml more than the right. The rate of introduction was deliberately kept slow, approximately 1 ml in 8 min, and monitor films were taken routinely. Injection was stopped before the thoracic duct was visualized. By adhering to this regimen, he had no clinical pulmonary complications in more than 1000 studies.

It should be pointed out that the method of cannulation of a tiny lymphatic channel in the foot to obtain a lymphangiogram is technically difficult, and the whole process is very time consuming. Thus, several new techniques and modifications have been tried. Hall and Krementz (1967) injected the contrast medium directly into the inguinal nodes, and Myhre (1971) dissected out the lymphatics in the groins, which are much larger in size than those in the foot. Newer methods of using radioisotope scanning to outline retroperitoneal nodes is discussed on page 74.

Indications

Presently, the indication for use of the lymphangiogram in non-Hodgkin's lymphomas is not as firm as that in Hodgkin's disease. The Committee on Hodgkin's Disease Staging Procedures at the Ann Arbor Conference listed bilateral lower extremity lymphogram as one of the "advisable radiological studies" under the heading of "Required Evaluation Procedures" (Rosenberg et al 1971).

Results of staging exploratory laparotomy showed that the lymphographic test could have a false negative rate of 12 percent and a false positive rate of 28 percent (p. 202). Despite these limitations, Glatstein (1971) pointed out that the lymphangiogram should not be abandoned. He gave three reasons: (1) It is frequently valuable in localizing nodes that are suspicious. A surgeon might have great difficulty in pinpointing a single suspicious node along the para-aortic chains. (2) The opacification of para-aortic and pelvic nodes is of great value to the radiotherapist when he maps out a subdiaphragmatic field. (3) The follow-up information obtained by sequential diagnostic abdominal and pelvic x-rays, especially during the first few post-treatment years, is an extremely important part of good medical management. Thus, Kaplan (1972) felt that the lymphangiogram remained an essential part of the diagnostic evaluation of all patients with Hodgkin's disease, except for those with specific contraindications.

However, others proposed more restricted use. Lee (1968) felt that the only indication for using the lymphangiogram was to outline the extent of disease in patients with clinically localized disease. Hall (1966) felt the lymphangiogram was not necessary if stage IIB (or more advanced) disease was present. Brickner et al (1968) found the lymphangiogram was positive only in 6 percent of 50 patients with stages II and IIA Hodgkin's disease. All 3 patients also had mediastinal disease. Thus, they felt, "Routine lymphangiography would seem to be of some value for delineation of treatment volumes in stage II cases when there is obvious mediastinal disease and the question of the extension into the abdominal lymph nodes is raised. In cases with stages III and IV disease, it is not very useful, since nearly all of these patients have disease within the abdominal lymph nodes."

In cases where the lymphangiographic picture is doubtful, and in cases where exploratory laparotomy is not planned, repeated radiographs of the suspicious nodes could be taken every 2 to 3 months to detect changes (Wallace 1970). The longest period after which a single lymphangiogram was still diagnostically adequate was 5 years. One patient had the lymphangiographic procedure repeated as many as 5 times over a period of 7 years without obvious ill effects.

Davidson et al (1967) used the lymphangiogram in the reassessment of treated patients for recurrent or new retroperitoneal disease. In 40 patients with Hodgkin's disease, they found 67 percent had abnormal lymphangiograms and only 4 out of the 27 had a palpable abdominal mass. Steiner et al (1970) conducted repeated lymphangiograms 11 to 40 months after radiotherapy. In patients without clinical suspicion of disease, only 1 of 13 had a positive lymphangiogram. In patients with systemic symptoms, abdominal or pelvic signs, 6 out of 14 had positive findings. In 30 percent of the cases, there was enough contrast material left 18 months after the lymphangiogram; in only 12 percent was opacification sufficient after 24 months. Thus, when necessary, they felt the lymphangiographic study should be repeated every 3 years after initial diagnosis and treatment. Lacher and Geller (1972) showed that follow-up abdominal films could also be used to monitor the effect of chemotherapy in treating persistent or recurrent lesions after radiotherapy.

The role of routine follow-up diagnostic radiographs in detecting relapse in Hodgkin's disease was assessed by Castellino et al (1973). Of 442 patients treated for cure between 1955 and 1970, 130 suffered relapse. The diagnosis of relapse was initiated by radiographic findings alone in 35 percent of the patients by clinical findings in another 35 percent, and by both radiographic and clinical findings in the remaining 30 percent. Of the 35 percent of patients who were symptomatically and clinically without the evidence of disease, the radiographic findings were equally divided between changes in retroperitoneal lymph nodes and in the mediastinum/lungs. These results emphasize the value of routine surveillance abdominal and chest films, as well as repeat lymphangiography in selected cases.

RADIOISOTOPE STUDIES

In the Report of the Committee on Hodgkin's Disease Staging Procedures (Rosenberg et al 1971) under the category of "Useful Ancillary Procedures Not Definitive for Diagnosis," several radioisotopic studies were listed: (1) Skeletal scintigrams should be performed in selected cases of roentgenological osseous abnormalities, unexplained osseous pain, or elevated serum alkaline phosphatase. (2) Hepatic and spleen scintigrams are of very limited value except when large filling defects are noted or when estimating the size of the spleen. Under the category of "Procedures Promising for Clinical Study at Selected Centers but Experimental at this Time," the Committee Report mentioned whole-body gallium and selenium scintigrams, especially for the demonstration of mediastinal disease.

The above recommendations regarding the use of radioisotope scintigrams appear to be valuable also for patients with non-Hodgkin's lymphomas. Recent reports demonstrating the clinical usefulness of these tests will be discussed in general terms here. It is enough to say that results of tissue biopsy taken at staging laparotomy and other surgical procedures have shown that scintigraphic abnormalities cannot be considered as diagnostic of lymphomatous involvement of the liver, spleen, or bone.

Spleen

Enlarged spleens weighing more than 400 g usually contained Hodgkin's disease (Kadin et al 1971). One simple method of estimating spleen size from routine abdominal films was to measure the vertical length from the tip of the spleen to its intercept with the diaphragm (Whitley et al 1966). In an average-size adult, when this height was more than 15 cm, there was a 98 percent probability that the spleen was also enlarged (more than 200 g). This finding appeared interesting, and Westin et al (1972) found a fairly good correlation between the spleen scan area and the length of the spleen on x-ray, but the standard deviation was rather large. Thus, they proposed the use of scan area as a criteria to measure spleen size. The upper limit of normal value was 81 cm^2.

Rollo and DeLand (1970) proposed a method to estimate splenic mass based on several measurements taken from the posterior and left lateral view of radioisotopic scans of the spleen. The method was independent of body configuration, required few measurements, and involved only one equation. The results were reproducible and correlated well with values determined at postmortem examination. Using this method, DeLand (1970) found that the normal spleen weight was relatively constant from age 30 to 59 years (male, 109 ± 27 g; female, 97 ± 24 g). After age 60, the spleen decreased in size.

Silverman et al (1972) reported a series of 42 Hodgkin's patients who had concomitant splenic and hepatic scans, exploratory laparotomy, and splenectomy. Positive criteria of involvement of the spleen included more than moderate enlargement in size, focal filling defects, or patchy distribution of radioisotope. The correctness of the reading was confirmed in 80 percent of the negative scans and in 40 percent of the positive scans. Searching for a better way to detect lymphomatous involvement of the spleen, Castellino et al (1972) performed selective splenic arteriograms in 33 patients prior to laparotomy. Although tumor nodules as small as 2 cm showed up on tomograms taken in conjunction with angiograms, the pictures seen in both normal and abnormal spleens were similar in general.

Milder et al (1973) reviewed 50 scans of the spleen and correlated them with clinical and pathologic findings in patients with Hodgkin's disease. Splenomegaly on scan was associated with advancing stage and tumor involvement of the spleen and liver. All 13 spleens measuring over 15 cm in length on scan and all 7 with filling defects were positive for tumor. In combination with the physical examination and lymphangiogram, however, the scan enabled accurate prediction of splenic involvement only in 43 percent of the cases.

Liver

Hepatic scintigrams, using radioactive tracers to demonstrate space-occupying defects in the liver, were first reported by Stirrett et al in 1954. Nagler et al (1963) reported an accuracy rate of 83 percent in 402 patients who had positive scans and 88 percent in 146 patients with negative scans.

The radioactive isotopes useful for liver scanning have changed over the years. Rose bengal iodine-131 was administered in the earlier studies, but greater uniformity of uptake pattern in normal and sharper delineation of defects in abnormal livers led to the employment of radioactive gold ^{198}Au in the 1960s. One valuable asset of colloidal gold is its retention by the Kupffer cells of the liver which permits repeated scans to be made if necessary. Its retention is independent of liver function. And when liver function is depressed, the spleen will occasionally concentrate the radioactivity. On the other hand, the clearance of the ^{131}I rose bengal is a reflection of the hepatic function, and maximum hepatic concentration occurred about 1 hr after administration. A repeated scan 2 hr later demonstrated the iodinated compound in the gall bladder, supplying an index regarding the function of that organ. By placing the collimator over the abdomen after the ingestion of a glass of cream or milk, one may determine the rapidity of excretion of the rose bengal via the common duct into the intestine. This method has proved valuable, for patients with jaundice, in the differentiation of parenchymal liver disease and extrahepatic obstruction as the cause of the jaundice.

Gollin et al (1964) found that abnormal liver scans were highly reliable in indicating localized disease because there was a false positive rate of only 2.5 percent. However, a normal scan was considerably less dependable, because this was seen in 27 percent of those who had documented disease. They considered this overall accuracy rate of 77 percent much better than any other single liver function test, since alkaline phosphatase which was almost as sensitive in detecting localized disease, yielded false positives twice as often. Using both radioisotopic scan and the alkaline phosphatase provided the most reliable index as to the presence or absence of localized hepatic disease. In 109 consecutive patients with primary extrahepatic carcinomas, Castagna et al (1972) found that scans correctly predicted the presence or absence of metastasis in 74.3 percent of the patients. Scan data were falsely positive in 14.7 percent and falsely negative in 11 percent. In patients without obstructive jaundice, the serum alkaline phosphatase appeared to be the most reliable blood test in predicting metastasis.

Molander et al (1967) reported the use of ^{131}I rose bengal scintiscan of the liver in 10 patients with malignant lymphomas. The most common pattern of hepatic involvement seen was that of diffuse, patchy infiltration. Others found that the typical picture of lymphomatous involvement of the liver was hepatomegaly with focal labeling defects. In cases where the liver was diffusely invaded, a generalized decrease in labeling rather than focal changes might be seen. In a series of 500 hepatic scans using rose bengal or gold, Ariel et al (1969) found that the diagnostic accuracy of detecting metastatic lesions was 85.2 percent. False positive diagnosis was made in 9.7 percent of the patients and false negative, in 5.1 percent. In 42 patients with lymphoma, the diagnosis was 100 percent correct, but "it was not possible, in most instances, to distinguish between parenchymal liver disease and lymphomatous involvement of the liver."

In the late 1960s, technetium-99 sulfide colloid was found to be superior to the radioactive gold because of improved counting statistics, reduced scanning time, lower radiation dose, and better spatial resolution. Spleen scan was easily obtainable in 77 percent of patients. Haynie et al (1970) compared the results using these two different isotopes. The false negative rate in abnormal livers with neoplastic or non-neoplastic disease was similar (20 percent), whereas in normal livers, technetium gave a lower false positive rate than gold (11 percent versus 26 percent). In 48 patients with suspected liver metastasis, Cantor et al (1970) found that the technetium scan demonstrated approximately 10 percent more intrahepatic lesions. Among the 5 patients, one had lymphosarcoma and 2 had Hodgkin's disease.

Some authors advocated the use of liver scintigraphy as part of the routine examination for the staging of patients with Hodgkin's disease (Smithers 1967). Ludbrook et al (1972) determined observer error in reading gamma camera-imaged technetium liver scans. On best performance, the average overall error rate was 20 percent, and this was similar among 7 observers. Thus, they emphasized that interpretations of liver scans should be used as an index of suspicion rather than as diagnostic findings. In a series of 49 patients who had technetium scans, staging laparotomies, and liver biopsies, 4 had proven Hodgkin's disease in the liver. Lipton et al (1972) showed that hepatic enlargement was not a valuable index. Focal filling defects were always associated with hepatic Hodgkin's disease, but this abnormality occurred only in 2 patients. A non-uniform uptake of radioactivity in the liver was the most common sign of liver disease, but this was not specific for Hodgkin's disease and was often associated with liver granulomas. No Hodgkin's disease was found in the livers when scintigraphs showed normal size and uniform uptake. Although this zero rate of false negatives was much lower than what was experienced by others, their conclusion was: "Laparotomy with liver biopsy remains the most specific means for staging abdominal Hodgkin's disease." Milder et al (1973) also found that filling defects or mottling were not a reliable sign of liver involvement and hepatomegaly in all ranges is more often associated with nonspecific factors than with tumor.

Since approximately 15 percent of intrahepatic metastases might be overlooked if reliance is based solely on inspection and palpation during surgery (Ozarda and Pickren 1962), and since the smallest lesion detectable by radioisotope liver scan is limited by the resolving power of the scanner or camera (Haynie et al 1970), several other experimental techniques have been tried to outline small lesions of the liver. Lawson (1962) obtained a detailed picture of the liver when oily contrast medium was injected accidentally into the portal vein system. Idezuki et al (1966) used this method intentionally in 37 cases and detected tumor masses as small as 1.5 cm in the liver. In order to obtain serial films to follow the response to therapy, Lee (1968) showed that in dogs the dose of oily contrast material given could be increased, and the radiopacity achieved persisted over 2 months.

By cannulating the reopened umbilical vein in adults, Piccone et al (1967) obtained transumbilical portal hepatography. Using water-soluble contrast medium, they demonstrated lesions as small as 1 cm in diameter. Under fluoroscopic control, they also injected iodinated oil, as much as 60 ml, into the umbilical vein and achieved what they called "angial residue hepatography" (Piccone et al 1968). This technique is contraindicated in patients with portosystemic vascular shunts or patent sinus venosus because of pulmonary oil embolism. The total number of patients who had this test was not given, but the authors said there was no death or complication from the use of lipid contrast medium. They felt this was a valuable adjunct to other x-ray procedures and commented that "angial residue hepatography provides the long-term radiologic visualization of the liver which makes possible hepatic tomography and fluoroscopically controlled liver biopsy."

Since most of the lymphomatous infiltration of the liver is diffuse, the technique of hepatography with oily contrast medium injected via the portal vein system appears to have limited value in the evaluation and staging of such disease. However, when malignant hepatic masses are found during abdominal operations, branches of the mesenteric vein can easily be cannulated and contrast medium administered. This technique could provide a simple and reliable record of the tumor size and offer an objective means for following the effectiveness of chemotherapy.

Other Sites

Radioisotopic bone scanning with strontium-85 is a well-documented technique for the detection of metastatic and primary bone tumors. It might reveal bone lesions prior to the development of roentgenographic changes (Charkes and Sklaroff 1964). Milner et al (1971) compared the value of bone scan and regular skeletal roentgenogram in 100 patients with metastatic bone lesions. They found bone scan gave a higher yield than that of roentgenogram alone (86 percent versus 73 percent), and in about 29 percent of the cases, additional lesions detected by the scan were not demonstrated by x-ray. Still, their data and other reports in the literature showed that there were significant false negative rates for both scans and routine x-rays (3–14 percent for scans and 27–52 percent for x-rays).

Edwards and Hayes (1969) reported striking localization of radioisotope gallium-67 in nonosseous tumors in patients with Hodgkin's disease and other lymphomas. Gallium appeared intracellularly, and it was associated with viable rather than fibrotic or necrotic tumor tissues. They scanned 41 patients with known diseases and outlined some tumor sites that were not detected by more conventional studies (Edwards and Hayes 1970). In particular, all 8 patients with non-Hodgkin's lymphomas showed good tumor localization, and the ratio of gallium in the tumor to that in the blood was greater than 100 : 1 at 15 days. In patients with Hodgkin's disease, only 6 of 11 scans demonstrate the known tumor site. Turner et al (1972) used gallium for whole-body scanning in 20 patients with Hodgkin's disease. Of 29 diseased sites, 23 (79 percent) were correctly identified and confirmed by pathological examination of tissues or chest radiographs and physical examination of superficial lymph nodes. However, 6 areas thought to be abnormal on the basis of the scan were found to be uninvolved at surgery.

Lomas et al (1972) studied the uptake of gallium by hepatic tissues in patients who had focal defects on routine colloid liver scans. Definite accumulation of the gallium was noted in 23 of 30 patients with hepatic cancer (including 2 of 2 patients with Hodgkin's disease). Twenty-six of 33 patients with benign or inflammatory lesions who had focal defects in colloid liver scans did not have an appreciable uptake of gallium.

When technetium-99 is administered into the body, 5–10 percent of the injected dose goes to the marrow, and the remainder is concentrated in the liver and spleen. Although the concentration in the bone marrow is not large, it can be useful in detecting marrow involvement in patients with malignant disease (Nelp and Bower 1969). Pinsky et al (1971) used 8 mci (millicuries) instead of the 3 mci usually given for liver and spleen scans, and used a colloid preparation which was passed through a 100-mm millipore filter first. Scanning of the marrow from the upper lumbar spine to the middle part of the femur was performed after the liver and spleen scans. In 22 patients with Hodgkin's disease, 18 marrows were interpreted as normal on scans, biopsies, and roentgenographic bone surveys. Four scans were interpreted as abnormal; of these, other tests were also positive in 3. The other patient, considered a false positive, had a normal bone survey and marrow biopsy, although the biopsy was not taken from the region of the abnormality seen on the scan.

Larson and Nelp (1971) described 4 abnormal scan patterns associated with malignancy involving the bone marrow. In Hodgkin's disease, they found the appearance of the scan reflected stages of the disease and prior radiotherapy. Focal scan defects were seen in 9 of 31 patients and were of 2 types: a small irregular defect due to infiltration of the tumor, and a sharply circumscribed defect due to radiotherapy. In patients with untreated early disease, the scan pattern was always normal. Among 17 patients with stages III or IV disease, regardless of previous therapy, scan patterns frequently showed peripheral expansion with central depression or greatly reduced intramedullary marrow uptake. Among 7 patients with lymphosarcomas, all 3 with biopsy or autopsy-proven tumors had abnormal scans of focal defects or peripheral expansion.

Since lower extremity lymphangiogram is a technically demanding and time-consuming procedure, several radioisotopic scanning procedures have been tested as possible alternatives. Pearlman (1970) injected radioactive gold into the feet and performed scintiscanning of the abdominal nodes. In 100 patients with known lymphomas, they found good anatomic and pathologic correlation between the scintiscan and the lymphangiogram. They suggested that this method could be used as a rapid screening procedure in the initial staging and subsequent evaluation of radiation response. When the scan is doubtful, further studies, including lymphangiograms, could then be carried out. Fairbanks et al (1972) used technetium-99 labeled colloid in 31 patients with various malignant lymphomas. They found an overall 66 percent agreement between interpretation of scintigrams and lymphangiograms. However, all of these tests are new, and radioisotope scans have the drawback of providing even less morphological details than lymphangiograms.

BONE-MARROW BIOPSY

The aspiration technique to obtain bone-marrow smears was first introduced by Arinkin in 1929. Snapper et al (1971) pointed out that smearing of the specimen not only ruined the entire topography of the bone marrow but also destroyed many white blood cells and immature reticulum cells. Liao (1971) tried to avoid the shortcomings of smears by using histologic sections of aspirated marrow simultaneously. He showed that sections were more valuable than smears in the diagnosis of granuloma, metastatic tumor, and lymphoma in the bone marrow. Among 1124 consecutive patients, 27 had malignant lymphomas diagnosed by sections, whereas only 9 of these patients had diagnostic smears. Specifically, in none of the 5 patients with Hodgkin's disease was the smear positive.

A Vim-Silverman needle biopsy of the bone marrow was reported as a simple procedure (McFarland and Dameshek 1958). Later, the larger Jensen-Westerman needle gained popularity and was used by Ellis et al (1964) in 1445 marrow biopsies. Studying a plug of bone measuring about 1 cm in length taken from the posterior iliac crest, Webb et al (1970) showed that 11 of 49 patients had positive evidence of Hodgkin's disease in the marrow, even though aspiration studies were unrevealing. The stages of 6 of the 11 patients were advanced from III to IV. However, biopsy failed to demonstrate marrow involvement in 5 of 39 patients who had disease proven at autopsy, suggesting that a negative biopsy could not exclude such possibility. Han et al (1971) showed that marrow specimens obtained by the Jensen-Westerman needle were superior to those obtained by the Vim-Silverman needle. The incidence of positive bone-marrow biopsies was higher in patients with late stages of disease (25 percent in stage III; 62 percent, stage IV) and with systemic symptoms (50 percent). None of the 12 patients with stages I or II Hodgkin's disease had positive marrow biopsies.

It is well known that the fibrotic and granulomatous nature of Hodgkin's disease prevents taking an adequate marrow specimen. When the biopsy specimen is small, the diagnosis of bone marrow involvement might be difficult. In such instances, Lukes (1971) suggested that proof of the lesion need not be as stringent as that required for the initial diagnosis of Hodgkin's disease. The presence of large, abnormal mononuclear cells with huge nucleoli was sufficient. The Committee on Histopathological Criteria said if there were only focal or diffuse areas of fibrosis which contained only the inflammatory cells characteristic of Hodgkin's disease, and when this microscopic picture was seen in an untreated patient with histologically proven Hodgkin's disease, it should be regarded as strongly suggestive of marrow involvement (Rappaport et al 1971).

Using the needle and/or open-bone biopsy technique, Rosenberg (1971) showed that about 9 percent of the untreated patients whose disease was more advanced than stage II had Hodgkin's disease of the bone marrow. Among 36 patients, 1 had positive aspiration, 12 had disease in the specimens obtained by the Jensen-Westerman needle, and 23 were diagnosed by open biopsy. Of the last 23, the aspiration test was negative in 16, and the Jensen-Westerman needle biopsy was negative in another 5. He found there was more involvement of the marrow in older male patients who had systemic symptoms and elevated alkaline phosphatase. The survival of patients with marrow involvement, whether discovered at the onset of the disease or developed later, did not appear to differ significantly when treated with the cyclical combination chemotherapy (MOPP). The actuarial survival rate at 2 years was 84 percent, although less than 20 percent were free of disease.

Thus, the Committee on Hodgkin's Disease Staging Procedures recommended that bone-marrow biopsy, either by a needle or open surgical technique, be carried out in the presence of any of the following conditions: (1) an elevated serum alkaline phosphatase; (2) unexplained anemia or other blood count depression; (3) roentgenographic or scintigraphic evidence of osseous disease; (4) generalized disease of the stage III category or greater (Rosenberg et al 1971). Open bone-marrow biopsies, as part of the staging laporatory, are discussed on p. 197 Ultmann and Moran (1973) pointed out that rarely bone marrow is inaded by extension from an involved contiguous lymph node; such cases should be considered as stage I_E, II_E, or III_E, but not as stage IV.

For patients with non-Hodgkin's lymphomas, many authors felt the bone-marrow biopsy was also an invaluable procedure in the initial staging and recommended that it be performed routinely in all patients. Vinciguerra and Silver (1971) used the needle biopsy in 75 patients: 47 (63 percent) had positive marrows and 40 had diseases of stage III or less. These included 44 percent of those with stage I disease; 75 percent, stage II; and 65 percent, stage III. Little correlation was found between the extent of the disease and/or abnormal blood tests, except hypogammaglobulinemia did seem to have more positive marrows.

Han et al (1971) felt aspiration and marrow biopsies appeared to be equally useful in the cases with lymphosarcomas, reticulum cell sarcomas, and chronic lymphocytic leukemia. Guller et al (1972) compared 79 simultaneous specimens of bone-marrow smears and histology sections taken with the Jensen-Westerman needle. In lymphosarcoma, they found an equal number of positive results.

However, similar to the experience in Hodgkin's disease, Jones et al (1972) felt the large and open bone-marrow biopsy were much superior to the aspiration method. In 218 previously untreated patients with non-Hodgkin's lymphomas, they found only 6 percent of the initial aspirates showed unequivocal lesions, whereas 18 percent of open and 16 percent of needle biopsies were positive. The incidence of initial bone-marrow involvement correlated with the histological subtypes of the lymphoma. Even with advanced disease (stages III and IV), histiocytic lymphomas involved the marrow uncommonly (5 percent), whereas 30 percent with poorly differentiated lymphocytic types did. Mixed histiocytic–lymphocytic types had an intermediate rate (15–20 percent). Nodular or diffuse histologic patterns per se did not influence the incidence of marrow involvement, but patients with nodular lymphomas and positive marrows survived significantly longer than those with diffuse lymphomas. In addition, they found that bone-marrow involvement correlated with advanced stages and the presence of spleno-megaly and constitutional symptoms. But contrary to the findings in Hodg-kin's disease, elevated serum alkaline phosphatase did not represent lymphomas in the marrow.

In the present EFSCH series, almost all of the bone-marrow tests were done by the aspiration technique, and the majority of patients were treated before the discovery of combination chemotherapy. Among 163 patients with Hodgkin's disease, only 1 had a positive bone marrow test in conjunction with a markedly enlarged liver. This is similar to what Rosenberg (1971) reported: only 1 out of 400 patients had a positive marrow by aspiration. Among 364 patients with non-Hodgkin's disease 37 had positive bone-marrow smears and in 15 of these, marrow was apparently the only extranodal site involved. Survival curves of these 37 and the other patients with stage IV disease, but without marrow involvement, were similar.

BLOOD TESTS

In the report of the Committee on Hodgkin's Disease Staging Proce-dures, the "required blood tests necessary for evaluation" listed only com-plete blood cell counts, platelet counts, erythrocyte sedimentation rates, serum alkaline phosphatase, and other tests for the evaluation of liver and renal functions (Rosenberg et al 1971). In addition, serum calcium and uric acid tests were useful for the overall management of patients. Under "procedures and tests promising for clinical study at selected centers but experimental at this time," there were 11 tests listed (p. 12). Several of the interesting and less-known tests and the controversy regarding their significance are mentioned here.

Sedimentation Rate

Hansen (1969) found that anemia, elevated sedimentation rates, and either neutropenia (< 4000) or neutrocytosis (> 10,000) at admission implied a lower survival rate in patients with reticulum cell sarcoma. Teillet et al (1971) called 5 abnormal blood tests (elevated sedimentation rate, sideremia, fibrinemia, alpha-2-globulinemia, and neutrocytosis) biological signs and found they had poor prognostic meaning for Hodgkin's disease. However, none of the blood tests was diagnostic, and similar abnormalities were encountered in a variety of other disease states, particularly in inflam-matory and infectious conditions. Kaplan (1971) felt the erythrocyte sedimen-tation rate was both the most reliable and the least expensive of these indicators. The sedimentation rate was elevated in 70 percent of patients with previously untreated, biopsy-proven Hodgkin's disease. Elevation of the serum ceruloplasmin was determined simultaneously in the same patients and was significantly less often elevated; the serum muramidase and leukocyte alkaline phosphatase were elevated in only one-third to one-fourth of the patients. But he warned that elevated sedimentation rate during the follow-up period was not diagnostic of recrudescence of disease, and it should never be taken as the basis for initiation of new programs of treatment in the absence of some other firm documentary evidence.

Rosenberg (1970) said that all patients with malignant lymphomas should have a serum protein electrophoretic pattern done, and those in the non-Hodgkin's group should have an immunoelectrophoresis as well. Parameters of hemolysin were also useful in selected patients; the determination of cutaneous anergy of the delayed hypersensitivity type is desirable and of interest in patients with Hodgkin's disease but cannot yet be used for prognostic or staging purposes.

Alkaline Phosphatases

Russell et al (1970) commented that bromosulfophthalein retention tests and alkaline phosphatase levels were the most sensitive tests to indicate liver involvement by Hodgkin's disease and lymphoma as well as other focal processes such as granulomas. There is now considerable evidence that in healthy persons the serum alkaline phosphatase is derived from three sources: liver, bone, and, in some cases, intestine (Kaplan 1972).

Aisenberg et al (1970) studied serum alkaline phosphatase in 111 patients at the onset of Hodgkin's disease. With each advancing stage, there was a progressive increase in the percentage of patients with elevated enzyme (14 percent in stages I and II; 65 percent, stage III; 81 percent, stage IV). In all stages, there was a very high incidence of elevated phosphatase in patients with fever but not in those with only pruritus. The most important cause of serum alkaline phosphatase elevation, especially in those with advanced disease, was due to high phosphatase which originated in the liver. In patients with localized disease and in patients younger than 21 years old, most of the elevated phosphatase appeared physiological and was of bone origin. Bodansky (1962) is of the opinion that, in the absence of a concomitant elevation of the serum 5-nucleotidase activity, an increased alkaline phosphatase activity indicates a skeletal lesion.

Bagley et al (1972) studied the clinicopathologic correlations in 127 patients who had liver biopsies (16 had open biopsies at laparotomy). Eight of the 89 previously untreated patients had positive biopsies, and all 8 had stage III disease and clinically enlarged spleens. Among these patients, positive biopsies were associated with older age and higher alkaline phosphatase. However, their overall data showed that alkaline phosphatase elevation, increased bromosulfophthalein retention, and hepatomegaly could all represent nonspecific reactions to the presence of Hodgkin's disease elsewhere in the patients and thus were of little value as indicators of hepatic involvement.

Among 26 Hodgkin's patients who had staging laparotomies, Levine (1972) did a prospective study of 9 patients who had persistent elevation of serum alkaline phosphatase, transaminase, or bromosulfophthalein retention levels. Findings during follow-ups of 12 to 28 months showed only 1 patient had histologically documented liver involvement. In particular, of the 8 patients with elevated alkaline phosphatase levels, 6 had returned to normal range within several months after completion of radiotherapy and remained so.

Stolbach et al (1972) also warned that the finding of an elevated alkaline phosphatase level did not necessarily indicate metastatic disease to bone or liver and should not constitute a contraindication to curative surgery. They presented a patient whose elevated serum alkaline phosphatase dropped following resection of a localized jejunel lymphocytic lymphoma. The patient showed no evidence of recurrence of disease 2 years after surgery and radiotherapy. The abnormal test was related to the presence of Regan isoenzyme of alkaline phosphatase which was probably produced by the tumor. This isoenzyme has been found in the serum of patients having a variety of malignancies involving different organs.

Trace Elements

Copper is present in the serum mainly in the form of ceruloplasmin, which behaves like an enzyme; a lesser proportion is carried by the serum proteins. Pagliardi and Giangrandi (1960) studied 23 patients with Hodgkin's disease and reported that the serum copper level was constantly increased during relapse. A drop to normal values always indicated an imminent remission, whether spontaneous or following treatment. Hrgovcic et al (1968) studied serum copper levels in 70 patients with lymphomas and leukemias. They confirmed its usefulness in the differentiation of active and inactive status in patients with Hodgkin's disease. However, they found this test was of doubtful value in patients with reticulum cell sarcomas. Warren et al (1969) found the persistence of serum copper levels of 150 mg or higher strongly suggested the presence of active disease. But they emphasized that many unrelated conditions, such as pregnancy, administration of estrogen and oral contraceptives, and chronic inflammation, could cause high serum copper levels.

Mortazavi et al (1972) evaluated the usefulness of serum copper measurement as a prognostic and therapeutic index. Of 42 patients with various lymphomas, 23 of 24 who had generalized disease had increased copper levels, and 6 of 18 with localized disease had raised concentrations. In all patients (Hodgkin's disease, lymphosarcoma, or reticulum cell sarcoma), the clinical results of treatments correlated well with the alterations in serum copper. Tessmer et al (1973) also confirmed the value of determining serum copper levels in 37 cases of Hodgkin's disease in children. The relationship is particularly pronounced in stage IV Hodgkin's disease with systemic symptoms. In the limited number of lymphocyte predominance cases, the relations of serum copper level to disease activity did not seem to be present (Hrgovcic et al 1973).

Ilicin (1971) reported that serum magnesium tended to move in the opposite direction from serum copper. In 22 patients with leukemia and 15 with malignant lymphomas, he found that the copper level was significantly lower and the magnesium significantly higher during therapy than before treatment. He suggested that the high magnesium levels were secondary to release of this element from damaged malignant cells. A low plasma zinc level has been recorded by Auerbach (1965), but it is not clear if this was secondary to anemia, leukopenia, or the lymphomatous process.

Antiviral Antibodies

The finding of high levels of antibodies to the Epstein-Barr virus in serum from patients with Burkitt's lymphoma stimulated the search for similar antibodies in patients with other tumors originating from the reticuloendothelial cells. Johansson et al (1970) reported that serum from patients with Hodgkin's disease contained a high titer against this virus. When the cases were grouped according to pathological subtypes, serum from patients with paragranuloma lesions did not show excess reactivity compared to the controls, whereas serum from patients with Hodgkin's sarcoma were highly reactive, reaching levels comparable to those seen in Burkitt's lymphoma and nasopharyngeal carcinoma. The granuloma group was intermediate. The percentage of sera with high antivirus titers was higher in the group whose peripheral lymphocyte counts were under 1000 than in the group with counts over 1000 (60 percent versus 31 percent), although there was no significant difference between the mean titers.

Levine et al (1970) also found that Hodgkin's patients have a higher titer against Epstein-Barr virus than non-Hodgkin's patients and normal controls. In untreated patients, higher titers were associated with a longer duration of symptoms, more generalized disease, shorter survival, and a histologic picture of the lymphocyte depletion type. Treated patients had significantly higher titers than untreated patients. When the same sera were tested for antibodies to four other herpes viruses (herpes simplex types I and II, cytomegalovirus and varicella), all were reported to be elevated in patients with Burkitt's lymphoma, but not in patients with Hodgkin's disease and control groups. They concluded that although this study suggested elevated antibody titers associated with a poor prognosis in patients with Hodgkin's disease, the data did not distinguish between an etiologic role for the virus and that of a passenger role which also could produce high titers as a result of the disease process.

A contradictory report was that of Goldman and Aisenberg (1970), who found that the titers and incidence of antibody to this particular virus and other herpes virus in 57 patients with Hodgkin's disease did not appear to differ from an age-matched control population. Thus, the importance of studying antibodies to virus in malignant lymphomas is presently unclear. It is interesting to note that Eisinger et al (1971) reported cells from lesions of Hodgkin's disease underwent changes in tissue culture accompanied by the emergence of an agent of the herpes virus group. This preliminary finding awaits confirmation from other researchers.

Order and Hellman (1973) have detected slow-migrating and fast-migrating tumor antigens in areas of spleen and nodal tissues which contained Hodgkin's disease. These antigens are antigenic in heterologous species (rabbit) but may not be antigenic in the patient. They are not sure whether these antigens were related to the patient's defense mechanisms, the neoplasm, or some other unknown factors. But they hypothesized that Hodgkin's disease probably resulted from a viral infection of some thymus-derived lymphocytes (T cells), and then other normal immunocompetent lymphocytes became reactive against abnormal viral-bearing T cells.

Lymphocyte Counts

Because of the personal interest of one of the authors (Y.N.L.) and the recent emphasis on the role of host immune response in neoplasia, we have studied the prognostic value of peripheral lymphocyte counts in patients with malignant lymphomas. In the EFSCH series of patients with Hodgkin's disease, the survival rate of those with lymphocyte counts of 2000–$3000/mm^3$ is better than those with counts between 1000 and 2000, and much better than those with less than 1000 or more than 3000 (Fig. 2-1). The corresponding adjusted 5-year survival rates are: 49 percent, 23 percent, and 0 percent; the 10-year survival rates are 30 percent, 18 percent, and 0 percent. The difference is statistically significant ($p < 0.02$). For comparison, those patients whose hemoglobin levels were more than 15 g-percent had the best survival rate, while those with hemoglobin less than 9 g-percent had the worst prognosis. Eosinphilia was recorded only in 11 patients and appeared to have no influence on survival.

For patients with non-Hodgkin's lymphomas, Figure 2-2 shows that those with lymphocyte counts of 3000–$4000/mm^3$ had the best prognosis; those with 1000–3000, intermediate; and those whose lymphocyte counts were below 1000 and above 4000, the worst. The corresponding adjusted 5-year survival rates are: 52 percent, 30 percent, and 16 percent; the 10-year rates are: 39 percent, 18 percent, and 5 percent. The cumulative differences are statistically significant up to 10 years ($p < 0.05$). This difference in survival rates is especially prominent for patients with the histological diagnosis of lymphocytic subtypes and not so obvious for patients with histiocytic, mixed cell, or pleomorphic patterns. Strangely enough, the favorable effect of this lymphocyte count level (3000–4000) manifested itself especially in patients with advanced disease (stages III and IV). The hemoglobin level

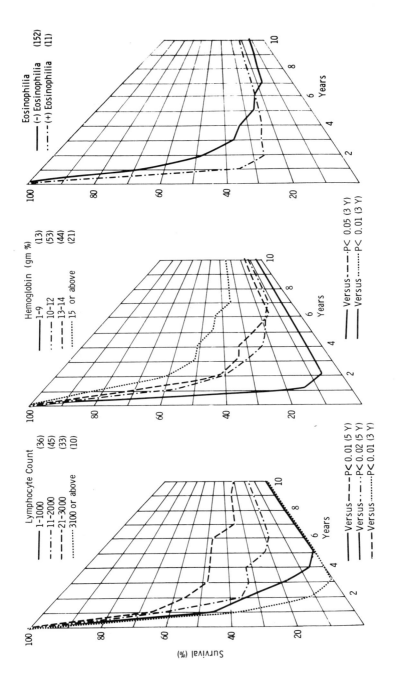

Fig. 2-1. Survival rates of patients with Hodgkin's disease versus (a) peripheral lymphocyte count (per mm³); (b) hemoglobin level (g-percent); (c) presence or absence of eosinophilia.

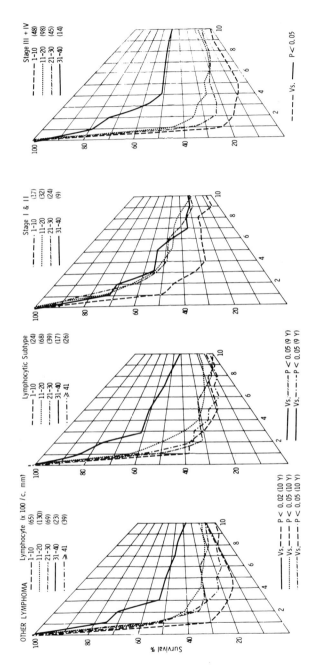

Fig. 2-2. Survival rates of patients with non-Hodgkin's lymphoma versus peripheral lymphocyte count (x100/mm³) (*a*) all patients; (*b*) patients with lymphocytic lymphoma, (*c*) patients with early disease; (*d*) patients with late disease.

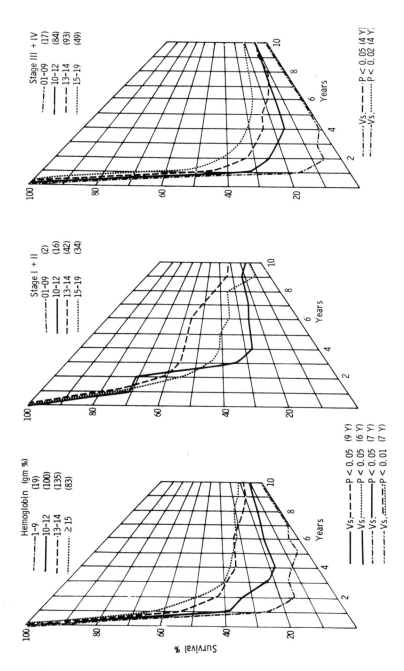

Fig. 2-3. Survival rates of patients with non-Hodgkin's lymphoma versus hemoglobin level (g-percent): (*a*) all patients; (*b*) patients with early disease; (*c*) patients with late disease.

at the time of diagnosis also has prognostic values (Fig. 2-3). Those patients whose hemoglobin was more than 13 g-percent did much better than those whose level was below 12 g-percent. This was true for patients with localized lymphomas (stages I and II) as well as for those with more advanced disease (stages III and IV).

Several reports correlating the prognosis of patients with cancer and the lymphocyte counts of peripheral blood have appeared in the literature. Among 589 patients with cancers of the uterine cervix, breast, and malignant lymphomas, Riesco (1970) reported a positive and significant correlation between 5-year curability of cancer and the total number of peripheral lymphocytes. Bill and Morgan (1970) found that there is a positive relationship of peripheral lymphocyte count at diagnosis and survival in patients with neuroblastoma in the first year of life. In 46 children studied, the mean count for 33 survivors is 7600, whereas the mean for 13 children who died is 5350. Pendergrast et al (1971) studied the peripheral lymphocyte counts of 61 patients before and after injection of a cancer vaccine. In patients who responded to immunization with the tumor homogenate, their peripheral lymphocyte counts increased while those who failed to respond decreased.

In patients with mammary cancer, Meyer et al (1970) found that the lymphocyte level tended to increase in patients whose metastases responded to hormonal therapy. On the other hand, there was a consistent drop in the lymphocyte count in those in whom the disease progressed. Holt and Lee (1972) studied peripheral lymphocyte counts and results of therapeutic castration for advanced breast cancer. Lymphocyte levels of patients who had an objective response stayed the same or showed a rise after castration, while lymphocyte counts of most of those who did not have objective response decreased.

Many reports showed that lymphocyte counts also had prognostic value in patients with malignant lymphomas. Rosenberg et al (1960) studied 1269 patients with non-Hodgkin's lymphomas. They found that if survival were analyzed as a function of the initial lymphocyte count, the 5-year survival rate of those with counts over 2000/mm^3 was about 15–25 percent better than those whose counts were below 1000 (median survival: 18 versus 3.2 months). The prognostic value of the total lymphocyte count was as great as for any other feature of the illness. Westling (1965) found that peripheral lymphocyte counts below 800/mm^3 at admission, in patients with Hodgkin's disease, reflected a bad prognosis. This factor had similar prognostic significance as fever, elevated sedimentation rate, and anemia. Meytes and Modan (1969) found that lymphocyte counts over 1800/mm^3 implied a longer survival for male patients but not for females.

Molander and Lacayo (1970) reported that recurrence rates for Hodgkin's patients after radiotherapy were correlated with the pretherapy lymphocyte counts (expressed as the percentage of lymphocytes in the total leucocyte count). Seventy-seven of 105 with recurrence had lymphocyte counts of 25 percent or less in differential count, whereas 49 of the 95 patients without recurrence had such low counts (p = 0.01). They saw no such correlation in 300 patients with lymphosarcomas. Swan and Knowelden (1971) reported a clear difference in prognosis among three lymphocyte groups of 328 patients with histologically diagnosed Hodgkin's disease. The worst prognosis was associated with lymphocyte counts of less than 1000/mm^3, and the best prognosis was in patients whose lymphocyte counts were above 1500 (5-year survival rate: 12 percent versus 35 percent).

Strum and Rappaport (1971) studied 40 Hodgkin's patients who survived 10 years or more. In about 80 percent of the cases, the initial lymph node biopsy showed nodular sclerosis; this histology was especially important in males. Among the laboratory tests, they found that the only hematologic feature that had prognostic value was the pretreatment lymphocyte count; the mean value was 2000/mm^3 for the long-term survivors versus 1750/mm^3 for patients who survived less than 5 years. The comparable figures for the hemoglobin were 13 g-percent versus 10.4 g-percent; and for eosinophil count, 280/mm^3 versus 150/mm^3. No mention was made of the level of statistical significance.

Tubiana et al (1971) studied prognostic factors in 454 patients with Hodgkin's disease. They found that the peripheral lymphocyte counts correlated with the histological subtypes. In patients with lymphocyte predominance lesions, 79 percent had lymphocyte counts more than 900/mm^3. The figure for patients with lesions of the lymphocyte depletion was 50 percent. The number of lymphocyte counts did not correlate with the results of tuberculin skin tests. Within each histological subtype, patients with lymphocyte counts higher than 900 had better survival rates than those with lesser counts. They said the differences in survival at 1 and 3 years after diagnosis (about 7–18 percent at third year) were statistically significant.

Impaired delayed hypersensitivity and prolonged skin homograft rejection have been demonstrated in patients with Hodgkin's disease. Defective lymphocyte functions have been implicated as the cause of the immunologic abnormalities, and lymphocytopenia probably contributes to further impairment. Aisenberg (1965) found that lymphocytopenia was characteristic of the terminal phase of Hodgkin's disease.

Brown et al (1967) were the first to evaluate immunologic functions in patients with Hodgkin's disease before they received any radiotherapy or chemotherapy. They found the impaired hypersensitivity was much less than previously reported; only 16 percent of 50 untreated patients failed to react to all skin tests. Patients with stage I disease had normal reactivity, but a significant decrease was observed in patients with more advanced disease. In addition, the peripheral lymphocyte counts in patients with stages III and IV disease were significantly lower than those in stages I and II (p < 0.02). And skin test reactivity was positively correlated with the peripheral lymphocyte counts: those patients who were positive to either chemical (DNCB) or intradermal antigens had significantly higher lymphocyte counts than did the unreactive patients (p = 0.02).

In a larger series of 103 patients with untreated Hodgkin's disease, Young et al (1972) further documented that absolute peripheral lymphocyte counts reflected different clinical staging, histological subtype, and skin test reactivity. In addition, in patients with stages III and IV disease, there was a significant difference between survival of those who presented with lymphocytopenia (lymphocyte counts of less than 1000/mm^3) and those who did not. This finding suggested that the peripheral lymphocyte count might be a more sensitive prognostic factor than the multitude of skin tests for checking delayed hypersensitivity.

It is obvious that, like multitudes of other neoplasms and diseases, there are many independent or interrelated clinical and pathological factors which influence the prognosis of patients with malignant lymphomas. According to Osgood (1954), peripheral lymphocytes accounted for only about 0.02 percent of the total lymphoid tissues scattered throughout the body. Aisenberg (1972) commented that blood lymphocyte counts are influenced by a variety of nonspecific factors, and the immunological testing of delayed hypersensitivity with intradermal antigens is by far the most useful to the practitioner.

In addition, there is now considerable evidence of the presence of two lymphocyte subpopulations with regard to origin, life-span and function: thymus-dependent (T) lymphocytes appear to be concerned with cell-mediated immunity, whereas bursa-equivalent (B) lymphocytes mediate humoral immunity. Fröland (1972) reported that the percentage of lymphocytes which form rosettes with sheep erythrocytes, probably a T cell property, and of lymphocytes which have surface-bound immunoglobin, probably a B cell marker, was within the normal range in five patients with Hodgkin's disease. Cohnen et al (1973) found that, in some patients with Hodgkin's disease, there might be a functional impairment of both T and B lymphocytes without a selective loss of T lymphocytes. Young et al (1973) reported that the results of lymphocyte blastogenic transformation by phytohemagglutinin, which stimulates predominantly T cells, did not correlate with survival, frequency of relapse, or remission duration in 43 patients with Hodgkin's disease. Ultmann and Moran (1973 have summarized many evidences that showed autoimmune mechanisms might play a part in the multitude of complications of Hodgkin's disease.

Thus, it is surprising that a simple test such as peripheral lymphocyte count could be correlated with final survival, although "lymphocytes are the major carriers of cell-mediated immune mechanisms, and the lymphocyte level is an index of cellular immune competence" (Burnet 1969). Fully realizing that the diagnosis of malignant lymphoma implies a complex disease with many heterogeneous and entangled facets, we present these data to stimulate further investigations of the role(s) of peripheral lymphocytes.

SUMMARY

For examination of retroperitoneal nodes, both intravenous pyelogram and inferior venacavogram were relatively ineffective. Lower extremity lymphangiogram can demonstrate retroperitoneal disease in more than one-third of the Hodgkin's patients clinically diagnosed as stages I and II, and in over 80 percent of those with early non-Hodgkin's lymphomas. Although lymphangiogram could have a false positive rate of 28 percent and a false negative rate of 12 percent, it remains a useful diagnostic procedure in the initial evaluation of Hodgkin's patients and in the follow-up reassessment of treated patients for recurrent or new diseases.

Radioisotopic studies of the liver, spleen, bone, marrow, and other soft tissues are useful ancillary procedures but the results are not definitive for diagnosis. With the discovery of new radioisotopes and improvement in the equipment and technique, such nondestructive procedures may attain more clinical significance in the future.

Bone-marrow biopsy with large needles has become an invaluable procedure in the initial staging of patients with malignant lymphoma. It was found that about 9 percent of untreated Hodgkin's patients whose disease was more advanced than stage II had marrow involvement. In patients with non-Hodgkin's lymphoma, marrow lesions were seen in 5 percent of those with histiocytic lesions and in 30 percent of those with poorly differentiated lymphocytic lymphoma.

Sedimentation rate, alkaline phosphatase level, and other liver function tests become more abnormal with progression of the Hodgkin's disease. Serum copper behaved the same way. However all these abnormal tests could represent nonspecific reactions to malignant and nonmalignant conditions. Recent findings of high levels of antibody titer to Epstein-Barr virus in patients with Hodgkin's disease are of interest. A simple test which was found to have prognostic significance in patients with both Hodgkin's disease and other malignant lymphoma is the peripheral lymphocyte count. It appears that both lymphocytopenia and lymphocytosis mean poor prognosis.

REFERENCE

Aisenberg AC: Current concepts in cancer 36. Updated Hodgkin's Disease, value of immunologic testing. JAMA 222:1301–1302, 1972

Aisenberg AC: Lymphocytopenia in Hodgkin's disease. Blood 25:1037–1042, 1965

Aisenberg AC, Kaplan MM, Rieder SV, et al: Serum alkaline phosphatase at the onset of Hodgkin's disease. Cancer 26: 318–326, 1970

Ariel IM, Molander DW, Galey D: Hepatic gammascanning: An aid in determining treatment policies for cancer involving the liver. Am J Surg 118:5–14, 1969

Arinkin MI: Die intravitale Untersuchungsmethodik des Knochenmarks. Folia haematol 38:233–240, 1929

Auerbach S: Zinc content of plasma, blood, and erythrocytes in normal subjects and in patients with Hodgkin's disease and various hematologic disorders. J Lab Clin Med 65:628–637, 1965

Bagley C M, Roth J A, Thomas L B, et al: Liver biopsy in Hodgkin's disease: Clinico-pathologic correlations in 127 patients. Ann Intern Med 76:219–225, 1972

Bill A H, Morgan A: Evidence for immune reactions to neuroblastoma and future possibilities for investigation. J Pediatr Surg 5:111–116, 1970

Bodansky O: New functional principles in diagnostic aspects of liver disease. Bull N Y Acad Med 38:712–726, 1962

Brown R S, Haynes H A, Foley H T, et al: Hodgkin's disease. Immunologic, clinical, and histological features of 50 untreated patients. Ann Intern Med 67:291–302, 1967

Brickner TJ Jr, Boyer CW Jr, Perry RH: Limited value of lymphangiography in Hodgkin's disease. Radiology 90:52–56, 1968

Burnet FM: Cellular Immunology. Cambridge, Cambridge University Press, 1969

Cantor RE, Cohn EM, Park CH, et al: Comparative liver scanning: Technetium sulfide Tc 99m vs gold Au 198. J A M A 211:1677–1680, 1970

Castagna J, Benfield JR, Yamada H, et al: The reliability of liver scans and function tests in detecting metastases. Surg Gynecol Obstet 134:463–466, 1972

Castellino R A, Blank N, Cassady J R, et al: Roentgenologic aspects of Hodgkin's disease: II. Role of routine radiographics in detecting initial relapse. Cancer 31: 316–323, 1973

Castellino R A, Silverman J F, Glatstein E, et al: Splenic arteriography in Hodgkin's disease: A roentgenologic-pathologic study of 33 consecutive untreated patients. Am J Roentgenol Radium Ther Nucl Med 114:574–582, 1972

Charkes N D, Sklaroff D M: Early diagnosis of metastatic bone cancer by photoscanning with strontium-85. J Nucl Med 5:168–179, 1964

Cohnen G, Douglas S D, König E, et al: In vitro lymphocyte response to phytohemagglutinin and pokeweed nitogen in Hodgkin's disease. An electron microscopic and functional study. Cancer 31:1346–1353, 1973

Davidson JW, Clarke E A: Influence of modern radiological techniques on clinical staging of malignant lymphomas. Can Med Assoc J 99:1196–1204, 1968

Davidson JW, Clarke E A: Significance of lymphographic appearances in Hodgkin's disease in Viamonte M, Koehler PR, Witte M, et al (eds): Progress in Lymphology, vol 2. Stuttgart, Thieme, 1970, pp 211–218

Davidson JW, Kaufman S D: Pulmonary complications of lymphography. N Engl J Med 285:237–238, 1971

Davidson JW, Saini M, Peters M V: Lymphography in lymphoma, with particular reference to Hodgkin's disease. Radiology 88:281–286, 1967

DeLand FH: Normal spleen size. Radiology 97:589–592, 1970

Dolan PA: Lymphography Br J Radiol 37:405–415, 1964

Edwards CL, Hayes RL: Scanning malignant neoplasms with gallium 67. J A M A 212:1182–1190, 1970

Edwards CL, Hayes RL: Tumor scanning with ^{67}Ga citrate. J Nucl Med 10:103–105, 1969

Eichner E: Problems of lymphangiography. Int Surg 55:196–199, 1971

Eisinger M, Fox SM, De Harven E, et al: Virus-like agents from patients with Hodgkin's disease. Nature 233:104–108, 1971

Ellis L D, Jensen WN, Westerman M P: Needle biopsy of bone and marrow: An experience with 1,445 biopsies. Arch Intern Med 114:213–221, 1964

Escobar-Prieto A, Gonzalez G, Templeton AW, et al: Lymphatic channel obstruction: Patterns of altered flow dynamics. Am J Roentgenol Radium Ther Nucl Med 113:366–375, 1971

Fairbanks V F, Tauxe WN, Kiely JM, et al: Scintigraphic visualization of abdominal lymph nodes with 99m Tc-pertechnetate-labeled sulfur colloid. J Nucl Med 13:185–190, 1972

Fallat RJ, Powell MR, Youker JE, et al: Pulmonary deposition and clearance of ^{131}I-labeled oil after lymphography in man: Correlation with lung function. Radiology 97:511–520, 1970

Fischer HW, Thornbury J R: Lymphography in the diagnosis of malignant neoplasms in Ariel IM (ed): Progress in Clinical Cancer, vol 1. New York, Grune and Stratton, 1965, pp 213–234

Froland SS: Binding of sheep erythrocytes to human lymphocytes. A probable marker of T lymphocytes. Scand J Immunol 1:269–280, 1972

Fuchs WA, Härtel M: Prognosis of Hodgkin's disease according to the radiographic pattern of lymph nodes, in Viamonte M, Koehler PR, Witte M, et al (eds): Progress in Lymphology, vol 2. Stuttgart, Thieme, 1970, pp 279–281

Glatstein E, Castellino RA, Blank N, et al: Defense of lymphangiography. N Engl J Med 285:1262–1263, 1971

Goldman JM, Aisenberg AC: Incidence of antibody to EB virus, herpes simplex, and cytomegalovirus in Hodgkin's disease. Cancer 26:327–331, 1970

Gollin FF, Sims JL, Cameron JR: Liver scanning and liver function tests: A comparative study. JAMA 187:111–116, 1964

Guller R, Senn HJ, Nagel GA, et al: Die Bedeutung der Knochenmarkund Leberpunktion bei malignen Lymphomen. Schweiz Med Wochenschr 102:318–323, 1972

Hall RD ,Krementz ET: Lymphangiography by lymph-node injection. JAMA 202: 1136–1139, 1967

Hall TC: New chemotherapeutic agents in Hodgkin's disease. Cancer Res 26:1297–1302, 1966

Han T, Stutzman L, Roque AL: Bone marrow biopsy in Hodgkin's disease and other neoplastic diseases. JAMA 217:1239–1241, 1971

Hansen HS: Reticulum cell sarcoma treated by radiotherapy: Significance of clinical features upon the prognosis. Acta Radiol [Ther]/(Stockh) 8:439–458, 1969

Haynie TP, Jhingran SG, Ilter RG, et al: Liver scintigrams in patients with cancer. Cancer Bull 22:33–36, 1970

Holt JE, Lee YN: Peripheral lymphocyte counts and results of therapeutic castration for advanced mammary cancer. Ann Surg 175:403–408, 1972

Hrgovcic M, Tessmer CF, Minckler TM, et al: Serum copper levels in lymphoma and leukemia: Special reference to Hodgkin's disease. Cancer 21:743–755, 1968

Hrgovcic M, Tessmer CF, Thomas FB, et al: Significance of serum copper levels in adult patients with Hodgkin's disease. Cancer 31:1337–1345, 1973

Idezuki Y, Sugiura M, Hatano S, et al: Hepatography for detection of small tumor masses in liver: Experiences with oily contrast medium. Surgery 60:566–572, 1966

Ilicin G: Serum copper and magnesium levels in leukemia and malignant lymphoma. Lancet 2:1036–1037, 1971

Johansson B, Klein G, Henle W, et al: Epstein-Barr Virus (EBV)-associated antibody patterns in malignant lymphoma and leukemia. I. Hodgkin's disease. Int J Cancer 6:450–462, 1970

Jones SE, Rosenberg SA, Kaplan HS: Non-Hodgkin's lymphomas. I. Bone marrow involvement. Cancer 29:954–960, 1972

Kadin ME, Glatstein E, Dorfman RF: Clinicopathologic studies of 117 untreated patients subjected to laparotomy for the staging of Hodgkin's disease. Cancer 27:1277–1294, 1971

Kaplan HS: Formal discussion of F. Teillet, et al's paper, "A reappraisal of clinical and biological signs in staging of Hodgkin's disease." Cancer Res 31:1730, 1971

Kaplan HS: Hodgkin's disease: Prognosis as related to pathology, staging, and treatment. Proc R Soc Med 65:62–64, 1972

Kaplan MM: Alkaline phosphatase. N Engl J Med 286:200–202, 1972

Kinmonth JB: Lymphangiography in man: Method of outlining lymphatic trunks at operation. Clin Sci 11:13–20, 1952

Kinmonth JB, Taylor GW, Harper RA: Lymphangiography: Technique for its clinical use in lower limb. Br Med J 1:940–942, 1955

Lacher MJ, Geller W: Radiologic follow-up after lymphangiography. NY State J Med 72:1743–1744, 1972

Larson SM, Nelp WB: The radiocolloid bone marrow scan in malignant disease. J Surg Oncol 3:685–697, 1971

Lawson GM: Hepatography with oily contrast agents: Preliminary report. Radiology 79:316–317, 1962

Lee BJ: Correlation between lymphangiography and clinical status of patients with lymphoma. Cancer Chemother Rep 52: 205–211, 1968

Lee BJ: Evaluation of the patient with lymphoma by means of lymphangiography: Comments on importance and complications, in Rüttimann A (ed): Progress in Lymphology, vol 1. Stuttgart, Thieme, 1967, pp 127–130

Lee BJ: Lymphangiography in Hodgkin's disease: Indications and contraindications. Cancer Res 26:1084–1089, 1966

Lee BJ, Nelson JH, Schwarz G: Evaluation of lymphangiography, inferior venacavography, and intravenous pyelography in the clinical staging and management of Hodgkin's disease and lymphosarcoma. N Engl J Med 271:327–337, 1964

Lee BJ, Stephenson P: Diagnostic and therapeutic implications of the lymphangiogram in the treatment and prognosis of Hodgkin's disease, in Viamonte M, Koehler PR, Witte M, et al (eds): Progress in Lymphology II. Stuttgart, Thieme, 1970, pp 281–288

Lee YN: Hepatography with oily contrast medium injected via the portal vein system. Surgery 63:948–953, 1968

Levine PH: Abnormal blood chemistry values in Hodgkin's disease: Lack of correlation with staging of disease. JAMA 220:1734–1735, 1972

Levine PH, Ablashi DV, Berard CW, et al: Elevated antibody titers to herpes-type virus in Hodgkin's disease. Proc Am Assoc for Cancer Res 11:49, 1970 (Abstr)

Liao KT: The superiority of histologic sections of aspirated bone marrow in malignant lymphomas: A review of 1,124 examinations. Cancer 27:618–628, 1971

Lipton MJ, DeNardo GL, Silverman S, et al: Evaluation of the liver and spleen in Hodgkin's disease. I. The value of hepatic scintigraphy. Am J Med 52:356–361, 1972

Lomas F, Dibos PE, Wagner HN Jr: Increased specificity of liver scanning with the use of 67 Gallium citreate. N Engl J Med 286:1323–1329, 1972

Ludbrook J, Slavotinek AH, Ronai PM: Observer error in reporting on liver scans for space-occupying lesions. Gastroenterology 62:1013–1019, 1972

Lukes RJ: Criteria for involvement of lymph node, bone marrow, spleen, and liver in Hodgkin's disease. Cancer Res 31:1755–1767, 1971

McFarland W, Dameshek W: Biopsy of bone marrow with the Vim-Silverman needle. JAMA 166:1464–1466, 1958

Meyer KK, Boselli BD, Weaver DR, et al: Cellular immune response to mastectomy and radiation. Guthrie Clin Bull 40:48–61, 1970

Meytes D, Modan B: Selected aspects of Hodgkin's disease in a whole community. Blood 34:91–95, 1969

Milder MS, Larson SM, Bagley CM Jr, et al: Liver-spleen scan in Hodgkin's disease. Cancer 31:826–834, 1973

Milner TH, Maynard CD, Cowan RJ: Evaluation of strontium 85 bone scans and roentgenograms in 100 patients. Arch Surg 103:371–372, 1971

Molander DW, Ariel IM, Pack GT: Hepatic gammascanning as an aid in the management of patients with malignant lymphomas. Am J Roentgenol Radium Ther Nucl Med 99:851–862, 1967

Molander DW, Lacayo G: Malignant lymphomas: Patterns of progression and factors influencing recurrence. Am J Roentgenol Radium Ther Nucl Med 108:348–353, 1970

Mortazavi SH, Bani-Hashemi A, Mozafari M, et al: Value of serum copper measurement in lymphomas and several other malignancies. Cancer 29:1193–1198, 1972

Musumeci R, Fossati-Bellani F, Damascelli B, et al: Usefulness of lymphography in childhood neoplasia. Cancer 29:51–57, 1972

Myhre O: Injection of contrast medium into unstained femoral lymph vessels for lymphography: A new technique and its indications. Acta Radiol [Diag] (Stockh) 11:604–608, 1971

Nagler W, Bender MA, Blau M: Radioisotope photoscanning of the liver. Gastroenterology 44:36–43, 1963

Nelp WB, Bower RE: The quantitative distribution of the erythron and the RE cell in the bone marrow organ of man. Blood 34:276–282, 1969

Oh KS, Greene RE, Wang CC: Lymphographic study of giant follicular lymphoma. Cancer 23:1325–1331, 1969

Order SE, Hellman S: Tumor-associated antigens: A new perspective of Hodgkin's disease. JAMA 223:174–175, 1973

Osgood EE: Number and distribution of human hemic cells. Blood 9:1141–1154, 1954

Ozarda A, Pickren J: The topographic distribution of liver metastases: Its relation to surgical and isotope diagnosis. J Nucl Med 3:149–152, 1962

Pagliardi E, Giangrandi E: Clinical significance of the blood copper in Hodgkin's disease. Acta Haematol 24:201–212, 1960

Pearlman AW: Abdominal lymph node scintiscanning with radioactive gold (Au[198]) for evaluation and treatment of patients with lymphoma. Am J Roentgenol Radium Ther Nucl Med 109:780–792, 1970

Pendergrast WJ Jr, Boehm OR, Humphrey LJ: Effect of immunotherapy on peripheral lymphocyte count. Arch Surg 103:184–188, 1971

Peters MV, Brown TC, Davidson JW, et al: The value of locating occult disease in the treatment of Hodgkin's disease, in Rüttimann A (ed): Progress in Lymphology, vol 1. Stuttgart, Thieme, 1967, pp 119–125

Peters MV, Brown TC, Rideout DF: Prognostic influences and radiation therapy according to pattern of disease. JAMA 223:53–59, 1973

Peters MV, Middlemiss KC: A study of Hodgkin's disease treated by irradiation. Am J Roentgenol Radium Ther Nucl Med 79:114–121, 1958

Piccone VA, Ferrante J, LeVeen HH: Angial residue hepatography versus direct transumbilical hepatography: A comparison of two new methods. Am J Surg 115:17–21, 1968

Piccone VA, LeVeen HH, White JJ, et al: Transumbilical portal hepatography, a significant adjunct in the investigation of liver disease. Surgery 61:333–346, 1967

Pinsky SM, Hoffer PB, Turner DA, et al: Place of ^{67}Ga in the staging of Hodgkin's disease. J Nucl Med 12:385, 1971

Rappaport H, Berard CW, Butler JJ, et al: Report of the Committee on Histopathological Criteria Contributing to Staging of Hodgkin's Disease. Cancer Res 31:1864–1865, 1971

Riesco A: Five-year cancer cure: Relation to total amount of peripheral lymphocytes and neutrophils. Cancer 25:135–140, 1970

Rollo FD, DeLand FH: The determination of spleen mass from radio-nuclide images. Radiology 97:583–587, 1970

Rosenberg SA: The clinical evaluation and staging of patients with malignant lymphoma, in Clark RL, Cumley RW, McCay JE, et al (eds): Oncology 1970, vol 4. Chicago, Year Book, 1971, pp 507–518

Rosenberg SA: Hodgkin's disease of the bone marrow. Cancer Res 31:1733–1736, 1971

Rosenberg SA, Boiron M, DeVita VT Jr, et al: Report of the Committee on Hodgkin's Disease Staging Procedures. Cancer Res 31:1862–1863, 1971

Rosenberg SA, Diamond HD, Craver LF: Lymphosarcoma: The effects of therapy and survival in 1269 patients in a review of 30 years experience. Ann Intern Med 53:877–897, 1960

Russell WO, Race GJ, Butler JJ, et al: Management of patients with lymphoma. Clinicopathological panel discussion, Leukemia-Lymphoma. Chicago, Year Book, 1970, pp 375–385

Silverman S, DeNardo GL, Glatstein E, et al: Evaluation of the liver and spleen in Hodgkin's disease. II. The value of splenic scintigraphy. Am J Med 52:362–366, 1972

Smithers DW: Hodgkin's disease. Br Med J 2:263–268, 1967

Snapper I, Flynn JT, Moumigis B: Clinicopathological Conference: Nodules and ulceration of skin with heart disease. NY State J Med 71:2760–2769, 1971

Steiner RM, Harell GS, Glatstein E, et al: Repeat lymphangiography in Hodgkin's disease. Radiology 97:613–618, 1970

Stirrett LA, Yuhl ET, Cassen B: Clinical applications of hepatic radioactivity surveys. Am J Gastroenterol 21:310–317, 1954

Stolbach L, Skillman J, Goodman R: Increase in serum alkaline phosphatase due to Regan isoenzyme in a patient with localized jejunal lymphoma. Arch Surg 105:491–493, 1972

Strum SB, Rappaport H: The persistence of Hodgkin's disease in long-term survivors. Am J Med 51:222–240, 1971

Swan HT, Knowelden J: Prognosis in Hodgkin's disease related to the lymphocyte count. Br J Haematol 21:343–349, 1971

Takahashi M, Abrams HL: The accuracy of lymphangiographic diagnosis in malignant lymphoma. Radiology 89:448–460, 1967

Teillet F, Boiron M, Bernard J: A reappraisal of clinical and biological signs in staging of Hodgkin's disease. Cancer Res 31:1723–1729, 1971

Tessmer CF, Hrgovcic M, Wilbur J: Serum copper in Hodgkin's disease in children. Cancer 31:303–315, 1973

Tubiana M, Attie E, Flamant R, et al: Prognostic factors in 454 cases of Hodgkin's disease. Cancer Res 31:1801–1810, 1971

Turner DA, Pinsky SM, Gottschalk A, et al: The use of ^{67}Ga scanning in the staging of Hodgkin's disease. Radiology 104: 97–101, 1972

Ultmann JE, Moran EM: Clinical course and complications in Hodgkin's disease. Arch Intern Med 131:332–353, 1973

Viamonte M Jr: Current status of lymphography. Cancer Res 31:1731–1732, 1971

Viamonte M Jr: Current Concepts in Cancer, No. 39. Updated Hodgkin's Disease. Current status of lymphography. JAMA 222:1299–1301, 1972

Vinciguerra V, Silver RT: The importance of bone marrow biopsy in the staging of patients with lymphosarcoma. Blood 38:804, 1971

Wallace S: Newer radiodiagnostic contributions to the study of the lymphoma patient. Leukemia-Lymphoma. Chicago, Year Book, 1970, pp 223–239

Warren RL, Jelliffe AM, Watson JV, et al: Prolonged observations on variations in the serum copper in Hodgkin's disease. Clin Radiol 20:247–256, 1969

Webb DI, Ubogy G, Silver RT: Importance of bone marrow biopsy in the clinical staging of Hodgkin's disease. Cancer 26:313–317, 1970

Westin J, Lanner L, Larson A, et al: Spleen size in polycythemia: A clinical and scintigraphic study. Acta Med Scand 191:263–271, 1972

Westling P: Studies of the prognosis in Hodgkin's disease. Acta Radiol [Diag] [Suppl] (Stockh) 245: 5–125, 1965

Whitley JE, Maynard CD, Rhyne AL: A computer approach to the prediction of spleen weight from routine films. Radiology 86:73–76, 1966

Wiljasalo S: Lymphographic polymorphism in Hodgkin's disease: Correlation of lymphography to histology and duration. Acta Radiol [Diag] [Suppl] (Stockh) 289:9–89, 1969

Young RC, Corder MP, Berard CW, et al: Immune alterations in Hodgkin's disease: Effect of delayed hypersensitivity and lymphocyte transformation on course and survival. Arch Intern Med 131:446–454, 1973

Young RC, Corder MP, Haynes HA, et al: Delayed hypersensitivity in Hodgkin's disease: A study of 103 untreated patients. Am J Med 52:63–72, 1972

3
Radiotherapy and Chemotherapy

RADIOTHERAPY

Once the diagnosis of malignant lymphoma is made by tissue biopsy, the most effective therapeutic modality is radiotherapy. When the disease is early and major organs are uninvolved, properly applied radiation can bring about a cure. On the other hand, if the lymphoma is disseminated, radiation becomes an effective adjunct to chemotherapy for the treatment of localized tumors in specific situations.

In the past decade, major advances have been made in the radiotherapeutic management of patients with Hodgkin's disease. This success has led to the application of similar therapeutic approaches to non-Hodgkin's lymphomas. Presently, the data are much more convincing and have been well accepted only for the Hodgkin's disease group.

Hodgkin's Disease

Historically, the first report of response of a lymphoma to radiation was that of Pusey (1902). In the early days, single cutaneous erythema doses were delivered to the lesions at repeated intervals using weak radiation sources. The 5-year survival rate was less than 10 percent. In 1925, Schwarz reported using fractionated irradiation by giving small doses daily, over a period of 2 to 3 weeks, to involved nodes.

Then Gilbert (1928) recommended segmental irradiation for patients with lymphomas and standardized a method of treating all the lymph node regions in succession. He achieved an average survival time of over 4 years and a 5-year survival rate of 34 percent (Gilbert, 1939). Hynes and Frelick

94

(1953) also used moderate doses of segmental radiation therapy to all the major lymphnode regions. They believed that malignant lymphomas were radiocurable because they achieved 5- and 10-year survival rates of 50 percent and 30 percent, respectively (Hynes 1955, 1969).

Peters (1950) reported 113 patients with histologically documented Hodgkin's disease treated over 18 years (1924–1942). After 1933, most of the patients received some prophylactic irradiation to contiguous clinically uninvolved nodal areas. Their overall 5-year survival rate was 51 percent and the 10-year rate, 35 percent. In this series, there was no difference in survival rates in those with stage I disease whether they received prophylactic irradiation or not. Later, Peters and Middlemiss (1958) reported 290 patients with Hodgkin's disease treated with radiotherapy from 1928 to 1954. The 10-year survival rate by stages was 58 percent for stage I; 35 percent, stage II; and less than 2 percent for others. They estimated that prophylactic irradiation of the adjacent lymph node regions increased the survival rates by at least 20 percent. With initial prophylactic irradiation, there was also prolongation of the survival of patients who later developed recurrent disease.

In 1962, Kaplan reported that about 77 percent of Hodgkin's patients who received palliative radiotherapy had recurrence or extension of their disease, while only 13 percent of those treated radically did so. With the availability of the linear electron accelerator, he was able to increase the tumor dose given to 3500–4000 rads in 3–4 weeks. He also described a new technique of giving high-dose radiotherapy to all the main lymphatics in two fields: (1) "mantle" field for the upper lymphatic chains of cervical, mediastinal, and axillary regions, and (2) "inverted Y" field for the lower trunk lymphatics of para-aortic, iliac, and femoral areas, with an optional extension to include the spleen. About the same time, lymphangiograms and inferior venacavograms became useful radiographic procedures in delineating retroperitoneal disease sites, and the new Luke's histological classification of Hodgkin's disease and the subtype of nodular sclerosis were described.

In 1963, Easson and Russell reemphasized the word "cure" in connection with patients who had localized Hodgkin's disease; this consisted of about one-third of all the patients. Their patients were treated from 1934 to 1957 at a dose of 2500–2750 rads in 3 weeks to a field covering gross adenopathy and a margin of 5–7 cm normal tissue. The patients were considered cured because their death rate after the tenth year was almost the same as that of the normal population. Similar results were seen in patients with early reticulum cell sarcomas and lymphosarcomas. Easson (1966a,b) also commented that over 50 percent of the patients with localized Hodgkin's disease survived 5 years, and about 40 percent might be expected to live 15 years. Patients with localized lymphosarcomas (about half of the total number) had a slightly better survival rate than those with Hodgkin's disease

(49 percent after 15 years). Thus, he concluded that although lesions of non-Hodgkin's lymphomas appeared differently on morphological grounds, their response to radiotherapy was remarkably similar, consistent, and encouraging. And all apparently localized cases should be treated with radical irradiation with curative intent.

Since reirradiation of recurrences is hazardous because of the poor tolerance of normal tissues, it is clear that the initial therapeutical decision is crucial and optimal dose levels should be given during the first course of treatment. Reviewing all of the available clinical evidence, Kaplan (1966a,c) demonstrated that the recurrence rate was inversely related to the dosage delivered: at a tumor dose of 3600 rads, the recurrence rate was 10 percent. This rate approached zero asymptomatically as the radiation dose delivered to involved nodes approached 4000 rads, administered at the rate of 1000 rads/week. Friedman et al (1967) found that Hodgkin's disease was capable of recovery from radiation effect and that its rate of recovery more closely resembled that of carcinoma than a radiosensitive lesion such as mycosis fungoids. The "equivalent single dose" for local control of Hodgkin's disease is 1750 rads. The actual dose employed by Kaplan (1970) was usually 4400 rads delivered over a 4-week period in increments of 220 rads per day. In a total of 317 involved lymph node areas at risk, he had a true recurrence rate of 1.3 percent and a marginal extension rate of 0.7 percent. For slower responding and more radioresistant but regionally localized disease, Rubin (1966) administered tumor doses up to a maximum of 5000 rads to assure complete regression.

In addition to survival data suggesting curability of patients with Hodgkin's disease, Kaplan (1962, 1968b) pointed out that the relapse-free interval was also an important indicator of long-term prognosis. He found that about 85 percent of all relapses occurred during the first 24 months after completion of initial radiotherapy, and the probability of developing a relapse later than 5 years was less than 5 percent. Acturarial analysis yielded annual relapse rates in stages I and II of 22 percent, 18 percent, 15 percent, 3.3 percent, and 5 percent in years one through 5, respectively; the corresponding figures in stages III and IV were 39 percent, 29 percent, 14 percent, 0 percent, and 0 percent, respectively. Musshoff and Boutis (1968) also found that patients without relapse were the only long-term survivors. At 14 years after radiotherapy, 20.9 percent of the patients remained in primary remission; and 21.2 percent of the entire series was alive (the difference was due to 1 single patient). Johnson (1968) pointed out that radiotherapy retarded growth rates of sublethally damaged cells, and recurrence in the nonirradiated areas usually appeared within 1 year whereas true recurrence within the volume of irradiation usually became apparent after 18 months.

Frei and Gehan (1971) reviewed 6 series reported in the literature and found higher relapse rates after radiation therapy. The recurrent rate from the 4th to the 10th year varied from 5 to 20 percent. Thus, they felt that

Hodgkin's patients who survived 4 years after radiotherapy without relapse had at least an 80 percent chance of cure, and those who were relapse free at 10 years had a chance in excess of 90 percent of being cured. However, Chawla et al (1970) reported that 3 of 23 patients (13 percent) who survived more than 10 years without recurrence still developed relapse.

The desirability of irradiating apparently uninvolved lymph node regions "prophylactically," long advocated by Gilbert (1939), Peters (1950, 1966), Hynes (1955), and Kaplan (1961), was put on solid scientific foundation by the detailed and systematic study of Rosenberg and Kaplan (1966). They found that about 90 percent of initial lesions, as well as later extensions of disease, involved lymph node chains that could be considered contiguous by the criterion of direct lymphatic communication. It was also pointed out that extension from nodes at the base of the neck to the abdomen could be by way of the "escape route" of the thoracic duct (Kaplan 1970). Later results from staging laparotomy and splenectomy also confirmed this predictable pattern of spread (Kaplan 1971a). Kaplan (1972) pointed out that the 10 percent unusual pattern might be accounted for by hematogenous spread in cases with histologic evidence of vascular invasion as described by Rappaport and Strum (1970). But Johnson (1969) felt that the rate of noncontiguous spread could be as high as 45 percent, and Smithers (1970, 1973) tried to propose an alternative hypothesis by suggesting that the disease could originate either unifocally or multifocally, depending on the varying lymph node susceptibility to the inciting factor or factors.

Since 1962, Kaplan and Rosenberg (1966) and Rosenberg and Kaplan (1970) have carried out several randomized clinical trials. Their results showed that: (1) In patients with stages IB and IIB disease, curative radiotherapy encompassing the involved area and the adjacent nodal chains was better than treatment to limited fields alone in decreasing relapse rate and in improving survival. (2) Even in patients with stages IA and IIA disease, total lymphoid radiotherapy covering all the major lymph node chains reduced the relapse rate. (3) In patients with stage IIIA disease, treated with total lymphoid radiotherapy, about 80 percent were continuously free of disease and 60 percent had survived 5 years (Kaplan 1968a). Even 41 percent of those with stage IIIB disease had control and possible cure after radical total lymphoid field radiotherapy (Kaplan 1970). (4) Favorable results could also be achieved in selected subgroups of patients with stage IV disease, in which the extralymphatic site of involvement was sufficiently localized and adjacent to the nodal disease to permit the utilization of intensive radiotherapy (Kaplan 1970).

Other cooperative clinical trials compared the value of treating the involved field alone (IF) versus involved areas and adjacent uninvolved areas (EF = extended field) for patients with stages I and II Hodgkin's disease (Nickson 1966). Preliminary results showed patients treated with EF therapy experienced approximately twice as many complaints related to radiotherapy as the IF patients; but the IF patients did show an extension of disease to adjacent nodes on the same side of the diaphragm almost 10 times in excess (Nickson and Hutchison 1972). Twelve of the 15 deaths reported were associated with extensions across the diaphragm which occurred with similar frequency in both EF and IF groups. Patients who were older than 60 showed an extremely poor prognosis, although females and those with lymphocyte predominance or nodular sclerosis did well regardless of age (Young et al 1972).

Johnson et al (1969, 1970c) compared extended field irradiation with total nodal irradiation for patients with stages I and II involvement. The results showed that total nodal irradiation was well tolerated, did improve survival, and prevented recurrences in noncontiguous lymph node areas. The result of total nodal radiotherapy for stage IIIA was as favorable as that for stages IA and IIA (better than 75 percent 5-year survival without recurrence), but patients with stage IIIB disease showed a high rate of extranodal spread within 6 months of initial treatment.

Thus, Kaplan (1971b) felt the evidence provided by a number of randomized clinical trials supported the view that intensive radiotherapy, in most instances utilizing the total lymphoid technique, was the treatment of choice, excluding exceptional cases, in all stages of I (A,B), II (A,B), II_E (A,B), IIIA, and III_EA, and quite possibly also in IIIB and III_EB. The exceptional cases mentioned by him included elderly, frail patients or those with serious cardiac, renal, pumonary, or other life-threatening medical conditions, as well as children under 5 years of age. They are not good candidates for either total lymphoid radiotherapy or quadruple combination chemotherapy. In elderly and medically debilitated patients, local radiotherapy is usually the treatment of choice in stages I and II, and single drug palliative chemotherapy in stages III and IV. In very young children, he has tried limiting the dose of total lymphoid radiotherapy to about 1500 rads, followed by the use of 6 cycles of quadruple chemotherapy (MOPP). Special problems with the irradiation of children were discussed by D'Angio and Nisce (1973). In addition to its effect on bone growth and damage to other tissues, they pointed out that the induction of secondary tumors is now a well-recognized complication of curative radiation therapy.

In carefully staged, optimally treated patients, physicians may now expect relapse-free 5-year survival rates of approximately 85–90 percent in stages I and II, 70 percent or more in stage IIIA, and 40–50 percent in stage IIIB, with an overall 5-year survival of 65–70 percent for all stages and all cases (Kaplan 1973). Rosenberg (1971) estimated that the survival rate of those with localized disease of the lung was similar to those with stages I and II. In order to approach such therapeutic results, the radiotherapy should not be attempted by inexperienced radiologists who do not devote their entire time to radiation therapy. The requirement for relatively high doses and very large fields in turn dictates the use of radiation beams generated by megavoltage apparatus, since comparable doses of 200 kV x-rays would elicit intolerably severe skin reactions and other radiation damage (Rosenberg and Kaplan 1970). Even in palliative radiotherapy for advanced lymphomas, the result of treatment with megavoltage x-rays is superior to that with kilovoltage (Kaplan 1966b).

In the presence of frank abdominal adenopathy, Fuller (1966) felt that the liver and spleen should be treated with radiotherapy prophylactically, because, in the majority of the patients, the disease eventually involved these organs. Rather than using the "inverted Y" field, they treated the entire abdomen and pelvis to 3000 rads tumor dose in 1 or 2 separate fields with shielding of the kidneys after 2000 rads (Fuller et al 1970). Because of the diversity of sites of origin, the number of patients who received total abdominal irradiation was too small for meaningful analysis of local control or complications (Gamble et al 1971). But for patients who presented with retroperitoneal disease, they achieved a 5-year survival rate of 50 percent.

At Memorial Hospital in New York, they have used a new "3 and 2" sequential treatment technique for administering total nodal radiotherapy to patients with stages IIIA and B Hodgkin's disease. In the first course, all lymph node bearing areas from the tips of the mastoid processes down to the femoral triangles are divided into 3 segments and each segment receives 2000 rads with daily increments of 250 rads. After 4 to 6 weeks rest, a second course of irradiation is given to the same nodal areas, but only 2 fields are used. Each field receives 1800 rads at a daily dose of 200 rads. The rationale of such sequential treatment is to minimize the dosimetry problem of field juncture, to allow bone marrow recovery between courses, and to administer larger daily doses initially in a smaller field to give prompt symptomatic relief for patients with stage IIIB disease (Young et al 1972). Johnson (1973) also felt that the tumoricidal effect of ionizing radiation in Hodgkin's disease does not depend strictly on the administration of tumor doses of 4000 rads within 4 weeks. He has observed equally satisfactory tumor sterilization with more protracted treatment. In particular, split-course irradiation has reduced not only the acute reactions and thereby improved tolerance to treatment, but also has virtually eliminated delayed complications in normal tissue.

Glicksman and Nickson (1973) described an inventory of the acute and late reactions to total nodal irradiation in the treatment of Hodgkin's disease. Most of the acute and subacute reactions are transient, a few of the late reactions are permanent and only a very small number are debilitating. The treatment of acute and subacute reactions is symptomatic, and the treatment of late complications is almost nonexistent. When megavoltage irradiation is delivered to the "mantle" field above the diaphragm, the following acute reactions may occur: dryness of the mouth, loss of taste, dysphagia, dry or moist desquamation and tanning of the skin, epilation, nausea and vomiting, apathy and lassitude. Almost all of these complaints will disappear by the third month. When irradiation is given to the periaortic nodes, nausea, vomiting, anorexia, lassitude, and, rarely diarrhea may occur. When the entire "inverted Y" technique is employed, the nausea and vomiting may be more pronounced and diarrhea is common, especially in patients who have spastic colitis, diverticulitis, or related conditions. The subacute reactions seen in patients who are treated by the "mantle" technique include radiation pneumonitis and Lhermitte's sign, which is numbness and tingling in the fingers and toes upon flexion of the neck; and those who are treated below the diaphragm may have artificial menopause, loss of libido or impotence. The late reactions of radiation therapy can affect all tissues that are in the path of the ionization rays. Although most of the acute and subacute reactions to irradiation tend to be of minor consequence, the later complications can be appreciably more formidable (see detailed discussions in Chapter 11, pp. 341–376).

Seydel et al (1969) have analyzed the results of secondary radiation treatment of postradiotherapy-relapsing Hodgkin's disease. In patients with localized relapse, 24 percent survived 8 years after adequate radiotherapy. In patients with generalized relapse, no long-term survivals were seen because only palliative treatment was given. Lacher (1969) reported that among patients who survived more than 10 years, repeated radiotherapy played an important role. Among another series of 58 long-term survivals, Chawla et al (1970) found 16 who received 10 or more courses of radiotherapy for recurring or new lesions. Moreover, patients who received "sterilizing" doses of radiation initially (3000 rads or more) required as many subsequent courses of treatment as did those whose first courses were "inadequate." Although they question the necessity of the current emphasis on aggressive initial therapy, these experiences pointed out that even a recurrent or new disease should be treated with curative intent whenever possible.

Although histopathologic features are known to influence both the pattern of spread and rate of progression of the disease, Kaplan (1971b) felt no consensus was possible with respect to modifications of therapeutic strategy for specific histopathologic subtypes of Hodgkin's disease. Rubin et al (1969) suggested that stage I cases of mixed cellularity and lymphocyte depletion might benefit from segmental sequential irradiation to all the lymphoid areas. Although Johnson (1969) confirmed others' findings that total nodal irradiation gave better survival results than extended field radiotherapy in patients with stages I and II disease (5-year, 90 percent versus 60 percent), he found that patients with nodular sclerosis did very well with extended field treatment alone, and total nodal irradiation appeared unnecessary.

Landberg (1969) and Johnson et al (1970b) reported that the incidence of extranodal relapse correlated not only with the initial clinical staging, but also with the histopathology in the original biopsy, i.e., high risk patients were those with a combination of constitutional symptoms and mixed cellularity or lymphocyte depletion histology. The diagnostic error in evaluating occult extranodal dissemination was higher for those patients with than those without constitutional symptoms (15 percent versus 4 percent). And the most frequent site of clinically unrecognized occult extranodal involvement was bone (Johnson 1971).

Peters (1970) and Peters et al (1973) also felt that the topographic–histologic pattern of presentation could be as important as the clinical stage. They even made treatment decisions according to the different patterns of presentation. In pattern 1, with lymphocyte predominant disease and occasionally mixed cellularity limited to one peripheral region (stage I) excluding the supraclavicular area, control was achieved by radiating only the region involved. In pattern 2, with nodular sclerosis lesions involving the mediastinum and supraclavicular regions (stage II), complete control of the disease followed treating the chest mantle and celiac regions. For lesions involving the inguinal and para-aortic areas of the mixed cellularity or occasionally other types, radiation was given to the "inverted Y" field if the spleen was not involved, and to the entire abdomen and pelvic nodes if the spleen was involved. In pattern 3, patients with stage III disease, (mostly mixed cellularity lesions), experienced long-term remission following treatment of all the main regions below and above the diaphragm but omitting the mediastinal field.

Non-Hodgkin's Lymphoma

Fuller and Fletcher (1962) found that local recurrences of non-Hodgkin's lymphomas were more frequent when the tumor dose given was less than 750 rads/week; and Paterson (1963) stated that recurrence appeared when only 2000 rads or less was given over 3 weeks. There is less consensus concerning the optimal time and dose factors for the radiotherapy of non-Hodgkin's lymphoma than exists for Hodgkin's disease because a wide variation in the radiosensitivity of lymphosarcoma and reticulum cell sarcoma has been observed and has resulted in reports of widely divergent treatment techniques. Johnson (1969) said that the general tumor dose for peripheral adenopathy is about 2500–3000 rads for lymphosarcoma and 4000–5000 for reticulum cell sarcoma. But Nobler (1968) felt that local recurrences of malignant lymphoma can be prevented more than 95 percent of the time if a tumor dose of 3500 rads is delivered in 3 to 4 weeks, or, rarely, 4000 rads in 4 to 5 weeks. Rosenberg and Kaplan (1970) used the same dose (4000–4400 rads) for all the non-Hodgkin's lymphomas except those of the diffuse histiocytic type, to which a dose of 5000 rads was normally delivered. Musshoff et al (1971) found that when 4500 rads was given in 4 to 5 weeks, the rate of local recurrence was about 1 percent. Prosnitz et al (1969) reported a high recurrence rate of 68 percent when 3000 rads or less of radiation therapy was given. Lipton and Lee (1971) reported no recurrence in 9 patients who received at least 3500 rads, in contrast to a recurrence rate of 42 percent in those who received less than 3500 rads. Seydel et al (1971) also found local recurrence was prevented in lymphosarcoma when 3500 rads or more was given in 4 weeks. For giant follicular lymphoma, a 2000-rad tumor dose given in 10 to 21 days was enough. Fridman et al (1972) found that short-term, high-increment therapy (2000-rad total dose delivered in 5 days) also gave good local control in patients with generalized reticulum cell sarcoma.

For localized non-Hodgkin's lymphoma, the 5-year survival rate was about 50 percent (Peters 1963). Prophylactic irradiation of clinically uninvolved nodes had not increased the 5-year survival rate nor decreased the reactivation of disease as it had for those with Hodgkin's disease (Peters 1963; Rosenberg and Kaplan 1968). One explanation could be the high rate of positive lymphangiograms and extranodal involvement in patients with these diseases. It was estimated that only about 10 percent of the total cases was truly confined to one anatomic region. It has been shown that the distribution of a recurrent or secondary disease after radiotherapy of a localized non-Hodgkin's lymphoma is more random and more widely disseminated than that of Hodgkin's disease (Scheer 1963; Prosnitz et al 1969). The chance of having contiguous or adjacent nodal recurrence of a lymphoma was twice as high in Hodgkin's disease as in non-Hodgkin's lymphomas (70 percent versus 40 percent) (Han and Stutzman 1967; Banfi et al 1968, 1969)

Peters et al (1968) also pointed out that at the time of diagnosis, 40–60 percent of the patients with non-Hodgkin's disease already had involvement of extranodal sites, compared to 9 percent of those with Hodgkin's disease. In other words, the scope of probable site involvement in early non-Hodgkin's lymphomas was wider than anticipated, and so-called "new" lesions might actually be the primary focus of disease which had previously been occult. Necropsy data also showed that 70 percent had widespread involvement of the intestinal tract and mesenteric nodes. In contrast, only one-third of the patients with Hodgkin's disease showed such involvement.

However, Hynes and Frelick (1953) obtained a high 5-year survival rate of 80 percent for early non-Hodgkin's lymphomas, probably because they routinely treated major lymph node stations on both sides of the diaphragm. Fuller and Fletcher (1962) claim an advantage with prophylactic irradiation of the mediastinum for patients with stage I lymphomas involving the lower neck and supraclavicular fossa.

Werf-Messing (1968) did a retrospective study of 142 patients who had local and regional non-Hodgkin's lymphomas of the nodes or the upper respiratory and digestive tract. All patients were treated with ortho-voltage radiotherapy to the involved areas; tumor doses varied from 2000 to 5000 rads. It was estimated that prophylactic irradiation to adjacent areas could probably increase the 5-year survival rate by 10 percent for those with stage I disease, and by 21 percent for stage IIs. And prophylactic irradiation to the liver–spleen–epigastrium could add another 17 percent. Rosenberg and Kaplan (1970) pointed out that the Waldeyer's ring should be irradiated routinely whenever there was lymphadenopathy in the neck because of the high frequency of involvement of structures in that area either primarily or secondarily during the course of the disease.

Hansen (1969) reviewed 265 patients with reticulum cell sarcoma, most of whom had received low dose radiotherapy (mean 2800 rads over 33 days or 600 rads/week). He found that fast disappearance of the tumor did not correlate with better survival. Recurrence occurred in all four stages. The overall local recurrence rate was 9 percent; recurrence at new site, 24 percent; and both, 6 percent. Forty percent of recurrences developed within 3 months, 70 percent within 6 months, and 85 percent within 1 year after the initial treatment. Newall and Friedman (1970a,b) studied the natural history and radiosensitivity of patients with reticulum cell sarcoma. They pointed out the unpredictability of routes of spread and occasional unexpected long survival in the presence of extensive disease. They stressed that new metastatic lesions should also be treated energetically with the aim of permanent control.

Musshoff et al (1971) showed that in three-quarters of the patients with non-Hodgkin's lymphomas, the disease began in lymph nodes (including Waldeyer's ring); and in one-quarter of the cases, in extranodular organs. When lymphoma originated in lymph nodes, the disease tended to be widespread (half of the patients belonged to stages I and II, and recurrence in distant nodes occurred four times as often as those with primary organ involvement). When lymphomas originated primarily in organs, the disease remained limited to local regions for a longer time and showed a greater tendency towards a continuous rather than discontinuous spread (two-thirds of the cases were stages I and II, and local and regional relapses were 1.5 times more frequent than in cases with primary lymph node involvement). However, Cox et al (1972) classified lesions of the Waldeyer's ring as extranodal tumors and reported just the opposite. Purely nodal lymphoreticular tumors had an indolent course, spread contiguously, and manifested further disease long after the initial treatment; extranodal tumors, which accounted for 30 percent of the total, spread to distant sites, and seemed either to be controlled permanently or to have very rapid progression.

Since patients with non-Hodgkin's lymphomas commonly had primary involvement of extranodal structures, and since recurrences in noncontiguous sites appeared to be much more common than in Hodgkin's disease, some felt that the addition of a more effective systemic therapy (either chemotherapy or total body irradiation) was indicated. Johnson (1969) used both total nodal irradiation and total body irradiation in patients with advanced lymphosarcomas. Total body irradiation was administered at a total dose of 100–300 rads, about 10 rads given on each of 3 to 5 days/week, with a 1-month interruption during treatment for some patients to permit partial bone marrow recovery. Subsequently, some patients received no additional treatment until relapse occurred, whereas others were given maintenance doses of total body irradiation on a monthly or biweekly basis. In certain cases of stage III involvement, total nodal radiotherapy with tumor doses of 2000–3000 rads was used either alone or following total body irradiation. Of 16 patients with stage III disease, 40 percent survived 5 years without recurrence (Johnson 1971). A similar treatment plan resulted in encouraging remission and survival rates in stage IV patients with generalized lymph node and bone marrow involvement, but not with extranodal dissemination to sites other than the bone marrow (Johnson et al 1970a). They also found that clinical staging correlated better with survival than did the histologic classification based on estimations of tumor cell differentiation.

However, Peters (1970) felt that histological types correlated with clinical presentation and should influence therapeutic plans. For the diffuse histological group in which the primary focus in most patients with early disease appeared to be intraabdominal, the whole abdomen was irradiated (total dose about 2000 rads). Radiation to all of the peripheral lymph node regions also could be indicated, but this decision depends on the sites of presentation. For nodular lymphomas, the advantage of active treatment of the asymptomatic patient was not clear because she had patients in this category whose disease did not become aggressive until 10 or more years later. Local radiation in patients with stage I disease was worthwhile because the lesion in many such patients appeared to be controlled for indefinite periods. For stages II and III disease, treatment should encompass all sites of suspected disease, which usually includes all the peripheral lymph node regions and the abdomen. For stage IV disease, if intrathoracic disease is identified or if there is local involvement of skin or skeleton, radiation could be used for palliation, when necessary, while administering chemotherapy.

Jones et al (1972) also found that the histopathological classification of Rappaport correlated very well with the results of radiotherapy. Their patients received high-dose radiotherapy, defined as at least 3000 rads in 3 weeks, either just to the involved field or to the adjacent noninvolved regions. The natural course of patients with localized diffuse histiocytic lymphomas was characterized by a median survival of 13 months and a high risk of relapse within 1 year of treatment. In contrast, patients with localized nodular mixed cell type or nodular lymphocytic poorly differentiated lymphomas exhibited a median survival of 80 months and a pattern of continued later relapse. Based on these preliminary findings, they are conducting new randomized clinical trials in which one of several treatment options will be selected according to the clinicopathological stage and histopathological subtype of the lymphoma involved.

CHEMOTHERAPY

Chemotherapy for the treatment of malignant lymphomas has developed significantly since 1946 when nitrogen mustard was the only agent available. In the 1950s, oral alkylating agents of chlorambucil and cyclophosphamide became available. About 1960, the purified alkaloids from the periwinkle plant (vinblastine and vincristine) were shown to have antimitotic activity. In 1962, methylhydrazine compound was introduced, and its mode of action was different from that of the alkylating agents, antimetabolites, and periwinkle alkaloids. Procarbazine was believed to act by generation of intracellular peroxide (Ultmann 1971).

Not infrequently, chemotherapy will eliminate all evidence of malignant lymphoma and achieve symptomatic relief; however, the disease inevitably recurs. Since there is no single, well-documented instance of the cure of a patient with Hodgkin's disease by treatment with any single drug alone, and since the curative potential of radiation therapy in patients with early disease is well documented, Kaplan (1971) emphasized that the practice of treating such potentially curable patients with single drug chemotherapy should be condemned. Moreover, there is suggestive evidence that the injudicious and inappropriate use of single drug chemotherapy might decrease the radio-responsiveness and increase the recurrence rate of Hodgkin's disease in patients subsequently treated with local radiotherapy (Johnson and Brace 1966).

Alkylating Agents

The principal alkylating agents are nitrogen mustard (Mustargen), chlorambucil (Leukeran), cyclophosphamide (Cytoxan), and thiotriethylene phosphoramide (Thiotepa). The mode of action of the alkylating agents is through an intramolecular conversion to a cyclic compound that forms a cross linkage between guanine moieties. This interferes with the replication of the deoxyribonucleic acid.

Nitrogen mustard has the advantage of rapid action, but it must be given intravenously. The usual dose is 0.2 mg/kg twice daily, with repeated courses at about 4 week intervals (Frei 1971). The initial remission rate is about 70 percent, but the duration is brief, and 9 percent of the patients relapse within 10 weeks (Ultmann 1971). As is true of other alkylating agents, bone marrow depression is the major toxic side effect. With mustard, the maximum depression is in 2–3 weeks and, therefore, is difficult to control.

The advantage of chlorambucil is that it may be given orally and its effects may be titrated more readily against both tumor and bone marrow response. A disadvantage is its slow rate of activity. It is useful in the maintenance therapy of patients previously treated with nitrogen mustard and can obviate the need for repeated courses of intravenous drugs. In both Hodgkin's disease and other lymphomas, response can be seen in about 60 percent of the cases, and the median duration of remission is 5 months.

Cyclophosphamide can be used both for induction (by intravenous administration) and maintenance (by taking orally). It is somewhat more predictably absorbed in the gastrointestinal tract than is chlorambucil. Patients who responded well to cyclophosphamide could be maintained at a dose of 50–100 mg/day orally. Although it has the advantage of having less toxicity to platelet formation, it does have two toxic manifestations not shared by other alkylating agents: alopecia and hemorrhagic cystitis. The former occurred in one-third of the cases and the latter, in about 5 percent. Approximately 65 percent of the Hodgkin's patients had objective response with a median duration of 8 months. Carbone et al (1968) administered cyclophosphamide intravenously at the rate of 15 mg/kg/week and found that about 50 percent of the non-Hodgkin's patients had remissions of 3–6 months with maintenance. Mendelson et al (1970) showed that larger doses (40 mg/kg/3–4 weeks) administered intravenously could be tolerated and resulted in longer durations of remission (median 20 months).

Thiotepa is active against Hodgkin's disease, but it has no special advantage over the other alkylating agents. Cytoxan or Thiotepa has been used in place of nitrogen mustard in combination chemotherapy to reduce nausea and vomiting (Young et al 1972).

Vinca Alkaloids

Vinblastine (Velban) provides significant objective improvement for the majority of patients with Hodgkin's disease, whereas vincristine (Oncovin) appears to be a useful agent in the management of non-Hodgkin's lymphomas. When compared to cyclophosphamide, vinblastine was shown to be superior as the initial agent in inducing remission in Hodgkin's disease (Stutzman et al 1966). In patients who did not receive previous therapy, vinblastine and nitrogen mustard seemed to be equally effective (Ezdinli and Stutzman 1968; Alison and Whitelaw 1970). But patients favored vinblastine because it had negligible side effects. In Hodgkin's patients previously treated, vinblastine and cyclophosphamide had about equal potential in inducing objective remission (Carbone et al 1968). In patients with non-Hodgkin's lymphomas, cyclophosphamide appeared superior (Stutzman et al 1966); and the mean duration of remission obtained with nitrogen mustard was longer than that obtained with vinblastine (Solomon et al 1969).

Solomon et al (1973) compared the relative efficacy of nitrogen mustard (Mustargen and vinblastine in 172 patients with advanced malignant lymphomas. In their protocol, response was defined as a reduction by at least 50 percent in the sum of the products of the bidimensional measurements of the tumor masses lasting at least 28 days and accompanied by subjective improvement. These two drugs gave an identical response rate (50 percent) in patients with Hodgkin's disease. The response to nitrogen mustard as first treatment has predictive value for response to vinblastine as second, but the converse is not true. In patients with non-Hodgkin's lymphomas, those with nodular, poorly differentiated lymphocytic lymphoma responded significantly better to nitrogen mustard than to vinblastine, and their response rate with the alkylating agent was also higher than that of the other persons with non-Hodgkin's lymphoma.

Vinblastine is used intravenously at a usual dose level of 0.05–0.20 mg/kg of body weight, titrated against the response of the disease and of the white blood cell count (Rosenberg and Kaplan 1970). Granulocytopenia is the major toxic effect, but recovery is rapid after cessation of the drug, and there is little or no depression of the platelet count. Another major side effect is neurologic in nature, eventually producing areflexia. Patients who respond well to vinblastine usually do so after the first or second injection. A remission rate of 65–80 percent can be expected with maintenance therapy. The mean remission duration was over 10 months, and occasionally lasted for several years (Flatow et al 1969).

Vincristine is slightly less effective in Hodgkin's disease, but has no cross resistance and can be used sequentially after vinblastine. In patients with diffuse non-Hodgkin's lymphomas of the poorly differentiated lymphocytic of histiocytic types, the first drug of choice might be nitrogen mustard or chlorambucil (Rosenberg and Kaplan 1970). When the disease becomes refractory to alkylating agents, vincristine is the second agent of choice. The dose needed is often small, 0.01–0.03 mg/kg of body weight at weekly intervals. The remission rate is about 40–50 percent and tends to be short (averaging about 4 months). It appears to be more effective in cases of reticulum cell sarcomas than in lymphosarcoma (Desai et al 1969). Neurotoxicity is more dose-limiting than that of vinblastine, and alopecia is also frequently observed with vincristine therapy. It was suggested that vincristine interferes with the metabolism of the nerve cell as well as of the Schwann cell (McLeod and Penny, 1969). Since neurological side effects occurred in 80 percent of the patients who received the usual dose, a lower dose of vincristine (0.0075 mg/kg) was tried, with slightly lower response rate obtained (Korbitz et al 1969).

Methylhydrazine

Procarbazine (Natulan, Matulene) is one of the methylhydrazine compounds and exhibits definite activity against Hodgkin's disease. The drug is known to inhibit the enzyme monoamine oxidase and interfere with pyridoxine metabolism (DeVita 1971). It can be used orally and is of special benefit because there is no cross resistance between it and the alkylating agents or the vinca alkaloids (Samuels et al 1967; Flatow et al 1969). However, when used as the third sequential drug for Hodgkin's disease, the response has been relatively short in duration (averaging 2 to 3 months). The younger patients and those with nodular sclerosis respond better, and the older patients do poorly no matter what the histologic type (Rapoport et al 1969). All responses were clinically evident 3 weeks after therapy was begun (DeConti 1971).

Procarbazine is given in gradually increasing doses to a tolerated dose of 150–300 mg/day. This is then continued on a daily basis until toxicity or tumor regression occurs. About 50 percent of the patients have neurotoxicity and bone marrow depression. The marrow toxicity is similar to that of mustard, affecting all of the formed elements. Neurotoxicity consists mainly of nausea, vomiting, peripheral neuritis, and, less commonly, sensorium change and hypotension (Samuels et al 1967). In several large groups of patients, the remission induction rate in Hodgkin's patients was approximately 60 percent, with an average duration of 6 months. Comparison of vinblastine with procarbazine suggests that both agents have similar remission induction rates (Bonadonna et al 1969), but that vinblastine is superior as a maintenance agent (Ultmann 1971). Aisenberg and Goldman (1971) showed that chemotherapy with either vinblastine or procarbazine has definitely prolonged the median survival of Hodgkin's patients from 18 to 42 months.

In non-Hodgkin's lymphomas, procarbazine has a response rate of about 30–40 percent (Brunner and Young 1965; Stolinsky et al 1969).

Other Agents

The lympholytic action of corticosteroids was utilized in treating patients with lymphocytic lymphomas, and a 75 percent response rate was obtained which lasted about 6 months (Burningham et al 1964). This drug is much less effective in Hodgkin's disease (the objective response rate is about 25 percent); but it is useful in cases of hemolytic anemia, thrombocytopenia, or bone-marrow supression (Rosenbaum 1970). Hall et al (1967) used high dose corticoid therapy in 36 patients with advanced lymphomas which were refractory to x-rays and alkylating agents and obtained worthwhile objective response in 66 percent of the cases. Ultmann and Nixon (1969) said steroid is especially useful in patients with systematic symptoms since it frequently produces lysis of fever, improved appetite, and a feeling of well being.

Carter and Livingston (1973) reviewed existing data on single drugs in the chemotherapy of Hodgkin's disease. They found that the complete remission rates using single alkylating agent were about 10 to 15 percent; and using vinca alkaloid or synthetic procarbazine, about 30 to 40 percent. Although combination chemotherapy has shown its superiority in the induction of complete remission of disease, many single agents, particularly those in the antimetabolite and antibiotic classes of antitumor drugs, have not had adequate evaluation, and may yet play important roles in the design of future combination therapies.

It is said that antimetabolite drugs (cytosine arabinoside, 5-fluorouracil, 6-mercaptopurine, and methotrexate) have not been too useful in adults with lymphomas. However, childhood non-Hodgkin's lymphomas may receive some satisfactory results (Karnofsky 1970). Of the antitumor antibiotics, dactinomycin was found to produce response in 9 out of 18 lymphoma patients (Carter and Livingston 1973). Mithramycin, mitomycin, adriamycin, and streptonigrin have all been reported to show some degree of activity. Another antibiotic, bleomycin, which showed effectiveness against squamous cell carcinoma of the skin, was tried in patients with malignant lymphomas. Although the enlarged lymph node shrank, the chief side effect was pulmonary toxicity (Kimura et al 1972). In 37 patients with disseminated and refractory lymphomas, Rudders (1972) reported an objective response rate of 49 percent.

BCNU (1,3-bis-β chlorethyl-l-nitrosourea) is a nitrosourea derivative. It has alkylating properties, but its mechanism of action is unknown. It affects both proliferating and nonproliferating cells. Some of the nitrosourea compounds pass the blood–brain barrier and are highly effective against intracranially transplanted leukemias (Loo, et al 1966). They produce objective response in approximately 50 percent of patients with advanced refractory Hodgkin's disease; the median duration of remission is 3–4 months (Lessner 1968; Young et al 1971). Responses were also noted, although to a lesser degree, in patients with non-Hodgkin's lymphomas. The drug appears to have no cross resistance with the vinca alkaloids or the alkylating agents (Marsh et al 1971). The usual dose is 150–250 mg/m^2 in a 3-day course every 6 weeks (Frei 1970). The agent is somewhat difficult to employ, since it produces leukopenia and thrombocytopenia 3–4 weeks after a single dose.

Combination Chemotherapy

The success of combination chemotherapy in the treatment of patients with acute leukemia has illustrated four points: (1) Patients who have partial response tend to have shorter remissions than those who have complete response. (2) It is possible to achieve a greater degree of tumor cell destruction by using drugs which have different modes of action. (3) Each agent has unique toxic manifestations, and a combination of agents does not necessarily result in additive toxicity. (4) Cyclic and repeated therapy permits destruction of tumor cells when they are in their most susceptible dividing phase. There is definite evidence that multiple drugs used in combination have materially advanced the treatment of human malignancies (Henderson and Samaha 1969).

Hodgkin's Disease

Seventy percent of the patients with Hodgkin's disease may have remissions with single agents; complete remissions, however, constitute only about one-third of this number; and the average duration of response to single agents is only approximately 6 weeks (DeVita and Carbone 1971). As soon as one combines two agents, for example vinblastine and chlorambucil, the complete remission induction rate increases to about 63 percent (Lacher and Durant 1965). Moxley et al (1967) found an even higher response rate (80 percent) when four drugs were used, some in combination with radiotherapy. Various combination chemotherapy has been tried in patients with Hodgkin's disease and other lymphomas. The results of eight published series have been summarized by Ultmann (1970).

Presently, the most successful and widely tested combination of drugs is that developed by DeVita and his coworkers (1967, 1969) at the National Cancer Institute, the so-called MOPP program. It consists of a 2-week therapy program of nitrogen mustard, vincristine (Oncovin), procarbazine, and prednisone, followed by 2 weeks of rest. The cycle is repeated every 4 weeks, and the entire course of treatment requires 6 months. The original MOPP program consisted of giving mustard (6 mg/m^2) and vincristine (1.4 mg/m^2) intensively on the first and eighth days in all 6 cycles; procarbazine (100 mg/m^2): orally daily for 14 days in all 6 cycles; and prednisone (40 mg/m^2): orally daily for 14 days during cycles 1 and 4 only.

The first group of 43 patients with advanced, but untreated, Hodgkin's disease who received the MOPP program showed a complete response rate of 81 percent (Carbone et al 1971). A complete response was defined as the disappearance of all tumors and a return to normal performance status. All but 2 of the patients completed the 6-cycle treatment, although 20 percent did require reduction of doses because of severe bone marrow depression. The duration of these responses was impressive; the median was between 29 and 42 months when the group was followed for 3 years. At the end of the fourth year, an overall survival rate of 63 percent was obtained; and of the responders, 77 percent were alive and 47 percent continuously free of disease (DeVita et al 1970). At the fifth year, 72 percent were alive and 41 percent remained free of disease with no further treatment (DeVita and Carbone 1971). The results of 35 patients who were at risk in excess of 5 years were similar. Of those who achieved complete remission, 70 percent were alive at 6 years, and the median duration of complete remission from the end of 6 cycles of MOPP was 36 months (DeVita et al 1972). As with radiotherapy, the relapse rate is highest in the first 2 years and then decreases with time. No relapse occurred in any patient who was free of disease for 42 months following MOPP therapy. Those who experienced relapse after a good remission lasting over 8 months could be easily retreated with the combination. Of the 8 patients who did not have complete remission, all were dead but one, with a median survival of 12 months (Canellos et al 1973).

The high complete response rate of MOPP therapy in previously untreated patients was confirmed by Nicholson et al (1970), Luce et al (1971), and Olweny et al (1971), who obtained a rate of 86 percent, 78 percent, and 76 percent, respectively. Nicholson et al (1970) substituted vinblastine for vincristine in order to alleviate the neurotoxicity, but noticed more leukopenia instead.

In patients who had received total nodal radiotherapy, a complete remission rate of 75 percent and a response duration comparable to patients previously untreated was achieved (Lowenbraun et al 1970a). Cooper et al (1972) reported a complete remission rate of 84 percent and a median duration of 28 months. Patients who had extensive prior chemotherapy, particularly with alkylating agents or chemotherapy plus irradiation, fared the worst. Nicholson et al (1970) reported a response rate of only 35 percent in such patients.

Since combination chemotherapy has proved to be so effective, there has been only one study comparing the use of the MOPP program with single agents. In this particular study, although the complete remission rate with MOPP was lower than reported by others, the difference between the MOPP complete remission rate (50 percent) and that obtained with nitrogen mustard (14 percent) was statistically significant (DeVita and Canellos 1972). It appears that, in general, all patients with stages IIIB and IV disease should be treated with the MOPP combination program. Aisenberg (1973) preferred to employ combination chemotherapy as the primary treatment of all patients with stage III disease, and use radiation in an adjuvant role.

Greenberg et al (1972) showed that the MOPP program has minimal toxic effects and can be safely administered by experienced and well trained physicians to outpatients with a minimum disruption of the family unit. However, there is an emotional strain on the patients because of the anticipation of vomiting, twice with each cycle of treatment, and alopecia in young patients (Rosenberg et al 1972). In addition, male patients treated with the MOPP program showed evidence of damage to spermatogenesis. Eight of the 10 patients who were studied showed either complete azoospermia or prolonged low sperm counts (DeVita et al 1972).

Nissen et al (1972) attempted to improve on the MOPP program by substitution of half of the vincristine doses by vinblastine and replacement of nitrogen mustard by chlorambucil. In patients who had no previous treatment, the results were similar. However, the MOPP routine was superior in all treated patients, although this program did have more neurotoxicity and hematologic toxicity. Later, in another protocol, they substituted carmustine (BCNU) for nitrogen mustard of the MOPP program. The early complete and partial response rate was 91 percent for the BOPP program and 88 percent for the MOPP program.

DeVita and Carbone (1971), in analyzing the response rates and survival results of patients who received MOPP therapy, showed that patients younger than 30 had a better overall prognosis than those in the older age group. Asymptomatic patients even with advanced disease never failed to achieve remission, and only one experienced relapse. In addition, all of the induction failures and all but one death were in the stage IVB category. The nodular sclerosis histology in patients with stage IVB disease adversely affected the duration of complete remission. Cooper et al (1972) found that excessive atypical histiocytes in the tissue biopsy reflected a shorter remission duration with combination chemotherapy.

Moore et al (1973) reported 81 patients who received MOPP chemotherapy for advanced Hodgkin's disease. They also found a decreased duration of remission in patients who were older, who had systemic symptoms, and bone marrow involvement. However, when patients under 30 years of age were compared to patients over 30 there was no significant difference found in the relapse rate or disease-free survival between the two groups. But the relapse rate in patients under 20 (4/15) was significantly less than in patients over 45(9/13); and the disease-free survival curves for these two groups were also significantly different. Similar analyses of results by sex and histology revealed no significant differences. It needs to be pointed out that the overall relapse rate for patients who achieved complete remission by the MOPP program was 28 percent. And in their series, reinduction with MOPP was unsuccessful in 8 of 8 instances. It was felt that in such cases resistance had developed to one or more of the agents used in the original combination therapy.

The proper approach to those patients who achieved a complete response is not clear, although in single-drug therapy with vinca alkaloids and cyclophosphamide, Carbone et al (1968) showed that the duration of maintained remission was 3–8 times as long as that for unmaintained remission. Data at the National Cancer Institute did not suggest any marked difference in patients who received maintenance therapy with intermittent MOPP or BCNU, as compared with patients who received no therapy. But Luce et al (1971) found that a median remission duration of 24 months could be prolonged to 36 months when patients were maintained on intermittent MOPP. Other maintenance therapy with single drugs of dactinomycin, methotrexate, vinblastine, chlorambucil, or prednisone showed conflicting results (DeVita and Canellos 1972). Frei (1973) pointed out that relapses after combination therapy usually occur at pretreatment sites of major tumor involvement and studies adding irradiation to these lesions are underway. Lenhard (1973) is evaluating the value of non-specific immunologic stimulation in extending the duration of disease-free remission after combination therapy through the use of BCG (Calmette-Guerin bacillus).

Non-Hodgkin's Lymphoma

With single-drug chemotherapy, about 66 percent of the patients with lymphocytic lymphomas were alive at one year, and 40 percent of those with histiocytic lymphomas survived the same period (Carbone 1972). Cytoxan is consistently better for the non-Hodgkin's lymphoma, and vincristine is probably better than Vinblastine (Carbone, 1973). The rate of complete remission with single drugs was usually less than 10 percent, and the duration of these remissions was less than 30 weeks, even with continued maintenance. Thus, several combination chemotherapy programs have been tried for non-Hodgkin's lymphomas.

Hoogstraten et al (1969) demonstrated the superiority of weekly combinations of cyclophosphamide, vincristine, and prednisone (COP program) over cyclophosphamide alone in achieving remissions. The combination therapy gave a higher complete response rate than single agents in both reticulum cell sarcoma (30 percent versus 10 percent) and lymphosarcoma (35 percent versus 21 percent). The addition of prednisone to the combination of cyclophosphamide and vincristine increased the complete response rate from 20 percent to 48 percent for the lymphocytic lymphoma patients and 7 percent to 41 percent for those with histiocytic lymphomas (Lenhard and Owens 1971). Luce et al (1971) used a different schedule of the COP program and achieved a complete remission rate of 50 percent and 39 percent, respectively, for reticulum cell sarcoma and lymphosarcoma. Bagley et al (1972) used COP in intensive 5-day cycles given every 3 weeks achieving complete remission in 57 percent and partial response in another 34 percent of cases. Eighty-nine percent of the complete remissions lasted more than one year. Survival of complete responders was significantly better than that of partial responders.

Lowenbraun et al (1970b) used the MOPP program in 23 patients with advanced non-Hodgkin's lymphomas. Complete remission was achieved in 7 of 15 with lymphosarcomas and 3 of 8 with reticulum cell sarcomas, with a disease-free duration of more than 36 months in 5 patients. These data showed that this combination chemotherapy can also produce remissions of substantial duration in non-Hodgkin's patients.

Mukherji et al (1971) questioned the efficacy of combination chemotherapy for patients with extranodal disease. They used a modification of the MOPP program, substituting cyclophosphamide for nitrogen mustard (COPP). Only 3 of 12 lymphosarcomas and 1 of 11 reticulum cell sarcomas achieved complete remission. However, DeVita and Canellos (1972) found that 50 percent of the patients who had visceral disease had complete remission with COP therapy. Kurnick and Robinson (1972) treated patients with stages III and IV lymphomas with the modified COPP program. They obtained a high complete remission rate of 90 percent. In patients who had relapses following previous therapy, the complete response rate was much lower (26 percent).

CHEMOTHERAPY AND RADIOTHERAPY

Soon after it became available, nitrogen mustard was used in conjunction with radiotherapy in the palliative management of patients with advanced Hodgkin's disease. Although some investigators concluded that this combination had merit, the general consensus was that nitrogen mustard did not add significantly to either the quality or duration of survival in these patients (Smithers 1969; Kaplan 1971).

With the discovery of newer chemotherapeutic agents, Tubiana et al (1966) conducted a cooperative randomized study of adding or not adding weekly vinblastine for 2 years after radical radiotherapy in patients with stages I and II Hodgkin's disease who were treated with either the "mantle" field or "inverted Y" technique. Their results showed that chemotherapy did decrease the annual recurrence rate from 24 percent to 8 percent for the first 4 years (Radiotherapy-Chemotherapy cooperative group, 1972). The difference remained statistically significant at the end of the fifth year, and patients treated with chemotherapy showed a trend toward higher survival rates (Tubiana and Amiel 1973). However, this beneficial effect of adding chemotherapy appeared to be important only for patients who were older than 30, and who had lesions of the mixed cellularity and lymphocyte depletion types. Bernard et al (1971) gave 154 Hodgkin's patients with untreated and localized disease nitrogen mustard before extended radiotherapy and vinblastine afterwards. Their preliminary report showed that the addition of 2 single chemotherapeutic agents did not improve the result of using radiotherapy alone. They then randomized patients into no treatment or treatment with MOPP chemotherapy programs for 3 months before radiotherapy. Four weeks after radiotherapy, the patients were randomized again into two groups; one received monthly vinblastine for 4 years and the other received the MOPP program every 6 months. Their preliminary results showed tolerance was good in 50 percent of the patients who received preradiation chemotherapy, and irradiation was well tolerated in all patients except one.

Presently, radiotherapy has shown its curative value in patients with stages I and II malignant lymphomas. But it is likely that the results of radiotherapy alone, though now greatly improved, will still leave plenty of room for further improvement in stages III and IV. DeVita and Canellos (1972) mentioned a controlled trail of combination chemotherapy (MOPP) versus total axial lymph node irradiation (TNI) in patients with stage IIIB Hodgkin's disease. They found chemotherapy was superior to radiotherapy in terms of median survival and the number of disease-free patients at 4 years. But failures following TNI tended to relate to extranodal dissemination, and failures after the MOPP program related to recurrence in previously involved nodes. Thus, their results suggested a rational approach of using both modalities in advanced cases, and many clinical trials have been initiated to assess the value of adding chemotherapy to radiotherapy.

In patients with stage III Hodgkin's disease, Bernard et al (1971) gave multiple drug chemotherapy (MOPP) before radiotherapy. On the whole, tolerance to this combination of intensive chemotherapy and extensive radiotherapy was good. However, they warned about the possibility of a chronic bone marrow insufficiency because this occurred in 7 of their 21 patients. Tubiana and Amiel (1973) gave a course of chemotherapy (usually procarbazine) and added radiotherapy (3500–4000 rads) to those who failed to achieve complete remission. Among 40 patients with sufficient follow-up studies, 5 complete and 34 incomplete remissions were obtained at the end of the course of chemotherapy, and 33 patients were in complete and 5 in incomplete remissions after radiotherapy. The median survival of these patients is 5 years and the median duration of first remission is 29 months. Thus, it appears that this type of combination is feasible and yields results that compare favorably with those of radiotherapy.

Gamble et al (1971, 1973) and Fuller and Gamble (1973) felt that preliminary chemotherapy was essential for control of local and systemic symptomatology before instituting radiotherapy. In patients with stage III Hodgkin's disease, they gave combination chemotherapy (currently MOPP) before definitive radiotherapy to all major lymphoid areas, including the whole abdomen. Two courses of MOPP were used initially; later the number of courses was changed to three. Their preliminary results were encouraging, although they warned of the possibility of immunologic suppression since, among 22 patients, 3 developed herpes zoster and 4 had pneumonia. Among 33 patients with stages IIIA and B disease who belonged to this ongoing study, the 3-year survival figure was 70 percent and the 5-year, 68 percent. In patients with stage III reticulum cell sarcoma or stages I and II disease of the abdomen, Gamble et al (1971) used a combination of Cytoxan, vincristine, and prednisone before giving intensive large volume radiotherapy to the involved region. Their survival figures for localized disease suggested that a combined approach using radiotherapy and chemotherapy was better than radiation therapy alone. For lymphomas involving the gastrointestinal tract, all patients had preliminary resections.

Others felt that since radiotherapy had demonstrated its curative effect in treating localized lymphomas, it should be given before combination chemotherapy (Bull et al 1970). Such an approach should have a 5-year survival rate of about 40–50 percent. Rosenberg (1971) reported that the patient's tolerance and the efficacy of chemotherapy given after radical radiation therapy were about the same as for those who received a lesser amount of radiation therapy. Moreover, they were able to give aggressive combination chemotherapy (MOPP) within 60 days of total lymphoid irradiation. Stutzman (1971) also found no evidence of increased toxicity; about 80 percent of the cases received the scheduled drug therapy and the complete response rate was high (56 percent). However, Curran and Johnson (1970) reported a poor tolerance of chemotherapy for approximately 12 months after radiotherapy in 50 percent of the patients who had heavy irradiation to more than 65 percent of their bone marrow.

Moore et al (1972) reported their early results of sequential radiotherapy and chemotherapy from Stanford University. Among 102 patients with previously untreated Hodgkin's disease, 4 had stage IB; 35, IIA or B; 37, IIIA; and 26, IIIB. They were randomized to receive either total lymphoid radiation alone (4400 rads delivered in 4 weeks) or followed by 6 cycles of MOPP therapy. The number of relapses in the group receiving sequential therapy was significantly less than that in the group receiving radiotherapy alone (1/48 versus 10/45). A subsequent report which included additional 6-month follow-up has slightly reduced the significance of the difference: the relapse-free 3-year survival rates became 88 percent versus 73 percent (Rosenberg et al 1972). However, the actual survival was not significantly different for the 2 groups; and when corrections for imbalance of both histology and sex were made, the disease-free survival from the end of all therapy was similar. Although the overall tolerance was surprisingly good, they considered it premature to recommend the general use of total lymphoid radiotherapy plus combination chemotherapy in patients with Hodgkin's disease.

In a double-blind study, Stutzman (1971) randomized 50 patients with advanced malignant lymphomas into receiving 3 weekly doses of either vincristine or placebo during the course of radiotherapy. There were 14 patients with Hodgkin's disease and 36 with other lymphomas. The tumor response within the radiation port at the end of the therapy was significantly better in the vincristine-treated group than in the placebo-treated group (55 percent versus 19 percent). The recurrence rate of the irradiated tumor was similar, but the survival of those treated with vincristine was better than for those receiving irradiation alone, suggesting the drug had systemic effects. However, in a retrospective study, Reilly et al (1972) found that chemotherapy with nitrogen mustard, chlorambucil, or prednisone, in conjunction with radiotherapy for reticulum cell sarcoma, showed no enhancement of local effects of radiotherapy nor improvement of survival rates.

In children with local and regional lymphosarcomas, the 5-year survival rate was much poorer than in adults (9 percent versus 33 percent) because of frequent recurrence and conversion to acute lymphocytic leukemia. Thus, Aur et al (1971) recommended a more aggressive approach utilizing both chemotherapy and radiotherapy. Initially, they gave prednisone and vincristine along with cobalt radiotherapy to clinically detectable tumor sites. This was followed by daily administration of 6-mercaptopurine, weekly methotraxate and cyclophosphamide, and a 15-day course of prednisone and vincristine every 10 weeks. Six of their 8 children attained remission and were well for 16–27 months.

Patients who developed new disease after receiving irradiation therapy to the mantle field offer special therapeutic challenges. The pattern of failure was consistent: the vast majority of patients had a transdiaphragmatic extension of the disease most often involving the para-aortic lymph nodes or the spleen. Attempts to control such "mantle failures" with radiation therapy alone were possible only in 18 percent of the cases; with added chemotherapy, in 37 percent. Thus, Rubin (1973) felt an integrated course of radiation therapy to the involved nodes, plus quadruple chemotherapy (MOPP) is indicated. He preferred to start with 3 cycles of MOPP therapy, followed by irradiation through an "inverted Y" field, and then 3 more cycles of MOPP.

Hoogstraten et al (1973) designed the most complete protocol to investigate the best way to use chemotherapy and radiotherapy in patients with stage III Hodgkin's disease. It was theorized that it would be possible to reduce the neoplastic cells in patients with advanced disease to a number equivalent to that in stage I or II with chemotherapy and that cures could be obtained in some of these patients with subsequent radiotherapy. Patients were randomly assigned into one of 5 treatment plans: (A) chemotherapy followed by radiation therapy to involved areas; (B) chemotherapy only; (C) total nodal radiation therapy followed by chemotherapy; (D) chemotherapy followed by total nodal radiation therapy; (E) total nodal radiation alone. The chemotherapy consisted of giving vinblastine (0.1 mg/kg/week) for 4 weeks, followed by nitrogen mustard (0.4 mg/kg) as a single dose on day 29. Total nodal radiotherapy consisted of 3000 to 3500 rads in 3½ to 4½ weeks to the "mantle" and "inverted Y" fields, while the spleen received 2500 to 3000 rads in 3 to 4½ weeks. Radiotherapy for patients in group A consisted of 3500 to 4000 rads given in 3½ to 5 weeks to the involved areas only. The results showed that the response rates for all the groups were similar (overall 88 percent), except that the rate of complete remission was low in group B (chemotherapy only) and the duration of remission for group B was only 3 months as compared to approximately two years for each of the other groups. Although the duration of remission for patients with nodular sclerosis lesion was longer than for those with the mixed cellularity type, the difference is not statistically significant. Neither sex nor the presence of symptoms had any influence on the remission duration and survival. But age and adequacy of therapy were found to be most important. The myelosuppression seen was progressively more severe with increasing age, and only one of every 6 patients 50 years or older was able to receive the prescribed amount of chemotherapy or radiotherapy or both. Among those who had adequate therapy (defined as receiving 75 percent or more of the prescribed chemotherapy and 3500 rads or more of the radiotherapy), all achieved a complete remission and 15 percent were dead; whereas only 25 of 35 inadequately treated patients achieved complete remission and 62 percent were dead. Thus, the median survival is 18 months for patients 50 years or older, 32 months for those patients between 30 and 49 years old, and more than 48 months for the youngest group.

A warning regarding the administration of both intensive chemotherapy and intensive radiotherapy was raised by Arseneau et al (1972). They reviewed the case records of 425 patients with Hodgkin's disease and found a significantly increased risk of developing second malignant tumors in the entire series (ratio of observed cases to expected = 3.5 : 1). The risk was similar for the subgroups who were treated with both radiotherapy and chemotherapy (ratio 3.3 : 1) and for those who had intensive radiotherapy without intensive chemotherapy (ratio 3.8 : 1). The greatest increase in risk was observed in 35 patients who received both intensive radiotherapy and intensive chemotherapy (ratio 29 : 1). In the last subgroup, 3 patients developed, respectively, virulent epidermoid carcinoma of the skin, widespread malignant mesothelioma or adenocarcinoma, and a poorly differentiated fibrosarcoma of the sternum. All 3 cases occurred in 8 patients who received both therapies within 12 months of each other. Subsequent to the publication of this paper, 2 more patients among the 35 developed leukemia. Rosenberg (1973) reported that he has treated 80 patients with the MOPP program after intensive radiation therapy, and 52 of these had their chemotherapy within 3 months of their irradiation as part of a protocol study. The median duration of follow-up is about 24 months. Fortunately, no nonlymphomatous malignant tumors have been recognized in these 80 patients.

SUMMARY

Once the diagnosis of malignant lymphoma is made, and when the disease is not widely disseminated, radiotherapy is the most effective therapy. The principle of prophylactic irradiation of clinically uninvolved nodal region and the concept of tumoricidal dose have been well demonstrated in Hodgkin's lesions. Thus Kaplan felt that intensive radiotherapy, in most instances utilizing the total lymphoid technique, was the treatment of choice for patients with all stages of I (A, B), II (A, B), and IIIA disease. The relapse-free 5-year survival rates should be over 85 percent for stages I and II, and 70 percent for stage IIIA. Even 40 percent of those with stage IIIB disease could be controlled with radical total lymphoid radiotherapy.

Radiotherapy for non-Hodgkin's lymphoma follows similar plan except there is less consensus concerning the optimal time–dose factor and less benefit seen with prophylactic irradiation. Since non-Hodgkin's lymphoma commonly presented with extranodal involvement, and since recurrence in noncontiguous sites is more common than in Hodgkin's disease, systemic therapy with either chemotherapy or total body irradiation has been tried.

The major chemotherapeutic agents useful in the treatment of malignant lymphoma included the alkylating agents, vinca alkaloids, methylhydrazine compounds, corticosteroids, antimetabolites, and nitrosoureas. Since the rate of complete remission with single agent was rather low and of relatively short duration, combination chemotherapy became a logical approach. Presently the most successful and widely tested combination of drugs is the MOPP program. In previously untreated patients with Hodgkin's disease, it can achieve complete remission in nearly 80 percent of the patients, with a median duration of 36 months. Younger patients and those without systemic symptoms responded better. Patients who had received prior chemotherapy or who had advanced nodular sclerosis lesions responded less well. The experience in using combination chemotherapy in treating non-Hodgkin's lesions was similarly encouraging.

With the discovery of newer chemotherapeutic agents, clinical trials testing the value of supplementing extended radiotherapy with drugs for patients with stage I and II Hodgkin's disease have appeared. Although preliminary results showed that the added chemotherapy might decrease the recurrence rate, the overall benefit is not proven. Several clinical trials utilizing combination chemotherapy and radiotherapy in patients with stages III and IV malignant lymphoma are in progress. On the whole, tolerance to such intensive chemotherapy and extensive radiotherapy was good, and the result showed that the combined approach might give better results than that for radiation therapy alone. However, a warning was raised recently when a report showed that there might be a 10-fold increase in the risk of developing a second malignant tumor if the patient received both therapies within 12 months of each other.

REFERENCES

Aisenberg AC: Malignant lymphoma. N Engl J Med 288:883–890, 935–941, 1973

Aisenberg AC, Goldman JM: Prolongation of survival in Hodgkin's disease. Cancer 27:802–805, 1971

Alison RE, Whitelaw DM: A comparison of nitrogen mustard and vinblastine sulfate in the treatment of patients with Hodgkin's disease. Can Med Assoc J 102:278–280, 1970

Arseneau JC, Sponzo RW, Levin DL, et al: Nonlymphomatous malignant tumors complicating Hodgkin's disease: Possible association with intensive therapy. N Engl J Med 287:1119–1122, 1972

Aur RF, Husto HO, Simone JV, et al: Therapy of localized and regional lymphosarcoma of childhood. Cancer 27:1328–1331, 1971

Bagley CM, De Vita VT, Berard CW, et al: Advanced lymphosarcoma: Intensive cyclical combination chemotherapy with cyclophosphamide, vincristine, and prednisone. Ann Intern Med 76:227–234, 1972

Banfi A, Bonadonna G, Carnevali G, et al: Malignant lymphomas: Further studies on their preferential sites of involvement and possible mode of spread. Lymphology 2:130–138, 1969

Banfi A, Bonadonna G, Carnevali G, et al: Preferential sites of involvement and spread in malignant lymphomas. Eur J Cancer 4:319–324, 1968

Bernard J, Boiron M, Teillet FR, et al: Combined radiotherapy and chemotherapy in human lymphomas in Clark RL, Cumley RW, McCay JE, et al (eds): Oncology 1970, vol 4. Chicago, Year Book, 1971, pp 538–545

Bonadonna G, Monfardini S, Oldini C: Comparative effects of vinblastine and procarbazine in advanced Hodgkin's disease. Eur J Cancer 5:393–402, 1969

Brunner KW, Young CW: A methylhydrazine derivative in Hodgkin's disease and other malignant neoplasms: Therapeutic and toxic effects studied in 51 patients. Ann Intern Med 63:69–86, 1965

Bull JM, de Kiewier JW, Rosenberg SA, et al: Cyclic chemotherapy (MOPP) combined with extended field radiotherapy for Hodgkin's disease. Clin Res 18:189, 1970

Burningham RA, Restrepo A, Pugh RP, et al: Weekly high-dosage glucocorticosteroid treatment of lymphocytic leukemias and lymphomas. N Engl J Med 270:1160–1166, 1964

Canellos GP, Young RC, Berard CW, et al: Combination chemotherapy and survival in advanced Hodgkin's disease. Arch Intern Med 131:388–390, 1973

Carbone PP: Non-Hodgkin's lymphoma: Recent observations on natural history and intensive treatment. Cancer 30:1511–1516, 1972

Carbone PP: Management of patients with non-Hodgkin's lymphoma. Arch Intern Med 131:455–459, 1973

Carbone PP, De Vita VT, Ziegler JL: Intensive therapy of patients with malignant lymphoma in Clark RL, Cumley RW, McCay JE, et al (eds): Oncology 1970, vol 4. Chicago, Year Book, 1971, pp 532–538

Carbone PP, Spurr C, Schneiderman M, et al: Management of patients with malignant lymphoma: A comparative study with cyclophosphamide and vinca alkaloids. Cancer Res 28:811–822, 1968

Carter SK, Livingston RB: Single-agent therapy for Hodgkin's disease. Arch Intern Med 131:377–387, 1973

Chawla PL, Stutzman L, Dubois RE, et al: Long survival in Hodgkin's disease. Am J Med 48:85–92, 1970

Cooper IA, Rana C, Madigan JP, et al: Combination chemotherapy (MOPP) in the management of advanced Hodgkin's disease: A progress report on 55 patients. Med J Aust 1:41–49, 1972

Cox JD, Laugier AJ, Gerard-Marchant R: Apparently localized and regionally advanced malignant lymphoreticular tumors in the adult: Early course following irradiation. Cancer 29:1043–1051, 1972

Curran RE, Johnson RE: Tolerance to chemotherapy after prior irradiation for Hodgkin's disease. Ann Intern Med 72:505–509, 1970

D'Angio GJ, Nisce LZ: Current Concepts in Cancer, No. 40. Updated Hodgkin's Disease, problems with the irradiation of children and pregnant patients. JAMA 223: 171–173, 1973

DeConti RC: Procarbazine in the management of late Hodgkin's disease. JAMA 215:927–930, 1971

Desai D, Ezdinli EZ, Stutzman L: Vincristine (VCR) therapy of lymphoma and chronic lymphocytic leukemia (CLL). Proc Am Assoc Cancer Res 10:18, 1969

De Vita VT: Chemotherapy of lymphomas, in Ultmann JE, Griem ML, Kirsten WH, et al (eds): Current Concepts in the Management of Leukemia and Lymphoma. New York, Springer, 1971, pp 159–171

De Vita VT Jr, Canellos GP: Treatment of the lymphomas. Semin Hematol 9:193–209, 1972

De Vita VT, Canellos GP, Moxley JH: A decade of combination chemotherapy of advanced Hodgkin's disease. Cancer 30:1495–1504, 1972

De Vita VT Jr, Carbone PP: Chemotherapeutic implications of staging in Hodgkin's disease. Cancer Res 31:1838–1844, 1971

De Vita VT, Serpick A: Combination chemotherapy in the treatment of advanced Hodgkin's Disease (HD). Proc Am Assoc Cancer Res 8:13, 1967

De Vita VT, Serpick A, Carbone PP: Combination chemotherapy of advanced Hodgkin's disease (HD): The NCI program, a progress report. Proc Am Assoc Cancer Res 10:19, 1969

De Vita VT Jr, Serpick AA, Carbone PP: Combination chemotherapy in the treatment of advanced Hodgkin's disease. Ann Intern Med 73:881–895, 1970

Easson EC: Long-term results of radical radiotherapy in Hodgkin's disease. Cancer Res 26:1244–1249, 1966b

Easson EC: Possibilities for the cure of Hodgkin's disease. Cancer 19:345–350, 1966a

Easson EC, Russell MH: The cure of Hodgkin's disease. Br Med J 1:1704–1707, 1963

Ezdinli EZ, Stutzman L: Vinblastine vs nitrogen mustard therapy of Hodgkin's disease. Cancer 22:473–479, 1968

Flatow FA, Ultmann JE, Hyman GA, et al: Treatment of advanced Hodgkin's disease with vinblastine (NSC-49842) or procarbazine (NSC-77213). Cancer Chemother Rep (Part 1) [Suppl] 53:39–47, 1969

Frei E III: Chemotherapy for lymphoma, in Clark RL, Cumley RW, McCay JE, et al (eds): Oncology 1970, vol 4. Chicago, Year Book, 1971, pp 526–532

Frei E III: Status and perspectives in chemotherapy of Hodgkin's disease. Arch Intern Med 131:439–445, 1973

Frei E III, Gehan EA: Definition of cure for Hodgkin's disease. Cancer Res 31:1828–1833, 1971

Fridman M, Stutzman L, Vongtama V, et al: Short-term radiation therapy of localized lymphoma. Radiology 102:413–416, 1972

Friedman M, Pearlman AW, Turgeon L: Hodgkin's disease: Tumor lethal dose and iso-effect recovery curve. Am J Roentgenol Radium Ther Nucl Med 99:843–850, 1967

Fuller LM: Results of large volume irradiation in the management of Hodgkin's disease and malignant lymphomas originating in the abdomen. Radiology 87:1058–1064, 1966

Fuller LM, Fletcher GH: The radiotherapeutic management of the lymphomatous diseases. Am J Roentgenol Radium Ther Nucl Med 88:909–923, 1962

Fuller LM, Gamble JF: Current concepts in cancer. 40. Updated Hodgkin's Disease, Combined chemotherapy-radiotherapy program. JAMA 223:168–169, 1973

Fuller LM, Gamble JF, Butler JJ: Results of definitive radiotherapy in localized Hodgkin's disease, as related to both clinical presentation and pathological classification. Leukemia-Lymphoma. Chicago, Year Book, 1970, pp 241–259

Gamble JF, Fuller LM, Butler JJ, et al: Combined chemotherapy and radiotherapy for advanced Hodgkin's disease and reticulum cell sarcoma: A preliminary report. South Med J 64:775–783, 1971

Gamble JF, Fuller LM, Ibrahim E et al: Combined chemotherapy: Radiotherapy management of stage III Hodgkin's disease. Arch Intern Med 131:435–438, 1973

Gilbert R: Radiotherapy in Hodgkin's disease (malignant granulomatosis); anatomic and clinical foundations; governing principles; results. Am J Roentgenol Radium Ther Nucl Med 41:198–241, 1939

Gilbert R: Le traitement de la granulomatose maligne par la roentgenthérapie pénétrante. Acta Radiol [Ther] (Stockh) 9: 552–581, 1928

Glicksman AS, Nickson JJ: Acute and late reactions to irradiation in the treatment of Hodgkin's disease. Arch Intern Med 131:369–373, 1973

Greenberg LH, Wong S, Richardson AP Jr, et al: Combination chemotherapy of Hodgkin's disease in private practice. JAMA 221:261–263, 1972

Hall TC, Choi OS, Abadi A, et al: High-dose corticoid therapy in Hodgkin's disease and other lymphomas. Ann Intern Med 66:1144–1153, 1967

Han T, Stutzman L: Mode of spread in patients with localized malignant lymphoma. Arch Intern Med 120:1–7, 1967

Hansen HS: Reticulum cell sarcoma treated by radiotherapy: Significance of clinical features upon the prognosis. Acta Radiol [Ther] (Stockh) 8:439–458, 1969

Henderson ES, Samaha RJ: Evidence that drugs in multiple combinations have materially advanced the treatment of human malignancies. Cancer Res 29: 2272–2280, 1969

Hoogstraten B, Holland JF, Kramer S, et al: Combination chemotherapy-radiotherapy for stage III Hodgkin's disease: An Acute Leukemia Group B study. Arch Intern Med 131:424–428, 1973

Hoogstraten B, Owens AH, Lenhard RE, et al: Combination chemotherapy in lymphosarcoma and reticulum cell sarcoma. Blood 33:370–378, 1969

Hynes JF: Curative treatment of Hodgkin's disease. Am J Roentgenol Radium Ther Nucl Med 105:629–635, 1969

Hynes JF: The radiocurability of malignant lymphoma. Acta Unio internat contra cancrum 11:514–525, 1955

Hynes JF, Frelick RW: Roentgen therapy of malignant lymphoma with special reference to segmental radiation therapy: Results 1935–1945. Am J Roentgenol Radium Ther Nucl Med 70:247–257, 1953

Johnson RE: Comparison of recurrence patterns in human lymphoma and experimental leukemia. Cancer 22:1137–1139, 1968

Johnson RE: The curative radiotherapy of lymphomas, in Ultmann JE, Griem ML, Kirsten WH, et al (eds): Current Concepts in the Management of Leukemia and Lymphoma. New York, Springer, 1971, pp 57–62

Johnson RE: Modern approaches to the radiotherapy of lymphoma. Semin Hematol 6:357–375, 1969

Johnson RE: Total nodal irradiation. JAMA 223:59–61, 1973

Johnson RE, Brace KC: Radiation response of Hodgkin's disease recurrent after chemotherapy. Cancer 19:368–370, 1966

Johnson RE, Kagan AR, Hafermann MD, et al: Patient tolerance to extended irradiation in Hodgkin's disease. Ann Intern Med 70:1–6, 1969

Johnson RE, O'Connor GT, Levin D: Primary management of advanced lymphosarcoma with radiotherapy. Cancer 25:787–791, 1970a

Johnson RE, Thomas LB, Chretien P: Correlation between clinico-histologic staging and extranodal relapse in Hodgkin's disease. Cancer 25:1071–1075, 1970b

Johnson RE, Thomas LB, Schneiderman M, et al: Preliminary experience with total nodal irradiation in Hodgkin's disease. Radiology 96:603–608, 1970c

Jones SE, Kaplan HS, Rosenberg SA: Non-Hodgkin's lymphomas. III. Preliminary results of radiotherapy and a proposal for new clinical trials. Radiology 103:657–662, 1972

Kaplan HS: Clinical evaluation and radiotherapeutic management of Hodgkin's disease and the malignant lymphomas. N Engl J Med 278:892–899, 1968a

Kaplan HS: Contiguity and progression in Hodgkin's disease. Cancer Res 31:1811–1813, 1971a

Kaplan HS: Evidence for a tumoricidal dose level in the radiotherapy of Hodgkin's disease. Cancer Res 26:1221–1224, 1966a

Kaplan HS: Hodgkin's Disease. Cambridge, Mass., Harvard University Press, 1972

Kaplan HS: Hodgkin's disease. Curr Probl Radiol 1:1–39, 1971b

Kaplan HS: Long-term results of palliative and radical radiotherapy of Hodgkin's disease. Cancer Res 26:1250–1252, 1966b

Kaplan HS: On the natural history, treatment, and prognosis of Hodgkin's disease. Harvey Lect 64:215–259, 1970

Kaplan HS: Prognostic significance of the relapse-free interval after radiotherapy in Hodgkin's disease. Cancer 22:1131–1136, 1968b

Kaplan HS: The radical radiotherapy of regionally localized Hodgkin's disease. Radiology 78:553–561, 1962

Kaplan HS: Radiotherapy of advanced Hodgkin's disease with curative intent. JAMA 223:50–53, 1973

Kaplan HS: Role of intensive radiotherapy in the management of Hodgkin's disease. Cancer 19:356–367, 1966c

Kaplan HS, Rosenberg SA: Extended-field radical radiotherapy in advanced Hodgkin's disease: Short-term results of 2 randomized clinical trials. Cancer Res 26:1268–1276, 1966

Karnofsky DA: Problems in the evaluation of chemotherapy for lymphomas. Leukemia-Lymphoma. Chicago, Year Book, 1970, pp 13–25

Kimura I, Onoshi T, Kunimasa I, et al: Treatment of malignant lymphomas with bleomycin. Cancer 29:58–60, 1972

Korbitz BC, Davis HL Jr, Ramire G, et al: Low doses of vincristine (NSC-67574) for malignant disease. Cancer Chemother Rep (Part 1) 53:249–254, 1969

Kurnick JE, Robinson WA: Combination chemotherapy of advanced lymphomas. Arch Intern Med 129:908–913, 1972

Lacher MJ: Long survival in Hodgkin's disease. Ann Intern Med 70:7–17, 1969

Lacher MJ, Durant JR: Combined vinblastine and chlorambucil therapy of Hodgkin's disease. Ann Intern Med 62:468–476, 1965

Landberg T: Clinical course of Hodgkin's disease treated with radiotherapy. Acta Radiol [Ther] (Stockh) 8:487–504, 1969

Lenhard RE Jr: Eastern Cooperative Oncology Group studies. Arch Intern Med 131:418–420, 1973

Lenhard RE Jr, Owens AH Jr: Prednisone in combination chemotherapy of lymphoma. Proc Am Assoc Cancer Res 12:35, 1971

Lessner HE: BCNU (1,3, Bis (β-chloroethyl)-1-nitrosourea): Effects on advanced Hodgkin's disease and other neoplasia. Cancer 22:451–456, 1968

Lipton A, Lee BJ: Prognosis of stage I lymphosarcoma and reticulum-cell sarcoma. N Engl J Med 284:230–233, 1971

Loo TL, Dion RL, Dixon RL, et al: The antitumor agent, 1,3-bis(2-chloroethyl)-nitrosourea. J Pharm Sci 55:492–497, 1966

Lowenbraun S, DeVita VT, Serpick AA: Combination chemotherapy with nitrogen mustard, vincristine, procarbazine and prednisone in previously treated patients with Hodgkin's disease. Blood 36:704–717, 1970a

Lowenbraun S, DeVita VT, Serpick AA: Combination chemotherapy with nitrogen mustard, vincristine, procarbazine and prednisone in lymphosarcoma and reticulum cell sarcoma. Cancer 25:1018–1025, 1970b

Luce JK, Gamble JF, Wilson HE, et al: Combined cyclophosphamide, vincristine, and prednisone therapy of malignant lymphoma. Cancer 28:306–317, 1971

Marsh JC, DeConti RC, Hubbard SP: Treatment of Hodgkin's disease and other cancers with 1,3-bis(2-chloroethyl)-1-nitrosourea (BCNU; NSC-409962). Cancer Chemother Rep (Part I) 55:599–606, 1971

McLeod JG, Penny R: Vincristine neuropathy: An electrophysiological and histological study. J Neurol Neurosurg Psychiat 32:297–304, 1969

Mendelson D, Block JB, Serpick AA: Effect of large intermittent intravenous doses of cyclophosphamide in lymphoma. Cancer 25:715–720, 1970

Moore MR, Bull JM, Jones SE, et al: Sequential radiotherapy and chemotherapy in the treatment of Hodgkin's disease: A progress report. Ann Intern Med 77:1–9, 1972

Moore MR, Jones SE, Bull JM, et al: MOPP chemotherapy for advanced Hodgkin's disease: prognostic factors in 81 patients. Cancer 32:52–60, 1973

Moxley JH III, DeVita VT, Brace K, et al: Intensive combination chemotherapy and X-irradiation in Hodgkin's disease. Cancer Res 27:1258–1263, 1967

Mukherji B, Yagoda A, Oettgen HF, et al: Cyclic chemotherapy in lymphoma. Cancer 28:886–893, 1971

Musshoff K, Boutis L: Therapy results in Hodgkin's disease: Freiburg i.Br., 1948–1966. Cancer 21:1100–1113, 1968

Musshoff K, Schmidt-Vollmer H, Merten D: Reticulum cell sarcoma: An oncologic model for a system of classifying the malignant lymphomas. Eur J Cancer 7:451–457, 1971

Newall J, Friedman M: Reticulum-cell sarcoma. Part II. Radiation dosare for each type. Radiology 94:643–647, 1970a

Newall J, Friedman M: Reticulum-cell sarcoma. Part III. Prognosis. Radiology 97:99–102, 1970b

Nicholson WM, Beard ME, Crowther D, et al: Combination chemotherapy in generalized Hodgkin's disease. Br Med J 3: 7–10, 1970

Nickson JJ: Hodgkin's disease clinical trial. Cancer Res 26:1279–1283, 1966

Nickson JJ, Hutchison GB: Extensions of disease, complications of therapy, and deaths in localized Hodgkin's disease: Preliminary report of a clinical trial. Am J Roentgenol Radium Ther Nucl Med 114:564–573, 1972

Nobler MP: Curative radiotherapy in the malignant lymphomas. Cancer 22:752–758, 1968

Olweny CL, Ziegler JL, Berard CW, et al: Adult Hodgkin's disease in Uganda. Cancer 6:1295–1301, 1971

Nissen NI, Stutzman L, Holland JF, et al: Chemotherapy of Hodgkin's disease in studies by Acute Leukemia Group B. Arch Intern Med 131:396–401, 1973

Paterson R: The Treatment of Malignant Disease by Radiotherapy (ed 2). Baltimore, Williams & Wilkins, 1963

Peters MV: Changing concepts in radiotherapy for the lymphomas. Leukemia-Lymphoma. Chicago, Year Book, 1970, pp 261–274

Peters MV: The contribution of radiation therapy in the control of early lymphomas. Am J Roentgenol Radium Ther Nucl Med 90:956–967, 1963

Peters MV: Prophylactic treatment of adjacent areas in Hodgkin's disease. Cancer Res 26:1232–1243, 1966

Peters MV: A study of survivals in Hodgkin's disease treated radiologically. Am J Roentgenol Radium Ther Nucl Med 63:299–311, 1950

Peters MV, Brown TC, Rideout DF: Prognostic influences and radiation therapy according to pattern of disease. JAMA 223:53–59, 1973

Peters MV, Hasselback R, Brown TC: The natural history of the lymphomas related to the clinical classification, in Zarafonetis CJ (ed): Proceedings of the International Conference on Leukemia-Lymphoma. Philadelphia, Lea & Febiger, 1968, pp 357–371

Peters MV, Middlemiss KC: A study of Hodgkin's disease treated by irradiation. Am J Roentgenol Radium Ther Nucl Med 79:114–121, 1958

Prosnitz LR, Hellman S, von Essen CF, et al: The clinical course of Hodgkin's disease and other malignant lymphomas treated with radical radiation therapy. Am J Roentgenol Radium Ther Nucl Med 105:618–628, 1969

Pusey WA: Cases of sarcoma and of Hodgkin's disease treated by exposures to x-rays: A preliminary report. JAMA 38:166–169, 1902

Radiotherapy-Chemotherapy Cooperative Group of E.O.R.T.C.: A randomized study of irradiation and vinblastine in stages I and II of Hodgkin's disease: Preliminary results. Eur J Cancer 8:353–362, 1972

Rapoport A, Cole P, Mason J: Correlates of survival after initiation of chemotherapy in 142 cases of Hodgkin's disease. Cancer 24:377–381, 1969

Rappaport H, Strum SB: Vascular invasion in Hodgkin's disease: Its incidence and relationship to the spread of the disease. Cancer 25:1304–1313, 1970

Reilly CJ, Han T, Stutzman L, et al: Reticulum-cell sarcoma: A review of radiotherapeutic experience. Cancer 29:1314–1320, 1972

Rosenbaum DL: The diagnosis and management of Hodgkin's disease: Current concepts. CA 20:286–297, 1970

Rosenberg SA: Other tumors complicating Hodgkin's disease. N Engl J Med 288:469, 1973

Rosenberg SA: Radiotherapy for lymphoma, in Clark RL, Cumley RW, McCay JE, et al (eds): Oncology 1970, vol 4. Chicago, Year Book, 1971, pp 518–525

Rosenberg SA, Kaplan HS: Evidence for an orderly progression in the spread of Hodgkin's disease. Cancer Res 26:1225–1231, 1966

Rosenberg SA, Kaplan HS: Hodgkin's disease and other malignant lymphomas. Calif Med 113:23–38, 1970

Rosenberg SA, Kaplan HS: The results of radical radiotherapy in Hodgkin's disease and other lymphomas, in Zarafonetis CJ (ed): Proceedings of the International Conference on Leukemia-Lymphoma. Philadelphia, Lea & Febiger, 1968, pp 403–408

Rosenberg SA, Moore MR, Bull JM, et al: Combination chemotherapy and radiotherapy for Hodgkin's disease. Cancer 30:1505–1510, 1972

Rubin P: Controversial issues in the treatment of Hodgkin's disease, in Brown EB and Moore CV (eds): Progress in Hematology, vol 5. New York, Grune & Stratton, 1966, pp 180–203

Rubin P: Current concepts in cancer. 39. Updated Hodgkin's Disease, comment: The mantle failure: The transdiaphragmatic extension. JAMA 223:65–67, 1973

Rubin P, Haluska G, Poulter CA: The basis for segmental sequential irradiation in Hodgkin's disease: Clinical experience of patterns of recurrence. Am J Roentgenol Radium Ther Nucl Med 105:814–829, 1969

Rudders RA: Treatment of advanced malignant lymphomas with bleomycin. Blood 40:317–332, 1972

Samuels ML, Leary WV, Alexanian R, et al: Clinical trials with N-isopropyl-alpha- (2-methylhydrazino)-P-toluamide hydrochloride in malignant lymphoma and other disseminated neoplasia. Cancer 20:1187–1194, 1967

Scheer AC: The course of stage I malignant lymphomas following local treatment. Am J Roentgenol Radium Ther Nucl Med 90:939–943, 1963

Schwarz G: Die forgesetzte Kleindosis und deren biologische Begründung. Strahlentherapie 19:325–332, 1925

Seydel HG, Bloedorn FG, Wizenberg MJ: Results of radiotherapeutic treatment of relapsing Hodgkin's disease. Cancer 23: 1033–1037, 1969

Seydel HG, Bloedorn FG, Wizenberg M, et al: Time-dose relationships in radiation therapy of lymphosarcoma and giant follicle lymphoma. Radiology 98:411–418, 1971

Smithers DW: Factors influencing survival in patients with Hodgkin's disease. Clin Radiol 20:124–134, 1969

Smithers DW: Hodgkin's disease: One entity or two? Lancet 2:1285–1287, 1970

Smithers DW: Patterns of spread of Hodgkin's disease. JAMA 222:1298–1299, 1972

Solomon J, Jacobs EM Jr, Batemen JR: Relative value of nitrogen mustard and vinblastine in treatment of lymphoma. Proc Am Assoc Cancer Res 10:85, 1969

Solomon J, Jacobs EM, Batemen JR, et al: Chemotherapy of lymphoma with mechlorethamine and vinblastine. Arch Intern Med 131:407–417, 1973

Stolinsky DC, Solomon J, Pugh RP, et al: Procarbazine HC1 in Hodgkin's disease, reticulum cell sarcoma, and lymphosarcoma. Proc Am Assoc Cancer Res 10:88, 1969

Stutzman L: Combined radiotherapy and chemotherapy of lymphomas and other cancers. Cancer Res 31:1845–1850, 1971

Stutzman L, Ezdinli EZ, Stutzman MA: Vinblastine sulfate vs cyclophosphamide in the therapy for lymphoma. JAMA 195:173–178, 1966

Tubiana M, Amiel J: Current concepts in cancer. No. 39. Updated Hodgkin's Disease, combined radiation therapy and chemotherapy. JAMA 223:61–64, 1973

Tubiana W, Mathe G, Laugier A: Current clinical trials in the radiotherapy of Hodgkin's disease at Institut Gustave Roussy. Cancer Res 26:1277–1278, 1966

Ultmann JE: The management of lymphoma. CA 21:342–359, 1971

Ultmann JE, Nixon D: The therapy of lymphoma. Semin Hematol 6:376–403, 1969

Werf-Messing, B van der: Reticulum cell sarcoma and lymphosarcoma: A retrospective study of potential survival in locoregional disease. Eur J Cancer 4:549–557, 1968

Young CW, Geller WG, Lieberman PH, et al: On the nature and management of Hodgkin's disease. Clin Bull 2:84–93, 1972 .

Young RC, DeVita VT Jr, Serpick AA, et al: Treatment of advanced Hodgkin's disease with 1,3 bis(2-chloroethyl)-1-nitrosourea BCNU. N Engl J Med 285: 475–479, 1971

4
Surgery for Diagnosis

The most frequent surgical procedure essential to the histological diagnosis of malignant lymphoma is a biopsy of the peripheral lymph nodes. This procedure established the diagnosis in 94 percent of the EFSCH patients with Hodgkin's disease, and in 77 percent of the patients with non-Hodgkin's lymphoma (Table 4-1). However, not uncommonly the intrathoracic or intraabdominal nodes are the first to become enlarged, and extranodal primary foci have been reported in almost every site and structure of the body. Thus, in some cases with malignant lymphoma, other major surgical procedures such as exploratory laparotomy, thoracotomy, and even laminectomy are utilized before the diagnosis is confirmed. The problem of undiagnostic or nondiagnostic node biopsy is also discussed in this chapter.

PERIPHERAL NODE BIOPSY

In a review of 618 cases of malignant lymphoma, Gall and Mallory (1942) noted that palpable, visible, or presumptive lymph node enlargement was present in over 90 percent of the subgroups with the exception of those with a diagnosis of reticulum cell sarcoma (20 percent of which had no evidence of lymph node disease).

In 316 patients with Hodgkin's disease reported by Pack and Molander (1966), peripheral lymphadenopathy was the initial manifestation in 57.2 percent of the patients. And over 25 percent of the patients had lymphadenopathy within the thoracic or abdominal cavities. Specifically, 16.4 percent presented as enlarged mediastinal nodes and 9.5 percent as mesenteric or para-aortic nodes. Initial enlargement of peripheral nodes occurred

Table 4-1
Methods of Establishing Diagnosis of Malignant Lymphoma
(EFSCH series)

	Hodgkin's disease	Other lymphomas
Peripheral node biopsy	154 (94%)	282 (77%)
Radical node dissection	2	5
Radical mastectomy	1	3
Exploratory laparotomy		
Biopsy only	3	34
With organ resection		20
Exploratory thoracotomy		3
Laminectomy		4
Non-nodal biopsy		
Soft tissue	1	6
Tonsil		1
Testes		1
Bone		1
Autopsy	2	4
Total patient number	163	364

in 63.5 percent of 1269 patients with non-Hodgkin's lymphoma (Rosenberg et al 1961). They commented that "though symmetrical enlargement may be seen, lymphosarcomatous adenopathy is usually asymmetrical."

The distribution of the first site of peripheral lymphadenopathy in the EFSCH series is given in detail in Table 4-2, and the sites of nodal biopsy which established the diagnosis are given in Table 4-3. The percentage figures do not correspond to each other because by the time a node was taken for diagnosis, the patient usually had adenopathy involving more than one site.

Table 4-2
Distribution of First Site of Lymphadenopathy (EFSCH series)

Hodgkin's Disease					
Stage	I	II	III	IV	Total
No. of patients	45	37	30	51	163
Neck					
Upper	16(36%)	6(16%)	13(43%)	21(41%)	56(34%)
Lower (right)	12(27%)	9(24%)	9(30%)	8(16%)	38(23%)
Lower (left)	17(38%)	16(43%)	12(40%)	17(33%)	62(38%)
Axilla	6(13%)	7(19%)	7(23%)	16(31%)	36(22%)
Groin	4 (9%)	4(11%)	8(27%)	5(10%)	21(13%)
Other					
Mesentery			1 (3%)		1 (0.6%)

Table 4-2 (con't)
Distribution of First Site of Lymphadenopathy (EFSCH series)

Other Lymphomas

Stage	I	II	III	IV	Total
No. of patients	66	36	91	171	364
Neck					
Upper	33(50%)	14(39%)	49(54%)	41(24%)	137(38%)
Lower (right)	10(15%)	7(19%)	17(19%)	23(13%)	57(16%)
Lower (left)	8(12%)	8(22%)	17(19%)	31(18%)	64(17%)
Axilla	10(15%)	2 (5%)	30(33%)	46(27%)	88(24%)
Groin	13(20%)	3 (8%)	43(47%)	50(29%)	109(30%)
Mediastinum		1 (3%)		4 (2%)	5 (1%)
Other					
Epitrochlear		1 (3%)		1 (0.5%)	2 (0.5%)
Tonsil	1 (2%)	1 (3%)	1 (1%)	4 (2%)	7 (2%)
Iliac		1 (3%)			1 (0.2%)
Mesentery		4(11%)	6 (7%)	13 (8%)	23 (6%)
Retroperitoneum	1 (2%)	3 (8%)		8 (5%)	12 (3%)
Soft tissue			1 (1%)		1 (0.2%)
Maxilla				1 (0.5%)	1 (0.2%)
Viscera				25(15%)	25 (7%)

Table 4-3
Biopsy of Lymphadenopathy for Diagnosis (EFSCH series)[*]

	Right	Left	Both	Unspecified	Subtotal	(%)
Hodgkin's Disease						
Neck						
Lower	29	34	4	1	68	52
Upper	12	8		2	22	17
Axilla	7	14			21	16
Groin	6	6			12	9
Soft tissue				1	1	1
Abdominal				3	3	2
Others	2		1	2	5	3
Subtotal	56	62	5	9	132	100
Other Lymphomas						
Neck						
Lower	17	23	1	2	43	17
Upper	30	36		3	69	28
Axilla	19	21	1	1	42	17
Groin	17	13	2	3	35	14
Soft tissue	1	1	1	3	6	2
Abdominal				34	23	13
Others	11	8	1	3	23	9
Subtotal	95	102	6	49	252	100

[*]Details of this study were taken from 132 patients with Hodgkin's disease and 252 patients with other lymphomas.

Peripheral node was present in 99.4 percent of the patients with Hodg-kin's disease at the time of diagnosis and biopsy of peripheral node alone established the diagnosis in 94 percent of the patients. In patients with non-Hodgkin's disease, peripheral adenopathy was present in 87 percent of the cases, and biopsy of peripheral node alone established the diagnosis in 77 percent. It appears that in Hodgkin's disease, when adenopathy first , appeared in the lower neck region, the left side was more commonly involved than the right in all stages (Table 4-2). In general, for diagnosis in both Hodgkin's disease and non-Hodgkin's lymphomas, 23 percent of the patients required more than one lymph node biopsy and the average number of biopsy per patient was 1.4.

Details of Taking Node Biopsy

Although nodal biopsy is usually a minor procedure, certain technical factors warrant emphasis. Moore (1968) commented that biopsy procedures of all kinds should be used far more frequently, not only for establishing initial diagnosis, but also for providing more accurate clinical surveillance of the disease process. The specimens should be handled with tender loving care. He listed seven "do's" and eight "don'ts" which all surgeons perform-ing biopsy procedures should know. (How many surgeons realize this: Don't put specimen on paper or in tubes with cotton plugs, because cellulose fibers ruin microtome knives?) Butler (1970) pointed out that when taking node biopsy for the diagnosis of malignant lymphoma, attention must be paid to the proper selection of the biopsy site, proper selection of the node at the chosen site, and proper removal of the node by the surgeon. The other three essential technical factors (proper fixation, correct cutting, and staining of the specimen) are the responsibilities of the pathologist and will not be discussed here.

1. When more than one anatomic area is involved, the site of biopsy should be carefully selected. It is better to remove a lower cervical or axillary lymph node and to avoid the submandibular, parotid, and inguinal nodes since the latter nodes often exhibit atypical changes secondary to the low-grade inflammatory processes that they commonly drain. Moreover, Scott (1958) pointed out that biopsy of axillary lymph nodes is sometimes followed by troublesome hematoma formation, and this group should be avoided if an alternative choice exists.

    On occasion, if the node which lies near the center of the sterno-mastoid muscle is excised, damage to the accessory spinal nerve may result, particularly if there is much periadenitis. Moore (1971) warned about this complication because it may cause disfigurement and dis-ability. In the EFSCH series, about 110 nodal biopsies were taken from the lower neck region and the accessory nerve was transected in only one case.

If a node in the groin is to be biopsied, this should be done prior to lymphangiography since tissue reactions to the dye distort microscopic morphology (Hall 1966). However, Dorfman (1971) stated the effects of lymphangiography did not interfer with his ability to detect microscopic lesions in the lymph nodes. In case of doubt, it seems prudent that the surgeon should consult the pathologist before any node biopsy is undertaken.

2.   If there are multiple nodes present in one region, the largest node, not the most accessible one, should be removed. Slaughter et al (1958) have shown that in patients with Hodgkin's disease normal lymph nodes may be found adjacent to diseased nodes and size is the only gross indication that a node is representative. This rule also applies in reactive processes of known and unknown etiology and in other types of lymphoma. However, Conley (1967) commented from experience that the largest node often became necrotic, and in certain instances, the critical nodes might be the fresh, smaller nodes about the periphery of the conglomerate mass.

3.   It is important that the entire node be removed in one piece and with the capsule intact since changes typical of benign hyperplastic lymph nodes are evaluated much more easily in the intact node than in segments of a fragmented node. And if a question arises between histiocytic reticulum cell sarcoma or metastatic poorly differentiated carcinoma, the presence of carcinoma in the subcapsular sinusoids will make diagnosis obvious in the latter. Wherever possible, two or three lymph nodes should be removed. Larsen et al (1972) reported two cases with reticulum cell sarcoma of the tonsils and maxillary sinus, both were misdiagnosed as undifferentiated carcinoma. They pointed out that when the diagnosis was made from a small piece of tissue removed by punch biopsy forceps, the distinction of these two diseases might be nearly impossible for the pathologist. Punch biopsy tends to squeeze and crush lymphoid cells until they resemble the cells of undifferentiated carcinoma.

4.   Thus, partial removal of a node is to be avoided and aspiration biopsy is condemned (Pack and Molander 1966). Other possible limitations of aspiration biopsy include necrotic liquification of the lymph node and the not uncommon extensive fibrotic reaction to lymphosarcoma and reticulum cell sarcoma which can cause an alteration in the microscopic picture (Conley 1967). However, Zajicek et al (1967) reported results of aspiration biopsy in 1200 lymph nodes of the neck; 10 percent of the cases were diagnosed as lymphoma or Hodgkin's disease. The overall agreement between cytologic and histologic findings was about 90 percent. But Butler (1969) commented that needle biopsies and frozen sections should be used to evaluate lymph nodes only if the presence of lymphoma was unlikely since both the smallness of the specimen and the distorted tissue make the diagnosis difficult.

5.   Daniels (1949) described the technique of scalene fat pad biopsy for the diagnosis of intrathoracic diseases. Schiff and Warren (1957) reported that scalene node biopsy was useful in diagnosis of obscure intrathoracic conditions and diseases involving lymph nodes. Even on nonpalpable scalene lymph nodes Shields et al (1958) found that about 12 percent of biopsies performed were diagnostic for Hodgkin's disease and lymphosarcoma in the presence of unilateral pulmonary or mediastinal lesions. Findings by Cooke and Glotzer (1964) also indicated that malignant lymphoma could be diagnosed by "blind" scalene fat biopsy in one-third of those cases with evidence of obscure systemic disease but without peripheral lymphadenopathy, mediastinal nodal enlargement, or pulmonary findings. A positive scalene node biopsy would certainly obviate the necessity for the more major diagnostic thoracotomy procedure.

Conn et al (1970) mentioned that all of the diagnostic scalene nodes obtained in their cases of malignant lymphoma were palpable. In cases with nonpalpable nodes, they recommended right scalene biopsy for lesions of the right lung, left scalene biopsy for lesions of the left upper lung, and bilateral scalene adenectomy for lesions of the left lower lung. Dorfman (1971) said that left scalene node biopsy has been included as part of the routine pretreatment staging procedures for Hodgkin's disease in order to better define the extent of involvement.

6.   Often the pathologist's report of the node biopsy is benign, nondiagnostic, or undiagnostic (see below). If the clinical picture of the patient warrants it, and if the pathologist cannot make a definite diagnosis from a biopsy specimen, the physician's thought should not be to "let time be the best therapy" (as suggested by Kurtz 1970), but "when and what to biopsy the second time" (Saltzstein 1971). A brief period of observation of the patient and his clinical course is justified if there is some suggestion that one is dealing with a benign process which will not advance. However, a word of caution must be added here, since a regressed adenopathy is not a guarantee that it is benign. As many as 8 percent of the patients with Hodgkin's disease gave a history that the lumps had fluctuated in size for several months and in some instances had disappeared completely although temporarily (Peters and Middlemiss 1958). And about 10 percent of the patients could give a history that their adenopathy was of chronic duration lasting over many years (Baker and Mann 1940). In the EFSCH series, 21 patients among the 163 (13 percent) with Hodgkin's disease gave a history of decreasing size of the adenopathy, and 18 patients did not even receive antibiotics.

When rebiopsy is necessary, it is better not to take nodes at or near the previous incision, since chronic inflammation and suture granulomatous reactions will make the histological interpretation difficult.

Undiagnostic or Nondiagnostic Node Biopsy

Hall and Olson (1956) mentioned that Mikuliz's disease and three sub-groups of Hodgkin's disease were diagnosed when the slide of a patient was seen by five nationally prominent pathologists in 1940. When the same slides were reviewed in 1954, a new diagnosis of lymphosarcoma was added. The patient was apparently free of disease after removal of the involved nodes and received no other therapy. Thus, it appears that when a diagnosis of malignant lymphoma is made, 20 percent of the cases could be in doubt.

Craver (1964) said that different nodes from the same patients or even different portions of the same node might show great variations in histologic type. The difficulties in diagnosis and subclassification of malignant lymphomas are well know. A single lymph node (or other) biopsy may not be sufficient to enable the pathologist to make a decision.

Dawson et al (1964) reviewed 158 difficult and doubtful node biopsies among 906 specimens seen over a 15-year period. All cases were followed for more than 3 years. Twenty-five of the 55 specimens originally diagnosed as reactive hyperplasia and 14 out of 28 of the equivocal groups were reclassified as malignant lymphoma, whereas only 3 out of 75 specimens originally diagnosed as lymphoma were rediagnosed as reactive. In 8 percent of all the cases, the pathological diagnosis was not substantiated by the clinical outcome.

Saltzstein (1965) studied the fate of 105 patients who had nondiagnostic lymph node biopsies and had follow-up for more than 5 years. About 53 percent of the patients eventually showed a disease related to the indications for biopsy and the others were living and well or had died of causes unrelated to the indications. If the original biopsy was done for lymphadenopathy, 1 patient out of 6 eventually was shown to have a malignant lymphoma. If the biopsy was done for other reasons, about one half of the patients developed a variety of diseases and in about 91 percent of these patients the specific diagnosis was established within 6 months.

Hartsock (1968) reviewed cases with histological pictures of postvaccinial lymphadenitis that had been misdiagnosed as malignant lymphoma. He pointed out that the history of vaccination was often overlooked at the time of surgery. If a biopsy is deemed necessary for a patient who has been vaccinated within 3 months, a lymph node that does not drain the vaccination site should be selected for removal.

Butler (1969) emphasized that every lymphoma may be simulated by a reactive process and that the diagnosis of lymphoma is based on morphologic features rather than clinical findings: on positive criteria rather than on the process of exclusion. Many non-neoplastic lesions and reactive processes of the lymph nodes need to be differentiated from lymphomas. Known etiologies such as rheumatoid arthritis, syphilis, toxoplasmosis, herpes zoster, dermatopathic lymphadenitis, etc., need to be ruled out.

Infectious mononucleosis may be diagnosed clinically as lymphoma or Hodgkin's disease since lymphadenopathy is a major feature, and the histology of node biopsies also suggests such a diagnosis (Salvador et al 1971; Agliozzo and Reingold, 1971). The Reed-Sternberg cell, a cytologic feature originally thought pathognomonic for Hodgkin's disease, has been described in cases of infectious mononucleosis (Lukes et al 1969; McMahon et al 1970; Tindle et al, 1972). Kaplan (1972) listed 37 Hodgkin's patients seen during an 8-year period who had infectious mononucleosis reasonably well-documented in their past history. He did not give the total number of patients seen during the same time, but quoted a study in progress by the Connecticut State Department of Health, which revealed data strongly suggesting that patients with a prior history of infectious mononucleosis are at an increased risk of developing malignant lymphomas. These results appear to confirm the suggestion by Lukes et al (1969) that "infectious mononucleosis on rare occasion may not be a self-limited lymphoid pro-liferation, but the initial infectious episode which precedes neoplastic trans-formation."

About 1 percent of the patients with Hodgkin's disease have the lesions of Kaposi's sarcoma (Higgins 1968) and lymphoma-like lymph node changes have been reported in Kaposi's sarcoma (Lubin and Rywlin 1971). Gilbert et al (1971) reported a case of Hodgkin's disease associated with Kaposi's sarcoma and malignant melanoma. Wilson and Nishiyama (1971) described a case who had Kaposi's sarcoma, leukemia, and possible Hodgkin's disease. These cases suggested the possibility of the existence of a general susceptibil-ity to tumor induction.

Since cells resembling Reed-Sternberg cells have been described in a variety of benign and malignant lesions other than Hodgkin's disease (Strum et al 1970), it is not surprising that Symmers (1968a) reported that the initial diagnosis of Hodgkin's disease was confirmed in only 53 percent of the 600 cases reviewed in a reference laboratory. The conditions most frequently confused with Hodgkin's disease, in decreasing order, were chronic nonspecific lymphadenitis, reticulum cell sarcoma, metastatic tumors, infectious mononucleosis, and dermatopathic lymphadenopathy. For the 226 cases originally diagnosed as reticulum cell sarcoma, Symmers (1968b) said the diagnosis was confirmed in 73 percent of the cases. The conditions most frequently misdiagnosed as reticulum cell sarcoma were Hodgkin's disease and metastatic tumors.

Drug-induced lymphadenopathy, especially those associated with anticonvulsants, is a special diagnostic problem, since there could be a spectrum of lymphoid reactions ranging from hyperplasia through neoplasia (Brown 1971). Alberto et al (1971) presented 3 cases to emphasize the diagnos-tic and prognostic difficulties presented by lymphoma or pseudolymphoma after Dilantin therapy. In the first case, the evolution was benign; in the second, it was malignant following the apparent benign onset of Hodgkin's disease; the third was diagnosed as Hodgkin's disease at the outset.

A new benign condition easily confused with malignant lymphoma both clinically and pathologically was described by Rosai and Dorfman (1972). They called it "sinus histiocytosis with massive lymphadenopathy," because it usually involves bilateral neck and sometimes the mediastinum. Most of the 27 patients were children and 13 of them were from Africa or the West Indies. Fever was almost always present and the clinical diagnosis was often Hodgkin's disease or leukemia. Two patients died, and in the remaining 25 patients, the lymphadenopathy slowly regressed, independently of therapy. Variakojis et al (1972) reported that an abundance of foamy macrophages, which was found only in the nodular sclerosis Hodgkin's lesions, could give rise to an erroneous diagnosis of lipid storage disease or the benign condition of massive sinus histiocytosis.

EXPLORATORY LAPAROTOMY

In a series of 240 patients hospitalized with Hodgkin's disease, Williams et al (1951) reported six laparotomies for the purpose of establishing the diagnosis. In these patients, the physical findings were those of chronic debilitating conditions with no peripheral adenopathy. In 4 of the 6 cases there was a palpable abdominal mass and in the other 2, jaundice. In the EFSCH series, 3 out of 163 patients with Hodgkin's disease had abdominal operations for the purpose of establishing a diagnosis, and 54 out of 364 patients with non-Hodgkin's disease lymphomas had abdominal operations for the purpose of establishing a diagnosis.

As Table 4-4 shows, abdominal involvement was the initial manifestation of Hodgkin's disease in 11.4 percent of 316 patients reported by Pack and Molander (1966). Mesenteric and para-aortic nodal involvement was present in 9.5 percent and gastrointestinal origin in 1.9 percent. The comparable figures for patients with non-Hodgkin's lymphoma as reported by Rosenberg et al (1961) in their large series of 1229 patients were 16.7 percent: 12.1 and 4.6 percent. In the EFSCH series, our percentages were very low for Hodgkin's disease (2 percent) and higher for other lymphomas—9.3 percent for abdominal nodal involvement and 5.5 percent for gastrointestinal involvement. The series reported by Banfi et al (1969) represented a selected series because all of these patients had lymphangiograms. Thus, it was not surprising that nearly 30 percent of the patients with malignant lymphoma had para-aortic involvement at the time of diagnosis.

Malignant lymphoma often is found when patients have exploratory laparotomy as a diagnostic procedure to search the cause of unexplained fever, abdominal mass, pain, hypersplenism, or jaundice.

Table 4-4

Percentage of Initial Manifestation of Disease in Malignant Lymphoma

	Hodgkin's Disease		Non-Hodgkin's Disease	
	No lymphography	*With lymphography*	*No lymphography*	*With lymphography*
Reference	Pack and Molander	Banfi et al	Rosenberg et al	Banfi et al
Year	1966	1969	1961	1969
No. of patients	316	99	1,269	67
Lymphadenopathy				
Cervical (%)	26.9	41.0	37.7	27.0
Axillary (%)	12.6	10.0	8.7	16.0
Mediastinal (%)	16.4	20.0	3.2	6.0
Abdominal*(%)	9.5	28.0	12.1	34.0
Inguinal (%)	10.7	1.0	12.3	17.0
Nasopharynx (%)	1.9		7.4	
Multiple (%)	7.0		4.8	
	85.0	100.0	86.2	100.0
Other tissue				
Skin/soft tissue (%)	1.3		0.5	
Lung, pleura (%)	1.9		0.1	
GI (%)	1.9		4.6	
Bone (%)	1.3		3.8	

*Abdominal lymphadenopahty includes spleen, iliac, mesenteric and paraaortic nodes.

Fever

Craver and Herrmann (1946) said enlargement of the retroperitoneal nodes might be accompanied by pyrexia with right lower quandrant abdominal pain. Three of their 406 patients with Hodgkin's disease were thought to have appendicitis. Two were subjected to laparotomy before coming to their clinic, and the third refused operation despite the fact that his physician made a diagnosis of ruptured appendix with peritonitis.

Geraci et al (1959) found 21 out of 70 patients with obscure fever of longer than 2 weeks duration had malignant disease on abdominal exploration. Ten out of the 21 patients had "lymphoblastoma," all without peripheral adenopathy and 7 with a palpable spleen. Williams (1966) found that 19 out of 46 patients with fever (temperature exceeded 38°C) of undetermined origin had cancer at laparotomy. Of these, 9 patients had lymphoma diagnosed. In the presence of organomegaly or abdominal masses, he felt laparotomy would be diagnostic in 80 percent of patients. Ben-Shoshan et al (1971) reported 23 patients who had exploratory laparotomy for fever of unknown origin with duration of more than 3 weeks. Of these, 70 percent had positive findings in the abdominal cavity. Three patients were found to have Hodgkin's disease.

Boggs and Frei (1960) studied fevers of so-called "undetermined origin" in 127 patients with neoplastic disease. They found the characteristics of the fever, with or without associated infection, were quite similar, although a low-grade fever, a regularly recurring fever, or a fever accompanied by relative bradycardia was more often not associated with infection. They proposed the term "fever of cancer" when the cause of fever could not be determined. Such fever was common in acute leukemia and Hodgkin's disease and not uncommon in chronic myelocytic leukemia, lymphosarcoma, and cancer of the lung, but was not seen in patients with chronic lymphocytic leukemia.

The cause of fever occurring during the course of malignant lymphoma is obscure. Fever is a frequent manifestation of Hodgkin's disease and occurred in 30 percent to 60 percent of the patients during the course of the disease (Hoster et al 1948). Baker and Mann (1940) commented that fever was unusual when superficial glands alone are involved, but it was the rule when the deeper structures became affected. Lobell et al (1966) found no evidence of bacterial infection in 50 percent of the febrile patients with Hodgkin's disease. Even in advanced diseases, fever of noninfectious etiology was almost twice as frequent as fever due to infections. Rosenthal and Talley (1971) suggested that the pathogenesis of such unexplained fever, in the absence of infection, is due to tissue necrosis with the release of endogenous pyrogen.

Mononuclear cells in vitro were found to be capable of more prolonged pyrogen production than the polymorphonuclear leukocytes. Thus Atkins and Bodel (1972) suggested that the shaking chill and rapid spiking fever of bacteremia may represent release of pyrogen from circulating leukocytes, whereas the slow, sustained fevers characteristic of many neoplastic and granulomatous diseases may result from the production of pyrogen by fixed mononuclear cells or by tumor cells themselves. Pyrogenic agents with biologic properties like endogenous pyrogen have been obtained in the urine of some febrile patients with Hodgkin's disease (Sokal and Shimaoka 1967; Wolstenholme and Birch 1971). Young et al (1972) demonstrated the presence of a cationic protein in the urine and plasma of febrile Hodgkin's disease patients but not in afebrile patients or normal individuals. This particular factor was observed to disappear from plasma following therapeutic response to vinblastine or procarbazine. The data strongly suggest that these trace proteins are pertinent to Hodgkin's disease activity and quite possibly to the disease-associated fever as well. Pinkard et al (1972) found Hodgkin's patients with features associated with poor prognosis also had elevated excretion of purine and pyrimidine in their urine, suggesting that the atypical histiocytes might be responsible for the fever of noninfectious etiology in this disease.

Abdominal Mass and/or Pain

For lymphoma of the gastrointestinal tract, many patients presented with symptoms related to the presence of the mass and in many instances the diagnosis could not be made until surgery was essentially complete (Klopp 1968). In a series of 50 exploratory laparotomies performed for obscure abdominal pain, mass, or both, 7 patients had lymphosarcoma or reticulum cell sarcoma diagnosed. In 4 of these, the lesion was located retroperitoneally and the other 3 patients had involvement of the gastrointestinal tract and ovary (Wroblewski et al 1954). It was pointed out that neither the type, location, nor severity of pain was helpful in deciding whether the lesions were benign or malignant; and at operation, lymphomatous disease might present a picture not unlike that of extensive and inoperable carcinoma. For primary lymphoma of the stomach, the surgeon might think he is dealing with a benign peptic ulcer (Azzopardi and Menzies 1960). Naqvi et al (1969) said gastrotomy should be performed whenever there is a suspicion of gastric lymphoma. Two patients were operated upon and no tumor was palpated in the stomach; following gastrotomy, hypertropic gastric rugae were seen and biopsied specimen established the diagnosis.

In a retrospective study of 49 patients with abdominal pain, Stonesifer and Cantrell (cited by Hubbard 1971) found an "organic" cause in 38.8 percent of the cases by diagnostic laparotomy. Hubbard reported that definite pathology was found on exploratory laparotomy in 41 of 100 patients studied prospectively who had no explanation after thorough investigation and whose pain did not respond to medical therapy. One patient had Hodgkin's disease. There was no mortality nor morbidity in his series; in particular, there was no patient who was psychologically worse after the surgery.

al-Bahrani and Bakir (1971) reported that a rare but not uncommon cause of persistent, unexplained abdominal pain in Iraq was primary intestinal lymphoma. They reported 45 patients who had abdominal pain which varied in its type (intermittent, 30; constant, 15), site (generalized, 11; umbilical, 13; epigastric, 12; others, 9), character (colicky, 26; aching, 15; hunger, 4), and relationship to meals (unrelated, 27; aggravated, 14; relieved, 4). All required laparotomy for the diagnosis. The most common site of lesion was the jejunum (16 patients) and 11 patients had lesions involving multiple sites. Extension of the tumor outside the intestinal wall was found in about half of the patients and mesenteric adenopathy was present in most patients.

In the literature, there are very few articles which deal with retroperitoneal tumors, despite its unique location. Pack and Tabah (1954) published a comprehensive collective review including 120 of their own patients who had primary retroperitoneal tumors. They pointed out that retroperitoneal tumors accounted for only 0.2 percent of all the malignant neoplasms. Because of its anatomical location, the urologist, the gynecologist, and the general surgeon all shared an interest.

Seventeen of these 120 had benign tumors, and 24 of the 103 malignant tumors were malignant lymphomas. There were 6 cases of Hodgkin's disease and 18, other lymphomas. All tumors presented in the abdomen first and all required laparotomy for biopsy and diagnosis. Pack and Tabah mentioned that malignant lymphoma presented in the retroperitoneum was not common since these cases came from the 2000 cases of lymphosarcoma and 1000 cases of Hodgkin's disease on file at the Memorial Cancer Center, New York. The sizes of the tumors were recorded in 23 cases: under 5 cm (1 case), between 6 and 10 cm (8 cases), between 11 and 20 cm (8 cases), and more than 21 cm (6 cases).

Splenomegaly and Hypersplenism

In the 240 patients with Hodgkin's disease reported by Williams et al (1951) 4 of the 6 patients who required laparotomy for diagnosis were thought, preoperatively, to have primary hypersplenism. The fact that the hypersplenism was secondary to Hodgkin's disease was first diagnosed at the time of the splenectomy. Scott (1958) mentioned 3 unusual patients with Hodgkin's disease: 2 presented with isolated splenomegaly, and another case, hemolytic anemia with splenomegaly. In the rare instance of primary Hodgkin's disease of the spleen, without abnormal blood counts, bone marrow changes, or peripheral lymph node enlargement, Pack and Molander (1966) said that the removal of the spleen might be done as an organ biopsy since needle aspiration of the spleen was not often diagnostic. If the patient did not have generalized Hodgkin's disease, there could be little objection to splenectomy as an initial measure.

For patients with non-Hodgkin's lymphoma, especially those with so called primary splenic lymphoma, splenectomy also is often the initial diagnostic procedure. In 18 patients who had splenectomy for leukemia and lymphoma, Fisher et al (1952) said that the diagnosis was made after splenectomy in 4. Two had leukemia, 2 had lymphosarcoma, and all had pancytopenia. Among a total of 254 splenectomies reported by Sandusky et al (1964), 7 had lymphomatous disease. In 5 the correct diagnosis was not established until after operation. Das Gupta et al (1965) reported 9 cases of primary splenic lymphoma; in 5 the diagnosis was not made preoperatively.

Among 52 patients who had splenectomy for the diagnosis of splenomegaly, Herrmann et al (1968) reported 1 patient with Hodgkin's disease and 14 had other malignant lymphomas. One of the 7 lymphosarcoma patients who had splenectomy for splenomegaly reported by Hyatt et al (1970) had a preoperative diagnosis of hypersplenism, secondary to portal hypertension from postnecrotic cirrhosis. Skarin et al (1971) reported 11 cases of lymphosarcoma of the spleen diagnosed by splenectomy. In 3 patients the only finding was splenomegaly and none initially had significant peripheral lymphadenopathy.

However, the overall incidence of patients who require splenectomy for diagnosis is low. In the 1269 cases of lymphosarcoma reviewed by Rosenberg et al (1961), 10 patients (or 0.8 percent) presented with a palpable spleen as an isolated manifestation of disease. Four of these patients had a histological diagnosis of giant follicle lymphosarcoma, or 2.5 percent of that particular group. But none of their cases had splenectomy. Ahmann et al (1966) found 49 of their 5100 patients with malignant lymphoma had the initial diagnosis made at splenectomy (an incidence rate of less than 1 percent). Of the 49, 12 had Hodgkin's disease. Symptoms of malignant lymphoma of the spleen included malaise, anorexia, weight loss (71 percent), abdominal pain (47 percent), and fever or night sweat (39 percent).

Jaundice

Very rarely, Hodgkin's disease may present with obstructive jaundice as the initial event (Scott 1958). In the 567 patients with lymphosarcoma, Molander and Pack (1963) reported 4 percent had jaundice as one of the first manifestations of the disease. Jaundice occurring in the course of malignant lymphoma may be a troublesome diagnostic and therapeutic problem. The incidence of jaundice in patients with Hodgkin's disease as reviewed by Hoster et al (1948) varied from 3 to 8 percent. In series dealing with deceased patients, this figure went up to 68 percent (Kilburn 1958). Among 1269 patients with non-Hodgkin's lymphoma, only 3 patients presented with jaundice, 91 patients developed this problem later on, and another 65 had jaundice preterminally (Rosenberg et al 1961).

In a large series of Hodgkin's disease patients (875), Levitan et al (1961) found jaundice developed in 3.8 percent of those patients who were still living and in 19.5 of the patients who died. Clinically, liver involvement and/or biliary ductal disease was the cause in 86.8 percent of the patients. Autopsy studies showed that intrahepatic involvement with Hodgkin's disease was responsible for 70 percent of the cases, hemolytic anemia for 5.2 percent, and extrahepatic obstruction due to tumor, 3.5 percent of the cases. In 14 percent, there was no satisfactory explanation and in 1.8 percent, choledocholithiasis was present. Bouroncle et al (1962) found similar incidences in 615 patients, except a higher percentage (9.7 percent) had extrahepatic obstruction and 12.9 percent had both intra- and extrahepatic biliary obstruction. In particular, jaundice unrelated to Hodgkin's disease occurred in 13 percent of the patients. Ehrlich et al (1968) found that extrahepatic biliary tracts were involved with tumor in less than 5 percent of those who had autopsy for Hodgkin's disease and lymphosarcoma, but in 25 percent of those with reticulum cell sarcoma.

The conventional liver function tests were not very helpful in establishing the cause of jaundice in malignant lymphoma. Liver biopsy, whenever feasible and not contraindicated by the danger of hemorrhage, should be done in order to establish the diagnosis. Therapy for cholelithiasis and choledocholithiasis in patients with malignant lymphoma should be similar to that in patients without such disease. Three patients with treated non-Hodgkin's lymphoma in the EFSCH series did have cholecystectomy for cholecystitis (pp. 388–389).

Rosenthal (1969) showed that when the liver was diffusely invaded with Hodgkin's disease, the liver scan showed generalized labeling rather than focal defects. Hardin and Johnston (1971) pointed out that liver and spleen scintigraphies are useful adjunctive procedures in the diagnosis and staging of Hodgkin's disease. Percutaneous transhepatic cholangiography is an additional useful procedure in the diagnosis of obstruction of the common bile duct at the porta hepatis (Wallace 1970).

Hodgkin's disease of the cystic node causing symptoms and signs suggestive of cholecystitis has been documented (Wee et al 1970). McNulty (1971) reported a patient who had obstructive jaundice secondary to Hodgkin's disease which was relieved after choledochojejunostomy and T-tube drainage for 18 months. Alpert and Jindrak (1972) reported an unusual case of sclerosing cholangitis involving the common bile duct and hepatic hilum, associated with, but physically separate from a rapidly enlarging paracholedochal mass of reticulum cell sarcoma.

Groth et al (1972) reported two patients who had laparotomy for obstructive jaundice. Normal extrahepatic bile ducts were found and the liver biopsy showed only marked cholestasis. At autopsy 1 to 3 months later, one of the patients was found to have Hodgkin's disease and the other, reticulum cell sarcoma. In both cases the lymphoma was localized mainly in the abdominal lymph nodes and spleen. They suggested that in all cases where the cause of the jaundice was not evident at laparotomy, biopsy specimens should be taken from these two tissues.

Summary of Abdominal Exploration at EFSCH

Among the 163 patients with Hodgkin's disease, 3 required abdominal exploration for diagnosis which was made by biopsy of the mesenteric and para-aortic nodes (Table 4-5). One patient (#23200) with back pain, fever, and an abnormal intravenous pyelogram was explored twice; the first time through a flank incision because of the presumptive diagnosis of a kidney tumor.

Among the 364 patients with other lymphomas, 54 required abdominal exploration. Almost all of the patients complained of abdominal pain and/or mass; one-fourth gave a history of weight loss, nausea, or vomiting. Only 4 patients presented with jaundice and 2 with hepatosplenomegaly. Fever as a complaint was rare in patients with non-Hodgkin's lymphomas (overall only 6 percent).

Thirty-four patients had exploration and biopsy for diagnosis but without resection of viscera. The diagnosis was made in 26 patients by biopsy of nodes and in 3, biopsy of stomach (Table 4-6). The predominant site of adenopathy was located in the mesentery in 8 patients; retroperitoneum, 9; both, 5; iliac region, 3; cecal and mesenteric mass, 1. In 5 additional patients, a bypass and decompressive operation was also done at the time of exploration (Table 4-7).

In the EFSCH series, 20 of the 364 patients with non-Hodgkin's lymphoma had abdominal exploration plus resection of various organs. Seven patients had subtotal gastrectomy, 4 had ileal resection, 4 had right hemicolectomy, 2 had hysterectomy, 1 had splenectomy, and another had radical nephrectomy. Details of these cases are presented elsewhere (pp. 252, 254, 372).

Since about 5 percent of the patients with malignant lymphoma had involvement of the gastrointestinal tract on admission, and about half of the tumors were primary lesions (Bush and Ash 1969), it is clear that "When laparotomy for biopsy is done, the surgeon, by the exercise of judgment and technical skill, may remove the bulk or all of the tumor, possibly relieving distressing symptoms and affording palliation" (Pack and Molander, 1966). Extranodal lesions originating in the viscera are much more common in patients with non-Hodgkin's lymphomas. Among 270 patients with reticulum cell sarcoma and 631 patients with lymphosarcoma. Peters et al (1968) reported that the gastrointestinal tract itself was one of the first recognized sites of involvement in 25 percent and 13 percent, respectively. The overall incidence for the combined series was 17 percent. This special problem will be discussed in more detail in Chapter 7.

Table 4-5
Abdominal Exploration for Hodgkin's Disease (EFSCH series)

Patient No.	Age	Sex	Date	Symptoms	Primary lesion	Pathological diagnosis	Postoperative		Survival (months)	Lymphoma at follow-up
							Radiation therapy (rads)	Chemo-therapy		
06569	14	M	6-44	Appendicitis	Mesenteric node (appendectomy)	LP	3500	–	15	+
23200	42	M	8-56	Back pain, fever, abnormal IVP	Kidney tumor					
			8-56		Para-aortic, mesenteric node	LD	1500	–	7	+
38946	41	F	2-70	Fever, abnormal IVP	Para-aortic, iliac node	LP	–	+	7	+

Table 4-6
Abdominal Exploration for Non-Hodgkin's Lymphoma (EFSCH series)

Patient No.	Age	Sex	Date	Other lesion	Primary lesion	Pathological diagnosis	Postoperative		Survival, months (*alive)	Lymphoma at follow-up
							Radiation therapy (rads)	Chemotherapy		
04043	45	F	4-42	Neck, upper	Mesenteric mass	LWN	1700	—	118	+
15779	63	F	9-50		Mesenteric mass	LPD	70 (TB)†	—	14	+
21257	50	F	7-55		Mesenteric mass	Und	2100	—	195*	—
22814	59	M	8-56		Mesenteric mass	UC	1200	—	2	+
24516	25	M	10-57		Mesenteric mass	MCN	3000	—	116	+
12818	69	M	7-60		Mesenteric mass	HWN	2800	+	13	+
31976	61	F	10-63		Mesenteric mass	LPN	4000	—	97*	— (lung cancer)
36319	40	F	2-65		Mesenteric mass	HPD	80 (TB)	+	44	—
09371	55	F	11-46	L. lower neck, chest & arm pain, RT: groin 2-45, neck 9-45	Retroperitoneal mass	HWD	4800	—	3	— (septicemia)
14490	62	M	11-50	Anemia	Retroperitoneal mass	UC		—	4	+ (septicemia)
17312	46	M	1-53		Retroperitoneal mass	LPD	4000	—	58	— (heart attack)
21242	73	M	8-55		Retroperitoneal mass	Und	500	—	2	+ (septicemia)
29826	75	M	12-61		Retroperitoneal mass	UC	2000	—	4	+
31116	48	M	1-63	Jaundice	Retroperitoneal mass	UC	1500	+	3	+
33679	54	F	1-65		Retroperitoneal mass	HWN	1300	—	75*	—
34864	77	M	12-65		Retroperitoneal mass	UC	2500	—	3	+
05367	60	F	7-43		Retroperitoneal and mesenteric mass	Und	1400	—	66	+
10028	72	M	8-47	Generalized	Retroperitoneal and mesenteric mass	LWD	710 (TB)	—	23	+

143

Table 4-6
Abdominal Exploration for Non-Hodgkin's Lymphoma (EFSCH series) cont'd

Patient No.	Age	Sex	Date	Other lesion	Primary lesion	Pathological diagnosis	Postoperative		Survival, months (*alive)	Lymphoma at follow-up
							Radiation therapy (rads)	Chemotherapy		
15488	60	F	8-51	Backache, ascites	Retroperitoneal and mesenteric mass	LPD	1800	−	2	+
19501	62	M	6-54		Retroperitoneal and mesenteric mass	Und	2300	−	6	+
37804	57	F	2-68		Retroperitoneal and mesenteric mass	LWN	2500	−	44*	−
20341	63	F	3-55		Stomach mass	UC	4700	−	127	− (hypertension)
24370	47	M	10-57		Stomach (antrum and body)	HWD	4000	−	14	+
04031	76	F	2-58		Stomach mass (liver biopsy positive)	Und	1000	−	104	− (old age)
02167	46	F	9-40	Axilla, groin	Pelvic mass	HPD	2000	−	6	+
19430	37	M	6-54	Leg edema	Iliac and mesenteric mass	LPD	2300	+	7	+
20837	16	M	6-55	Jaundice, hepatosplenomegaly	Liver tumor retroperitoneal and mesenteric mass	LPD	−	+	1	+
27290	74	M	12-59	Leg edema	Iliac and mesenteric mass	LWD	−	−	1	+ (heart attack)
32236	58	F	12-63		Cecal and mesenteric mass	Und	3000	−	11	+

* TB = total body irradiation.

Table 4-7

Abdominal Exploration and Decompression for Non-Hodgkin's Lymphoma (EFSCH series)

Patient No.	Age	Sex	Date	Indication	Operation	Diagnosis	Other lesions at operation	Postoperative Radiation therapy (rads)	Chemotherapy	Survival	Lymphoma at follow-up
18907	54	M	2-54	Rectal and omental mass	Colostomy	HWD	Jaundice and ascites	—	—	9 days	+
20463	65	M	3-55	Cardiac mass	Gastrostomy	HWD	neck	4000	—	66 months	?
20453	49	M	4-55	Pyloric mass	Gastrojejunostomy	UC		700	—	11 months	+
32144	45	M	8-63	Retroperitoneal mass	Cholecysto-jejunostomy	HPD	Jaundice	3200	—	5 months	+
40607	66	M	12-71	Retroperitoneal mass and ileocecal intussusception	Ileocolostomy	LWD		—	—	2 months	+

OTHER OPERATIONS FOR DIAGNOSIS

Thoracotomy

In addition to abdominal explorations, thoracotomy may be required to obtain tissues for the diagnosis of malignant lymphoma. Blades (1946) described 109 patients who had thoracotomy for mediastinal tumors. Among the 15 patients with malignant tumors, 4 had Hodgkin's disease and 2 had lymphoblastoma. In 3 Hodgkin's patients the tumor was resected before the true nature of the lesion was established. Quinlan et al (1963) presented 110 patients who required thoractomy for diagnosis of intrathoracic lesions. During the same period, 1600 major thoracotomy operations were performed. There were 3 patients with Hodgkin's disease and 3 with sarcoma in his group of 110. The operative mortality of diagnostic thoracotomy was 3.5 percent since 1950. Burke et al (1967) reported a series of 296 thoracotomies performed for mediastinal tumors over a 14-year period. In 12 patients, a diagnosis of Hodgkin's disease was made on microscopic examination of excised tissues. Van Heerden et al (1970) reviewed a series of 97 cases of malignant lymphoma clinically presenting in the mediastinum: 35 of these had thoracotomy and biopsy, 16 had thoracotomy with curative resection, and 5 had palliative resection.

Grosfeld et al (1971) reported a series of primary mediastinal tumors observed in 62 infants and children. Forty-seven patients had malignant tumors and 20 of these were lymphomas. Thoracotomy was required for diagnosis in 9 patients. They pointed out that because of the high incidence of malignancy in this age group, all childhood mediastinal lesions should be explored. Oh et al (1971) reported 3 cases of large, but normal, thymus in late childhood. Since there was no accurate method for differentiating this lesion from tumors and other lesions, exploratory thoracotomy was necessary for all 3. La Franchi and Fonkalsrud (1973) reported 14 malignant lymphomas of the mediastinum in children. Thoractomy was necessary to establish the diagnosis in 5. None of the lymphatic tumors was resected.

Ellman and Bowdler (1960) reported a case of Hodgkin's disease presented as a rounded shadow in the left lower lobe requiring diagnosis by thoracotomy. In cases of lymphoma of the lung, Klopp (1968) commented that the lesions usually presented as asymptomatic shadows on chest x-rays and the diagnosis was usually established postoperatively, after complete removal had been accomplished.

However, occasionally, various minor procedures other than thoracotomy can establish the diagnosis of intrathoracic malignant lymphoma. When the lymphomatous lesions presented intrabronchially, the diagnosis could be established by bronchoscopy (Higginson and Grismer 1950). When pleural disease is present with or without the presence of fluid, pleural biopsy might yield a histological diagnosis (Scerbo et al 1971). A new technique using bronchial brush biopsy established the presence of pulmonary Hodgkin's disease in 3 patients who had negative cytology (Variakojis et al 1972).

Statistically, about 1 percent of the patients with malignant lymphoma required thoracotomy for diagnosis. In 240 patients with Hodgkin's disease, Williams et al (1951) reported 3 who had thoracotomy with lung and/or mediastinal node biopsy for initial diagnosis. Fisher et al (1962) found lung parenchyma was involved in about 30 percent of their 154 patients during the course of Hodgkin's disease. In 2 patients, thoracotomy was done because the lesions could not be differentiated from bronchial carcinoma. Steel (1964) presented 4 patients with Hodgkin's disease of the lung with cavitation, and 3 required exploratory thoracotomy. The lesions simulated other cavitated lesions such as tuberculosis, lung abscess, congenital cyst, especially in the absence of extrathoracic and mediastinal adenopathy. Rubin (1968) said that correct diagnosis was established by thoracotomy in 10 of his 11 cases with various malignant lymphomas of the lung. Levinsky et al (1971) reported a Hodgkin's disease patient who had bilateral thoracotomy for excision and diagnosis of left and right hilar lymphadenopathy.

In "Progressive Pulmonary Insufficiency and Malignant Lymphoma," Dr. Arnold Seitam discussed a patient with the diagnosis of malignant lymphoma who required thoracotomy and lung biopsy for coexisting sarcoidosis. Another case presented at a clinicopathological conference also had bilateral thoracotomy because (1) the pathologists could not decide whether the pulmonary process was a form of lymphoma or a limited form of Wegener's granulomatosis, and (2) a second thoracotomy and right lower lobectomy had to be done because of massive bleeding after insertion of a chest tube for empyema (Castleman and McNeely 1971). Castellino and Blank (1972) pointed out that Hodgkin's disease could cause enlargement of the lymph nodes located at the cardiophrenic angle. They presented 5 cases and in 2, thoracotomy and biopsy were done to define the nature of these asymptomatic masses which appeared on routine chest x-rays.

Munnell (1971) reported a total of 146 thoracic operative procedures for diagnosis and palliation done on 104 out of 1036 patients with malignant lymphoma. Their entire series included 401 patients with leukemia. Thus, about 88 out of 653 nonleukemic patients underwent 131 thoracic procedures (or 13.5 percent of the lymphoma patients had an average of 1.5 operations per patient). The 146 thoracic surgical procedures included 92 for scalene fat pad biopsy, 15 for bronchoscopy and/or mediastinoscopy, and 39 procedures for palliation or, on occasion, cure. Apparently 9 exploratory thoracotomies were done: 2 patients (1 lymphosarcoma, 1 Hodgkin's disease) had thoracotomy for pleural effusion and lung mass, and 7 other patients (3 Hodgkin's disease, 3 non-Hodgkin's lymphoma, 1 leukemia) required thoracotomy for diagnosis.

In the EFSCH series, about 52 percent of the patients with Hodgkin's disease and 17 percent of those with other lymphomas had diagnostic biopsy of lower neck adenopathy. No case had diagnosis established either by bronchoscopy or mediastinoscopy. None of the 163 Hodgkin's disease patients had thoracotomy, while 3 of the 364 non-Hodgkin's disease patients had thoracotomy as one of the initial diagnostic procedures (Table 4-8). All had pleural effusion; one is still living and another, who had chylous effusion treated only with nitrogen mustard instilled in the chest cavity, lived nearly 8 years.

Mediastinoscopy and Mediastinotomy

Scalene fat pad biopsy was described by Daniels (1949). Harken et al (1954) extended this operation to include the examination of homolateral superior mediastinal nodes with a laryngoscope. Carlens (1959) improved on this technique and described mediastinoscopy. In addition to its usefulness as a method to determine resectability of pulmonary cancers, this procedure may provide the only source of histological diagnosis in certain intrathoracic disease and reduce the number of unnecessary exploratory thoracotomies.

The morbidity and mortality rates of mediastinoscopy appeared to be low. Among 9543 patients who had this procedure, Ashbaugh (1970) found only 9 deaths (0.09 percent) and 140 complications (1.5 percent). Specifically, there was hemorrhage in 48, pneumothorax in 43, recurrent nerve injury in 22, infection in 12, tumor implantation in 8, phrenic nerve injury in 3, and less commonly, esophageal injury, chylothorax, air embolism, and transient hemiparesis.

Akovbiantz and Senning (1967) reported a series of 400 patients who had mediastinoscopy. Among these, 58 required this procedure for diagnosis and 5 had Hodgkin's disease. Among another 400 cases, Sarin and Nohl-Oser (1969) reported 12 cases of Hodgkin's disease. Redding et al (1971) reported the use of mediastinoscopy in 2 patients with Hodgkin's disease to determine the presence or absence of mediastinal involvement. They surveyed 7 surgeons who had wide experience with this procedure and collected 32 patients in whom mediastinoscopy established the diagnosis of Hodgkin's disease not made otherwise. They also reviewed 9 series reported in the literature (Hosie and Ford 1967; Jepsen 1966; Kirschner 1967; Lincoln and Provan 1970; Nielsen and Olsen 1966; Nohl-Oser 1965; Pinkham and Torgerson 1969; Trinkle et al 1968; Ward et al 1969). Among the reported total of 1309 mediastinoscopies, there were 13 cases of Hodgkin's disease and 12 other lymphomas diagnosed by this method. Thus, about 2 percent of the patients who had mediastinoscopy had malignant lymphoma.

Munnell (1971) reported that 5 out of 46 mediastinoscopies they performed showed evidence of some type of malignant lymphoma. Unsuspected second neoplasms were found in 2 patients (rhabdomyosarcoma in a patient with reticulum cell sarcoma; thyroid cancer in another with lymphatic

Table 4-8
Thoracotomy for Diagnosis of Non-Hodgkin's Lymphoma (EFSCH series)

Patient No.	Age	Sex	Date	Indication	Operation	Pathological diagnosis	Postoperative		Survival months (*alive)	Lymphoma at follow-up
							Radiotherapy	Chemotherapy		
39192	62	M	10-62	Pleural effusion (chylous)	L-Thoracotomy, pleura + lung biopsy	UC	–	NH₂ (IP)	93	+
37009	19	M	3-68	Pleural effusion, hilar node	Thoracotomy, pleural biopsy	LWD	+	NH₂ (IP), Cytoxan MOPP	8	+
38126	30	M	5-69	Pleural effusion, medi-astinal node	R-Thoracotomy, needle biopsy of liver	LWD	+	COP	30*	?

leukemia). He even suggested that mediastinoscopy should be part of the operative staging procedures like exploratory laparotomy, and that it should be more commonly used in the future care of lymphoma. At EFSCH, we have used mediastinoscopy only since 1970. Our pathologists had difficulty in making the diagnosis of Hodgkin's disease because the forcep-biopsied tissues were usually too small, crushed, and distorted.

Stemmer et al (1965) described the technique of anterior transthoracic, extrapleural mediastinotomy via a parasternal incision. Calvin et al (1971) reported 93 patients who required such exploration because it had not been possible to establish a tissue diagnosis by the more conventional techniques of bronchoscopy, cytology, and scalene node biopsy. In a later report, Stemmer et al (1971) reported that 3 out of 134 explorations were done for tumors other than bronchogenic, esophageal, and metastatic lesions; presumably, these 3 could include malignant lymphomas. This procedure obtained correct biopsy in 95 percent of the patients, but in his series there were 9 complications and 1 death.

Laminectomy and Non-Nodal Biopsy

Love et al (1954) presented 39 patients who had "lymphoblastomas" primarily of the spinal extradural space without clinical evidence of tumor elsewhere. All required laminectomy for diagnosis. Lymphosarcoma of the small cell type was the most prevalent tumor (14 patients) followed by reticulum cell sarcoma (11 patients), Hodgkin's disease (7 patients), and mixed cell type. Fisher et al (1962) reported that dural deposits, causing partial or complete obstruction on myelography, occurred in 4 of their 154 patients with Hodgkin's disease. Almost all of the dural lesions had concomitant vertebral involvement. Cooper (1970) reported a series of 80 patients with reticulum cell sarcoma. Three patients presented with back pain and paresthesia in the lower extremities or perineal region. Two patients had laminectomy and the third died before surgery could be instituted.

In the EFSCH series, 4 of the 364 non-Hodgkin's disease patients had laminectomy as one of the initial diagnostic procedures (Table 4-9). All patients had neurological impairment and bony lesions. Two lesions could not be classified (UC), one was lymphocytic poorly differentiated nodular type (LPN), and the other, histiocytic well-differentiated diffuse type (HWD). One patient (#16101) lived 14 years without recurrence after laminectomy and radiotherapy.

Since Rubin et al (1969) showed that high-dose radiotherapy alone could give quick spinal cord decompression, and Silverberg and Jacobs (1971) pointed out that intravenous chemotherapy followed promptly by radiotherapy could produce rapid regression of the neurological symptoms, it is apparent that the need of performing therapeutic laminectomy for extradural metastases of malignant lymphoma might diminish in the future.

Table 4-9
Laminectomy for Diagnosis of Non-Hodgkin's Lymphoma (EFSCH series)

Patient No.	Age	Sex	Date	Indication	Level of laminectomy	Pathological diagnosis	Postoperative Radiation therapy (rads)	Postoperative Chemo-therapy	Survival (months)	Lymphoma at follow-up
16101	53	F	4-50	Leg paralysis	T2-5	UC	2210	–	168	? (old age)
31140	57	M	2-63	Leg paralysis	T3-5	UC	3200	–	4	+
35936	57	F	12-66	Leg paralysis	T9-11	LPN	4200	–	3	+
38720	29	M	8-69	Arm pain, paresthesia	C7-T1	HWD	4500	–	8	+

However, diagnostic laminectomy may still be required in occasional cases.

Regarding non-nodal tissue biopsy for diagnosis in the EFSCH series, among the 163 patients with Hodgkin's disease only 1 patient (#37956) presented with an isolated non-nodal lesion (subcutaneous nodule over the sternum). Four of the 364 patients with other lymphomas presented only with skin nodules. This special presentation is discussed on pp. 322–324. Another Hodgkin's patient (#13154) had radical mastectomy as did 3 patients with non-Hodgkin's lymphoma (p. 183).

Other unusual non-nodal presentations of malignant lymphomas included lesions of the tonsil, testes, and bone. Details regarding these specific sites are given on pp. 287, 268, and 317). In the EFSCH series, among the 364 patients with non-Hodgkin's lymphoma (Table 4-10), 1 patient each had tonsillectomy and orchiectomy, respectively, before the true nature of the mass was known. A third patient had open bone biopsy for a lesion of the femur. At the time of diagnosis, 5 out of the 364 patients had testicular mass, 7 had enlarged tonsils, and 15 had bony lesions.

SUMMARY

The diagnosis of malignant lymphoma can only be made by histological examination of tissue biopsies. Biopsy of enlarged peripheral nodes established diagnosis in 94 percent of the cases with Hodgkin's disease, and in 77 percent of those with other lymphomas. When taking a biopsy, surgeons should pay particular attention to the proper selection of the biopsy site, proper selection of the node at the chosen site, and proper removal of the node. It is difficult to make a diagnosis on a partially removed node or a small specimen taken by punch or needle biopsy. If clinically indicated, rebiopsy should be done if the first biopsy report was benign or nondiagnostic. Many reactive and infectious processes can simulate lymphoma and the diagnosis of malignant lymphoma can be a challenging problem even for the experienced pathologist.

Exploratory laparotomy, excluding staging operations, may be required to establish diagnosis in 2 percent of the patients with Hodgkin's disease and in 15 percent of those with other lymphomas. In over half the cases, biopsy of mesenteric or retroperitoneal nodes established the histological identity, whereas resection of the visceral organs may be required in others. Often malignant lymphoma was diagnosed when patients had exploratory celiotomy to find the cause of unexplained fever, abdominal mass and/or pain, hypersplenism, or jaundice. The cause of fever occurring during the course of malignant lymphoma is often obscure, although pyrogenic substances have been isolated in febrile patients with Hodgkin's disease. Abdominal mass and pain are the common presenting signs and symptoms of gastrointestinal and retroperitoneal lymphomas. Splenectomy was the initial diagnostic

Table 4-10
Non-Nodal Biopsy for Diagnosis of Non-Hodgkin's Lymphoma (EFSCH series)

Patient No.	Age	Sex	Date	Indication	Operation	Pathological diagnosis	Postoperative		Survival (*alive)	Lymphoma at follow-up
							Radiation therapy (rads)	Chemo-therapy		
38567	66	M	10-66	Tonsilar mass	Tonsillectomy	LWD	4000	+	61 months*	?
	70	M	9-70	Breast mass	Breast biopsy	LWD	–	+		?
23207	85	M	1-57	Tonsil and testicular mass	Bilateral orchiectomy	HPD	–	–	6 months	
21667	9	M	1-56	Osteolytic lesions	Femur biopsy	HWD	–	–	9 days	+ (aspira-tion)

procedure in about 1 percent of the patients with lymphoma. Jaundice occurring initially or during the course of malignant lymphoma may be a troublesome diagnostic and therapeutic problem.

Malignant lymphoma, especially Hodgkin's disease, may present as mediastinal masses or less likely, pulmonary lesions. Even using bronchoscopy, scalene fat pad biopsy, or mediastinoscopy, thoracotomy may still be required for diagnosis in about 1 percent of the patients. Another 1 percent may need laminectomy as one of the initial diagnostic procedures because of neurological impairment and bony lesion without peripheral adenopathy. Other non-nodal tissues which are often biopsied for diagnosis include bone, subcutaneous tissue, testes, and tonsils.

REFERENCES

Agliozzo CM, Reingold IM: Infectious mononucleosis simulating Hodgkin's disease. Am J Clin Pathol 56:730–735, 1971

Ahmann DL, Kiely JM, Harrison EG Jr, et al: Malignant lymphoma of the spleen: A review of 49 cases in which the diagnosis was made at splenectomy. Cancer 19: 461–469, 1966

Akovbiantz A, Senning A: Mediastinoscopy, in Rüttimann A (ed): Progress in Lymphology, vol 1. Stuttgart, Thieme, 1967, pp 264–266

Alberto P, Cougn R, Maurice P, et al: Trois cas de lymphome malin ou pseudo-lymphome chez dez epileptiques traites par la diphenylhdantoine. Schweiz Med Wochenschr 101:1173–1174, 1970

Alpert LI, Jindrak K: Idiopathic retroperitoneal fibrosis and sclerosing cholangitis associated with a reticulum sarcoma: Report of a case. Gastroenterology 62: 111–117, 1972

Ashbaugh DG: Mediastinoscopy. Arch Surg 100:568–573, 1970

Atkins E, Bodel P: Fever. N Engl J Med 286:27–34, 1972

Azzopardi JG, Menzies T: Primary malignant lymphoma of the alimentary tract. Br J Surg 47:358–366, 1960

al-Bahrani ZR, Bakir F: Primary intestinal lymphoma: A challenging problem in abdominal pain. Ann R Coll Surg Engl 49:103–113, 1971

Baker C, Mann WN: Hodgkin's disease. Lancet 1:23–25, 1940

Banfi A, Bonadonna G, Carnevali G, et al: Malignant lymphomas: Further studies on their preferential sites of involvement and possible mode of spread. Lymphology 2:130–138, 1969

Ben-Shoshan M, Gius JA, Smith IM: Exploratory laparotomy for fever of unknown origin. Surg Gynecol Obstet 132:994–996, 1971

Blades B: Mediastinal tumors: Report of cases treated at army thoracic surgery centers in United States. Ann Surg 123:749–765, 1946

Boggs DR, Frei E III: Clinical studies of fever and infection in cancer. Cancer 13: 1240–1253, 1960

Bouroncle BA, Old JW Jr, Vazques AG: Pathogenesis of jaundice in Hodgkin's disease. Arch Intern Med 110:872–883, 1962

Brown JM: Drug-associated lymphadenopathies with special reference to the Reed-Sternberg cell. Med J Aust 1: 375–378, 1971

Burke WA, Burford TH, Dorfman RF: Hodgkin's disease of the mediastinum. Ann Thorac Surg 3:287–296, 1967

Bush RS, Ash CL: Primary lymphoma of the gastrointestinal tract. Radiology 92:1349–1354, 1969

Butler JJ: Histopathology of malignant lymphoma and Hodgkin's disease. Leukemia-Lymphoma. Chicago, Year Book, 1970, pp 123–142

Butler JJ: Non-neoplastic lesions of lymph nodes of man to be differentiated from lymphomas. Natl Cancer Inst Monogr 32:233–255, 1969

Calvin JW, Stemmer EA, Steedman RA, et al: Clinical application of parasternal mediastinotomy. Arch Surg 102:322–325, 1971

Carlens E: Mediastinoscopy: A method for inspection and tissue biopsy in the superior mediastinum. Dis Chest 36:343–352, 1959

Castellino RA, Blank N: Adenopathy of the cardiophrenic angle (diaphragmatic) lymph nodes. Am J Roentgenol Radium Ther Nucl Med 114:509–515, 1972

Castleman B, McNeely BU: Case records of the Massachusetts General Hospital: Weekly clinicopathological exercises: Case 10-1971. N Engl J Med 284:544–551, 1971

Conley J: Biopsy in the head and neck, in Rüttimann A (ed): Progress in Lymphology, vol. 1. Stuttgart, Thieme, 1967, pp 294–299

Conn JH, Fain WR, Chavez M, et al: Scalene lymphadenectomy in 500 patients: Critical evaluation, in Viamonte M, Koehler RP, Witte M, et al (eds): Progress in Lymphology II. Stuttgart, Thieme, 1970, pp 144–148

Cooke WB, Glotzer DT: Scalene node biopsy for the diagnosis of obscure systemic disease. Am J Surg 107:769–772, 1964

Cooper IA: Clinical presentation of reticulum-cell sarcoma: A disease with many faces. Med J Aust 1:697–704, 1970

Craver LF: Treatment of Hodgkin's disease, in Pack GT, Ariel IM (eds): Treatment of Cancer and Allied Diseases (ed 2). New York, Hoeber, 1964, pp 168–191

Craver LF, Herrmann JB: Abdominal lymphogranulomatosis. Am J Roentgenol Radium Ther Nucl Med 55:165–172, 1946

Daniels AC: Method of biopsy useful in diagnosing certain intrathoracic diseases. Dis Chest 16:360–366, 1949

Das Gupta T, Coombes B, Brasfield RD: Primary malignant neoplasms of the spleen. Surg Gynecol Obstet 120:947–960, 1965

Dawson PJ, Cooper RA, Rambo ON: Diagnosis of malignant lymphoma: A clinicopathologic analysis of 158 difficult lymph node biopsies. Cancer 17:1405–1413, 1964

Dorfman RF: Formal discussion of Robert J Lukes' paper "Criteria for Involvement of Lymph Node, Bone Marrow, Spleen, and Liver in Hodgkin's Disease." Cancer Res 31:1768–1769, 1971

Ehrlich AN, Stalder G, Geller W, et al: Gastrointestinal manifestations of malignant lymphoma. Gastroenterology 54:1115–1121, 1968

Ellman P, Bowdler AJ: Pulmonary manifestations of Hodgkin's disease. Brit J Dis Chest 54:59–71, 1960

Fisher AM, Kendall B, Van Leuven BD: Hodgkin's disease: A radiological survey. Clin Radiol 13:115–127, 1962

Fisher JH, Welch CS, Dameshek W: Splenectomy in leukemia and leukosarcoma. N Engl J Med 246:477–484, 1952

Gall EA, Mallory TB: Malignant lymphoma: Clinico-pathologic survey of 618 cases. Am J Pathol 18:381–429, 1942

Geraci JE, Weed LA, Nichols DR: Fever of obscure origin: The value of abdominal exploration in diagnosis. Report of 70 cases. JAMA 169:1306–1315, 1959

Gilbert TT, Evjy JT, Edelstein L: Hodgkin's disease associated with Kaposi's sarcoma and malignant melanoma. Cancer 28:293–299, 1971

Grosfeld JL, Weinberger M, Kilman JW, et al: Primary mediastinal neoplasms in infants and children. Ann Thorac Surg 12:179–190, 1971

Groth CG, Hellström K, Hofvendahl S, et al: Diagnosis of malignant lymphoma at laparotomy disclosing intrahepatic cholestasis. Acta Chir Scand 138:186–189, 1972

Hall CA, Olson KB: Prognosis of the malignant lymphomas. Ann Intern Med 44:687–706, 1956

Hall TC: Summary of informal discussion on: General considerations. Cancer Res 26:1095–1096, 1966

Hardin VH, Johnston GS: Liver and spleen scintigraphy in staging Hodgkin's disease. J Surg Oncol 3:109–115, 1971

Harken DE, Black H, Clauss R, et al: A simple cervicomediastinal exploration for tissue diagnosis of intrathoracic disease. N Engl J Med 251:1041–1044, 1954

Hartsock RJ: Postvaccinial lymphadenitis: Hyperplasia of lymphoid tissue that simulates malignant lymphomas. Cancer 21:632–649, 1968

Hermann RE, DeHaven KE, Hawk WA: Splenectomy for the diagnosis of splenomegaly. Ann Surg 168:896–900, 1968

Higgins GK: Pathologic anatomy, in Molander DW, and Pack GT (eds): Hodgkin's Disease. Springfield, Ill., Thomas, 1968, pp 20–63

Higginson JF, Grismer JT: Obstructing intrabronchial Hodgkin's disease: Case report. J Thorac Surg 20:961–967, 1950

Hosie RT, Ford HS: Mediastinoscopy. Am Surg 33:594–596, 1967

Hoster HA, Dratman MB, Craver LF, et al: Hodgkin's disease: 1832–1947. Cancer Res 8:1–48, 49–78, 1948

Hubbard TB Jr: Answers to questions on diagnostic laparotomy. Hospital Medicine 7:71–80, June 1971

Hyatt DF, Skarin AT, Moloney WC, et al: Splenectomy for lymphosarcoma. Surg Gynecol Obstet 131:928–932, 1970

Jepsen O: Mediastinoscopy: Bioptic Mediastinal Exploration by the Method of Carlens. Copenhagen, Munksgaard, 1966

Kaplan HS: Hodgkin's disease. Cambridge, Mass, Harvard University Press, 1972, pp 32–39

Kilburn KH: Secondary Amyloidosis and hepatic failure in Hodgkin's disease. Am J Med 24:654–658, 1958

Kirschner PA: Mediastinoscopy: Experiences with fifty cases. Mt Sinai J Med NY 34:559–573, 1967

Klopp, CT: Surgical treatment of primary lymphoma. Cancer Management: A special graduate course on cancer. Sponsored by American Cancer Society. Philadelphia, Lippincott, 1968, pp 393–397

Kurtz DM: To biopsy or not to biopsy. JAMA 214:1888, 1970

La Franchi S, Fonkalsrud EW: Surgical management of lymphatic tumors of the mediastinum in children. J Thorac Cardiovasc Surg 65:8–14, 1973

Larsen RR, Hill GJ II, Ratzer ER: Reticulum cell sarcoma in head and neck surgery. Am J Surg 123:338–342, 1972

Levinsky L, Lewinski U, Vries A de, et al: Bilateral thoracotomy for Hodgkin's disease involving the hilar nodes. Chest 59:446–448, 1971

Levitan R, Diamond HD, Craver LF: Jaundice in Hodgkin's disease. Am J Med 30:99–111, 1961

Lincoln JC, Provan JL: Mediastinoscopy in the diagnosis of nonmalignant thoracic disease. J Thorac Cardiovase Surg 60:144–148, 1970

Lobell M, Boggs DR, Wintrobe MM: The clinical significance of fever in Hodgkin's disease. Arch Intern Med 117:335–342, 1966

Love JG, Miller RH, Kernohan JW: Lymphomas of spinal epidural space. Arch Surg 69:66–76, 1954

Lubin J, Rywlin AM: Lymphoma-like lymph node changes in Kaposi's sarcoma. Arch Pathol 92:338–341, 1971

Lukes RJ, Tindle BH, Parker JW: Reed-Sternberg-like cells in infectious mononucleosis. Lancet 2:1003–1004, 1969

McMahon NJ, Gordon HW, Rosen RB: Reed-Sternberg cells in infectious mononucleosis. Am J Dis Child 120:148–150, 1970

McNulty JG: Diagnosis of extrahepatic jaundice in Hodgkin's disease. Br Med J 4:26–27, 1971

Molander DW, Pack GT: Lymphosarcoma: Choice of treatment and end-results in 567 patients. Role of surgical treatment for cure and palliation. Rev Surg 20:3–31, 1963

Moore CV: Surgical experience with laparotomy in 125 patients with lymphoma. Presented at the Symposium on Hodgkin's Disease at St. Louis, October 7–9, 1971

Moore GE: The importance of biopsy procedures. JAMA 205:917–920, 1968

Munnell ER: Current concepts of thoracic surgery in the management of lymphoma. Ann Thorac Surg 11:151–159, 1971

Naqvi MS, Burrows L, Kark AE: Lymphoma of the gastrointestinal tract: Prognostic guides based on 162 cases. Ann Surg 170:221–231, 1969

Nielsen EG, Olsen H: Mediastinoscopy: An analysis of 223 cases. Danish Med Bull 13:193–197, 1966

Nohl-Oser HC: Mediastinoscopy. Br Med J 1:1167–1169, 1965

Oh KS, Weber AL, Borden S IV: Normal mediastinal mass in late childhood. Radiology 101:625–628, 1971

Pack GT, Molander DW: The surgical treatment of Hodgkin's disease. Cancer Res 26:1254–1263, 1966

Pack GT, Tabah, EJ: Primary retroperitoneal tumors: A study of 120 cases (Part I & II). Int Abst Surg 99:209–231, 313–341, 1954.

Peters MV, Hasselback R, Brown TC: The natural history of the lymphomas related to the clinical classification, in Zarafonetis CJ (ed): Proceedings of the International Conference on Leukemia-Lymphoma. Philadelphia, Lea & Febiger, 1968, pp 357–371

Peters MV, Middlemiss KC: A study of Hodgkin's disease treated by irradiation. Am J Roentgenol Radium Ther Nucl Med 79:114–121, 1958

Pinkard KJ, Cooper IA, Motteram R, et al: Purine and pyrimidine excretion in Hodgkin's disease. J Natl Cancer Inst 49:27–38, 1972

Pinkham RD, Torgerson AC: Mediastinoscopy: An important adjunct in the diagnosis and treatment of intrathoracic lesions. Am J Surg 118:562–566, 1969

Progressive pulmonary insufficiency and malignant lymphoma. Postgrad Med 49:221–226, 1971

Quinlan JJ, Schaffner VD, Hiltz JE: Thoracotomy for the diagnosis of intrathoracic lesions: A review of 110 cases. Can J Surg 6:322–332, 1963

Redding ME, Anagnostopoulos CE, Ultmann JE: The possible value of mediastinoscopy in staging Hodgkin's disease. Cancer Res 31:1741–1745, 1971

Rosai J, Dorfman RF: Sinus histiocytosis with massive lymphadenopathy: A distinct clinicopathologic entity simulating malignant lymphoma. Lab Invest 26:489, 1972

Rosenberg SA, Diamond HD, Jaslowitz B, et al: Lymphosarcoma: A review of 1269 cases. Medicine 40:31–84, 1961

Rosenthal SL, Talley RW: Fever in neoplastic disease. Henry Ford Hosp Med J 19:15–20, 1971

Rosenthall L: The Application of Radioiodinated Rose Bengal and Colloidal Radiogold in the Detection of Hepatobiliary Disease. St. Louis, Green, 1969

Rubin M: Primary lymphoma of lung. J Thorac Cardiovasc Surg 56:293–303, 1968

Rubin P, Mayer E, Poulter C: Extradural spinal cord compression by tumor. I. High daily dose experience without laminectomy. Radiology 93:1248–1260, 1969

Saltzstein SL: The fate of patients with nondiagnostic lymph node biopsies. Surgery 58:659–662, 1965

Saltzstein SL: Value of biopsy Hodgkin's disease. JAMA 215:984, 1971

Salvador AH, Harrison EG Jr, Kyle RA: Lymphadenopathy due to infectious mononucleosis: Its confusion with malignant lymphoma. Cancer 27:1029–1040, 1971

Sandusky WR, Leavell BS, Benjamin BI: Splenectomy: Indication and results in hematologic disorders. Ann Surg 159:695–710, 1964

Sarin CL, Nohl-Oser HC: Mediastinoscopy: A clinical evaluation of 400 consecutive cases. Thorax 24:585–588, 1969

Scerbo J, Keltz H, Stone DJ: A prospective study of closed pleural biopsies. JAMA 218:377–380, 1971

Schiff P, Warren BA: Scalene node biopsy: Its value as a diagnostic aid in chest diseases. Dis Chest 32:198–206, 1957

Scott RB: The surgical aspects of the lymphomata. Ann R Coll Surg Engl 22:178–196, 1958

Shields TW, Lees WM, Fox RT: The diagnostic value of biopsy of nonpalpable scalene lymph nodes in chest diseases. Ann Surg 148:184–188, 1958

Silverberg IJ, Jacobs EM: Treatment of spinal cord compression in Hodgkin's disease. Cancer 27:308–313, 1971

Skarin AT, Davey FR, Moloney WC: Lymphosarcoma of the spleen: Results of diagnostic splenectomy in 11 patients. Arch Intern Med 127:259–265, 1971

Slaughter DP, Economou SG, Southwick HW: Surgical management of Hodgkin's disease. Ann Surg 148:705–710, 1958

Sokal JE, Shimaoka K: Pyrogen in the urine of febrile patients with Hodgkin's disease. Nature 215:1183–1185, 1967

Steel SJ: Hodgkin's disease of the lung with cavitation. Am Rev Respir Dis 89:736–744, 1964

Stemmer EA, Calvin JW, Chandor SB, et al: Mediastinal biopsy for indeterminate pulmonary and mediastinal lesions. J Thorac Cardiovasc Surg 49:405–411, 1965

Steemmer EA, Calvin JW, Steedman RA, et al: Parasternal mediastinal exploration to evaluate resectability of thoracic neoplasms. Ann Thorac Surg 12:375–384, 1971

Strum SB, Park JK, Rappaport H: Observation of cells resembling Sternberg-Reed cells in conditions other than Hodgkin's disease. Cancer 26:176–190, 1970

Symmers WS Sr: Survey of the eventual diagnosis in 600 cases referred for a second histological opinion after an initial biopsy diagnosis of Hodgkin's disease. J Clin Pathol 21:650–653, 1968a

Symmers WS Sr: Survey of the eventual diagnosis in 226 cases referred for a second histological opinion after an initial biopsy diagnosis of reticulum cell sarcoma. J Clin Pathol 21:654–655, 1968b

Tindle BH, Parker JW, Lukes RJ: "Reed-Sternberg cells" in infectious mononucleosis? Am J Clin Pathol 58:607–617, 1972

Trinkle JK, Bryant LR, Malette WG, et al: Mediastinoscopy-diagnostic value compared to bronchoscopy: Scalene biopsy and sputum cytology in 155 patients. Am Surg 34:740–743, 1968

Van Heerden JA, Harrison EG Jr, Bernatz PE, et al: Mediastinal malignant lymphoma. Chest 57:518–529, 1970

Variakojis D, Fennessy JJ, Rappaport H: Diagnosis of Hodgkin's disease by bronchial brush biopsy. Chest 61:326– 330, 1972

Variakojis D, Strum SB, Rappaport H: Foamy macrophages in Hodgkin's disease. Arch Pathol 93:453–456, 1972

Wallace S: Newer radiodiagnostic contributions to the study of the lymphoma patient. Leukemia-Lymphoma. Chicago, Year Book, 1970, pp 223–239

Ward PH, Stephenson SE, Harris PF: Mediastinoscopy: A new challenge for the endoscopist. Eye Ear Nose Throat Mon 48:159–161, 1969

Wee GC, Hagen G, Torres A, et al: Hodgkin's disease of the cystic node as a cause of nonvisualization of the gallbladder. Am J Gastroenterol 54:272–276, 1970

Williams RD: Abdominal cancer and fever of undetermined origin. CA 16:83–85, 1966

Williams RD, Andrews NC, Zanes RP Jr: Major surgery in Hodgkin's disease. Surg Gynecol Obstet 93:636–640, 1951

Wilson PR, Nishiyama RH: Lymph nodal Kaposi's sarcoma and chronic lymphocytic leukemia associated with a hepatic nodule simulating Hodgkin's disease. Cancer 27:1419–1425, 1971

Wolstenholme GE, Birch J (eds): Pyrogens and Fever. Edinburgh, London, Churchill Livingston, 1971

Wroblewski F, Pack GT, LaDue JS: Indications for exploratory laparotomy in obscure clinical abdominal disease. NY State J Med 54:2073–2077, 1954

Young CW, Hodas S, Bittar E: Studies on fever in Hodgkin's disease. Clin Bull 2:72, 1972

Zajicek J, Engzell U, Franzén S: Aspiration biopsy of lymphnodes in diagnosis and research, in Rüttimann (ed): Progress in Lymphology, vol 1. Stuttgart, Thieme, 1967, pp 262–264

5

Major Surgery
in Malignant Lymphoma

OVERALL ROLE

Surgery as treatment for malignant lymphoma has never been practiced widely. Peters (1968) reviewed the historic evolution of the clinical concepts and modes of treatment of Hodgkin's disease and described four phases (similar accounts could also be given for the non-Hodgkin's lymphoma). During the early period before 1900, the majority of observations depicted Hodgkin's disease as a fatal illness of suspected infectious origin. From 1900 to 1930, the prevailing attitude was still one of hopelessness in spite of reported improved survival rate and occasional patients who had long-term survival following either a radical lymphadenectomy or radiation therapy. During the third period (1930–1960), there were two advancements in the treatment of malignant lymphomas: (1) the change of radiotherapy from the status of a technical art to that of a precise medicophysical science; (2) the introduction of chemotherapy as a palliative treatment in advanced cases and as supplemental treatment following or prior to radiotherapy in patients who had rapidly progressive disease. The limitations of surgery in the treatment of malignant lymphoma were recognized. Long-term survivors following radical surgery were found only when the patients happened to present with localized lesions, or if early disease was discovered accidentally in extranodal sites. During the period since 1960, the attitude toward Hodgkin's disease has transformed gradually into one of optimism, and physicians now speak of "cures" in spite of an element of uncertainty. In addition to technical advances of radiotherapeutic equipment, which made aggressive treatment plans possible, newer chemotherapeutic agents and combination drug therapy programs have achieved dramatic gains in objective and subjective responses.

159

Since the report of Glatstein et al (1969), use of the exploratory laparotomy and splenectomy as a pretherapy staging technique to delineate the intraabdominal involvement has been widely accepted and practiced in patients with Hodgkin's disease. Hass et al (1971) and Hanks et al (1972) also utilized staging laparotomies in patients with non-Hodgkin's lymphomas.

Present therapy of lymphomas involving lymph-node-bearing areas (stages I, II, III) consists of various schedules of intensive and extensive irradiation. Patients with stage IV disease and many of those with stage III non-Hodgkin's lymphoma are usually treated by chemotherapy (Fridman and Ezdinli 1971). Although surgery is rarely employed now as the definitive treatment of these disorders, pretreatment surgical staging has been gaining popularity. This aspect tends to overshadow the other roles of surgery in the management of patients with malignant lymphoma. We believe major surgical procedures will always be essential in the diagnosis of lesions that present initially in the abdominal or thoracic cavities, especially the extranodal malignant lymphomas. In addition, surgery also is important in the treatment of complications and new conditions encountered in the course of the diseases.

Ellis Fischel State Cancer Hospital Experiences

To have an overall balanced view and to define the role of surgery in the management of patients with Hodgkin's disease and other malignant lymphomas, a retrospective and all-inclusive study of 527 patients seen and treated in our hospital (EFSCH) from 1940 to 1971 was carried out. There were 163 patients with Hodgkin's disease and 364 with other lymphomas. Clinical characteristics and pathological details were described in Chapter 1.

The indications for surgery and the types of operations performed are listed in Table 5-1. It can be seen that almost 1 out of every 5 patients with Hodgkin's disease and 1 out of every 3 patients with other lymphomas had various major procedures. In patients with non-Hodgkin's lymphoma, a high proportion (50 percent) had more than one operation. Also in patients with other lymphomas, the percentage of patients who required major surgery for diagnosis is high (20 percent). Since this is a retrospective study, and since we do not have a protocol to use staging laparotomy routinely (1969–1971 only 15 patients had staging operation), the experiences reported here essentially represent the multiple roles of surgery excluding exploratory laparotomy with multiple tissue biopsies and splenectomy.

Thirty of the 163 patients with Hodgkin's disease (18.4 percent) had 32 operations, and 109 of the 364 patients (29.9 percent) with non-Hodgkin's disease had 146 major surgical procedures (excluding peripheral node biopsy and including procedures requiring more than local anesthesia). A total of 178 separate operations were performed on 139 patients (average 1.3/patient).

Table 5-1
Surgical Operations in Patients with Malignant Lymphoma (EFSCH series)

	Hodgkin's disease	Lymphoma
Operation for diagnosis		
Celiotomy and biopsy	4	29
Celiotomy and by-pass		5
Celiotomy and resection		21
Radical mastectomy	1	3
Radical node dissection	2	5
Laminectomy		4
Thoracotomy		3
Non-nodal biopsy	1	4
	7	74
Operation for staging		
Pretherapy	8	2
Posttherapy	4	1
	12	3
Operation as therapy		
Wide excision		8
Postradiotherapy nodal dissection		2
		10
Operation for complication		
Nonmalignant	3	20
Malignant		
GI complication	2	11
Splenectomy	4	—
Others	3	9
Radiotherapy complication		8
	12	48
Operation for second cancer	1	11
Total	32 (30)*	146(109)

*Number of patients in parenthesis.

According to organ sites and surgical specialties, these 178 operations can be listed as 116 abdominal operations (including 4 operations on the uterus), 6 radical mastectomies, 11 radical node dissections, 5 laminectomies, 4 thoracotomies, 3 bone operations, and 33 various other surgical procedures.

A total of 101 procedures were carried out initially for diagnosis and 42 of these had radical excision (Table 5-2). Of the 86 operations done initially on 84 patients with non-Hodgkin's lymphoma, there were 2 for staging, 34 diagnostic celiotomies and biopsies, 11 other diagnostic operations, and 39 for diagnosis and resection. Among the 39 resections, 9 were gastrectomes; 4 each of resections of small bowel or colon; 2, splenectomies; 2, hysterectomies; 3, radical mastectomies; 7, radical node dissections, and 8, wide excisions. Fifteen operations done before therapy on patients with

Table 5-2

Distribution of Initial Major Operations for Diagnosis of Malignant Lymphomas (EFSCH series)

		Non-Hodgkin's Lymphoma		Hodgkin's Disease	
		Diagnosis	*Diagnosis and resection*	*Diagnosis*	*Diagnosis and resection*
Abdominal operations					
Biopsy					
Mesentery	8 ⎫				
Retroperitoneum	8 ⎪				
Both	5 ⎬	29		1	
Stomach	3 ⎪				
Others	5 ⎭			2	
Staging		3*		12*	
Gastrectomy			9		
Bowel resection			4		
Colon resection			4		
Decompression		5			
Splenectomy			2		
Hysterectomy			2		
Appendectomy				1	
		37	21	16	0
Nonabdominal operations					
Radical mastectomy			3		1
Radical node dissection			7		2
Laminectomy		4			
Thoracotomy		3			
Bone operation		1			
Wide excision		3	8		
		11	18	0	3
Total		48	39	16	3
Postoperative complication		3	5	1	
Postoperative death		3	1		

*One patient with non-Hodgkin's disease and 4 with Hodgkin's disease had staging laparotomy after receiving therapy.

Hodgkin's disease included 8 for staging, 4 exploratory celiotomies for diagnosis, 2 radical node dissections, and 1 radical mastectomy.

After the diagnosis was established, another 77 operations were performed either for disease complications or for additional cancer (Table 5-3). Seventeen operations were carried out among the patients with Hodgkin's disease; 9 for malignant complications, 4 for staging of recurrent lesions, 3 for nonmalignant lesions, and one for secondary cancer. Among the non-Hodgkin's patients 60 operations were performed: one laparotomy for late staging, 20 operations for malignant complications, 8 for radiotherapy complications, 20 for nonmalignant lesions, and 11 for secondary cancers. Among the secondary cancers there were 2 patients each with cancers of the lung, breast, and uterine cervix, and 1 patient each with neoplasms of the bladder, lip, rectum, pyriform sinus, and thyroid.

The postoperative morbidity and mortality are related to the indication and type of operation performed. There were 14 morbidities among the 178 operations representing an incidence of 7.9 percent. The individual morbidity rate was 3 percent for those with Hodgkin's disease and 9 percent for the other lymphomas. The overall mortality rate was 7.2 percent (10/139). Three of the 30 Hodgkin's patients who had operations died postoperatively, and 7 of the 109 non-Hodgkin's patients expired. Details of the postoperative complications and deaths are listed in Table 5-4. It is apparent that diagnostic resection of the colon or decompression for obstructive lymphomatous lesions of the gastrointestinal tract carried the highest chance of wound complications. Operations for malignant complications in general carried more morbidities and mortalities (5 of 29 [17 percent] had morbidity and 6 of 29 [21 percent] died postoperatively). To put the data differently, all 6 postoperative deaths occurred in patients who had surgery for malignant complications.

Literature Review

There are very few reports dealing with the overall role of surgery in the management of patients with malignant lymphoma. Data from the literature are compared with our present series and presented in Table 5-5.

Since radiotherapy has now become the standard treatment for localized malignant lymphoma, it is surprising that Hellwig (1947) reported surgical therapy was initially employed with the intention of effecting a cure in 67 of 130 cases with various subtypes of lymphoma. Williams et al (1951) reported 31 of 240 patients with Hodgkin's disease needed 35 major surgical procedures (an incidence rate of 12.9 percent). Only 1 patient had radical neck dissection for cure, whereas 11 had surgery for diagnosis, 16 for treatment of malignant complications, and 7 for unrelated conditions. Included in the 34 major operations were 23 celiotomies, 6 thoracotomies, 3 laminectomies, 1 mastectomy, and 1 drainage of abscess. They pointed out that major surgery did not accelerate the course of Hodgkin's disease and such patients tolerated operative procedures well, except in those cases in which the disease is generalized or terminal.

Rosenberg et al (1961) reported a large series of 1269 patients with non-Hodgkin's lymphoma. Seventy-six patients underwent radical operations for possible cure with 13.1 percent developed postoperative complications. Among the 76 cases treated surgically, 29 were node dissections, 21 were gastrectomies, 6 were bowel resections, 1 was pelvic exenteration,

Table 5-3
Distribution of Major Operations for Subsequent Complications and Additional Cancers (EFSCH series)

| | | Non-Hodgkin's Lymphoma | | | Hodgkin's Disease | | |
| | | Complication | | | Complication | | |
	Radio-therapy	Malignant	Non-malignant	Second cancer	Malignant	Non-malignant	Second cancer
Abdominal operations							
Biopsy	1	2			1		
Bowel resection		2	2		1		
Colon resection		1					
Decompression		9	1	1			
Splenectomy		1			4		
Operation on uterus						1	
Cholecystectomy			4	1			
Adhesionolysis			3				
Appendectomy			1			1	
Vagotomy and pyloroplasty			1			1	
Aortic aneurysmectomy			1				
Clipping internal vena cava			1				
	1	15	14	2	6	3	0
Nonabdominal operations							
Radical mastectomy				2			
Radical node dissection				2			
Laminectomy					1		
Thoracotomy				1			
Bone operation		2					

Others							
Wide excision	6	3	6		1		1
Tracheostomy/bronchoscopy					1		1
Herniorrhaphy	1						
B-K amputation				1			
Thyroid lobectomy					1		
Cone cervix	$\frac{7}{}$	$\frac{5}{}$	$\frac{6}{}$	$\frac{1}{9}$	$\frac{3}{}$	$\frac{0}{}$	$\frac{1}{1}$
Total	8	20	20	11	9	3	1
Postoperative complication	5	5			3		
Postoperative death	3	3			3		

Table 5-4
Postoperative Complications in Operations for Malignant Lymphoma (EFSCH series)

Category	Operation	No. of Operations	Complication		Postoperative death	
			No.	Type	Internal (days)	Cause
Hodgkin's disease						
Diagnosis	Appendectomy	1	1	Wound infection		
Malignant complication	Late splenectomy	4			8	Carcinomatosis
	GI perforation	1			14	Septicemia (moniliasis)
	Jaundice	1			14	Pneumonia, pancreatitis
	Others	3				
Non-Hodgkin's lymphoma						
Diagnosis	Exploration	29	1	Wound infection	8	Myocardial infarction
	Staging	3	1	Pneumothorax	9	Carcinomatosis
	Decompression	5	1	Wound dehiscence	9	Aspiration
	Bone biopsy	1			1	GI bleeding
Diagnosis and resection	Gastrectomy	9	1	Wound infection		
	Colectomy	4	1	abdominal abscess		
	Other abdominal resection	8	1	Subphrenic abscess		
	Wide excision	8	1	Lymph leakage for 3 weeks		
	Radical mastectomy	3	1	Wound abscess		
	Splenectomy	1	1	Re-explore for bleeding		
Malignant complication	GI operation	12	2	Wound infection	3	GI bleeding
	Other complication	7	2	Wound infection	14	Bleeding
					7	Septicemia

166

and 19 were other procedures. There was no mention of how many patients needed surgical consultation for complications, but they commented that intestinal or tracheal obstruction, perforation of abdominal viscus, gastrointestinal hemorrhage, obstructive jaundice, and radiation ulcerations of skin and eye needed surgical intervention.

Molander and Pack (1963) reported that in a series of 567 patients with non-Hodgkin's disease, 42 patients had curative surgical resections for unifocal disease and 10 had palliative surgery. The 42 surgical treatments for non-Hodgkin's lymphoma included 19 radical node dissections, 9 gastric resections, 6 small bowel and 3 large bowel resections, 2 segmental operations on lungs, 1 hysterectomy, 1 splenectomy and 1 partial hepatic lobectomy. Pack and Molander (1966) reported another series of 316 patients with Hodgkin's disease, 12 of whom had curative and 12 of whom had palliative surgical procedures. Eleven of the 12 surgical procedures for treatment of unicentric Hodgkin's disease were radical node dissections, and the 12th was segmental excision of the lung. In both series almost all the palliative procedures were related to malignant lymphomas and included 11 for intestinal obstruction, 4 for gastric hemorrhage, 4 for removal of bulky retroperitoneal mass, 2 splenectomies, and 1 portacaval shunt.

By the use of lymphangiography, inferior venacavography and intravenous pyelography, Lee et al (1964) found unifocal lymphosarcoma and reticulum cell sarcoma appeared to occur more frequently in patients with the following clinical patterns of disease: reticulum cell sarcoma presenting in a single bone; lymphosarcoma or reticulum cell sarcoma in a solitary focus high in the neck or in the head; and lesions primary in an extranodal site, most commonly the gastrointestinal tract. In such cases, they felt that obliterative local radiotherapy, and occasionally surgery with intent to cure, should be carried out. Peters (1965) also commented that the treatment of choice for stages I and IIA Hodgkin's disease involving groups of lymph nodes is radical irradiation. But if the site happens to be extranodal, e.g., the intestinal tract, a salivary gland, or extradural involvement, the treatment of choice might be radical surgery. For some of the latter sites it is probably wise to supplement the surgical excision with irradiation to areas of immediate lymphatic drainage.

Newall et al (1968) showed that 69 of 91 (more than 75 percent) of the patients with the diagnosis of reticulum cell sarcoma had extranodal lesions as sites of first presentation. Even among the 22 patients who had lymph node disease before treatment, 6 presented with mesenteric or retroperitoneal nodes and 4 required laparotomy for diagnosis (Newall and Friedman 1970). The prognosis of patients who had abdominal nodes at the onset was much better than those who had superficial nodes.

Banfi et al (1968a,b) studied 500 consecutive untreated patients with malignant lymphoma. Initially 99.5 percent of those with Hodgkin's disease, had involvement of the nodes and spleen (11 percent were of para-aortic nodes). But in patients with non-Hodgkin's lymphoma, about 12 percent had extranodal disease, 6 percent had para-aortic disease and 11 percent had iliac disease. They pointed out that extranodal disease was more common in children. Jenkin et al (1969) reported that about one-third of children with non-Hodgkin's lymphoma had primary lesions of the gastrointestinal tract.

According to several of the largest series of malignant lymphomas reported in the literature (Table 5-5), about 11.4 to 16.7 percent of the patients had abdominal nodes or gastrointestinal lesions as the initial focus of disease and up to 9.1 percent had disease in intrathoracic organs or bone. In patients with Hodgkin's disease, Peters et al (1968) reported that 4 percent had paraaortic node lesions and 9 percent had lesions of the extranodal organs as first recognized sites of involvement (including gastrointestinal tract and pharynx, 4 percent). For patients with non-Hodgkin's lymphoma 7 percent had paraaortic nodes. Among 270 reticulum cell sarcoma and 631 lymphosarcoma patients, 61 percent and 40 percent, respectively, had extranodal presentations, including those of gastrointestinal tract and pharynx, 37 percent and 22 percent. Details of extranodal involvement as reported by Peters et al (1968) and in the present EFSCH series are presented in Table 1-7 on pp 30–31.

In 340 biopsy-proven, untreated Hodgkin's patients who had the most exhaustive evaluative procedures of lymphangiogram, bone-marrow biopsy, pulmonary and mediastinal tomogram, liver function tests, and in some instances, laparotomy and biopsy of the liver and retroperitoneal nodes, Kaplan (1972) reported that the number of patients who had involvement of extranodal sites were as follows: lung parenchymas 20; pleura, 11; liver, 9; marrow, 7; pericardium, 5; bone, 4; and epidural space, 2. In addition to staging laparotomy, he commented that thoracotomy might be required in an occasional patient for biopsy of mediastinal nodes or for biopsy of pleural or pulmonary nodules. Laminectomy is usually indicated for decompression in patients with progressive spinal cord compression or in occasional instances in which neurologic abnormality was the initial presenting manifestation and no prior tissue diagnosis exists. In rare cases of apparently primary extranodal Hodgkin's disease arising in organs such as the stomach, small intestine, or thyroid, he felt that surgical resection followed by radiotherapy appeared to be the treatment of choice. Regarding surgical procedure for complications, 8 of 41 of his patients who received 2 or more courses of radiation therapy over the mediastinum developed radiation-induced heart disease. Pericardectomy for alleviation of constrictive manifestation was required in 2 of the 5 cases with severe symptoms.

An overall view of the distribution of extranodal lesions occurring in patients with non-Hodgkin's lymphoma can be obtained from the largest series reported by Freeman et al (1972) and presented in Table 5-6. These data were collected by the End Results Group of the National Cancer

Table 5-5
Major Surgery and Sites of Unusual Presentations in Patients with Malignant Lymphoma

	Hodgkin's disease			Non-Hodgkin's lymphoma		
	Williams et al	Pack and Molander	EFSCH	Molander and Pack	Rosenberg et al	EFSCH
Period of study	1940–1950	1945–1957	1940–1971	1945–1957	1928–1952	1940–1971
No. of patients	240	316	163	567	1,269	364
No. of patients who had operations	31		30			109
No. of operations	35	24	32	52	76	146
No. of early operations						
Staging	0	0	8	0	0	2
Diagnosis	11	ND*	4	ND	ND	45
Curative	1	12	3	42	76	39
No. of follow-up operations						
Staging	0	0	4	0	0	1
Palliative	16	12	9	10	ND	28
Unrelated	71	ND	3	ND	ND	20
Second Cancer	0	ND	1	ND	ND	11
Percentage with unusual presentations						
Abdominal nodes (%)		9.5	0.6	7.0	12.1	9.3
Gastrointestinal tract (%)		1.9	0	8.8	4.6	5.5
Lung/pleura (%)		1.9	0	8.1	0.1	0.8
Bone (%)		1.3	0	1.0	3.8	1.4

*ND = No data reported.

169

Table 5-6
Localized Extranodal Non-Hodgkin's Lymphoma: Specific Sites and Survival Rates (Freeman et al 1972)

					Survival Rates (%)	
System	No. of patients	%	Site	No.	*5-Year*	*10-Year*
Gastrointestinal	541	37	Esophagus	3		
			Stomach	346	39	32
			Small intestine	110	28	28
			Large intestine	82	37	34
Head and neck	417	28	Tonsil	162	40	29
			Adenoid	37	29	28
			Salivary gland	69	67	21
			Thyroid	36	48	25
			Nose	33		
			Orbit	32		
			Larynx	8		
			Oral cavity	40		
Bone and soft tissue	302	20	Bone	69	31	22
			Skin	110	70	64
			Connective tissue	90		
			Breast	33	35	31
Chest	88	6	Lung	53	57	8
			Mediastinum	35		
Urinary	12	1	Kidney	10		
			Bladder	2		
Male genital	28	2	Testis	23	21	31
			Other	5		
Female genital	16	1				
CNS	23	2				
Other sites	40	3				
Total	1467	100			41	33

Institute from 100 hospitals of various types, sizes, and locations in the United States. From 1950 to 1964, a total of 12,447 patients were reported to have malignant lymphoma. In 2194 (18 percent) the lymphomas were said to have originated in sites other than lymph nodes. In 1467 patients with non-Hodgkin's lesions, the extranodal involvement appeared to be localized. Hodgkin's disease was represented by only 90 extranodal tumors. If one-third of the whole series of 12,447 were of Hodgkin's disease, this represented an incidence of 2 percent with extranodal lesions. The incidence rate for non-Hodgkin's lymphoma would be about 25 percent. Detailed discussions of each of the extranodal lesions are presented in Chapters 7–10. The overall survival rates of patients with some of the more common extranodal sites are also presented in Table 5-6. It is to be noted that in this series of 1467 patients, initial treatment was distributed as follows: 35 percent had surgical therapy alone, 31 percent had radiotherapy alone, 25 percent had surgery plus radiotherapy, and 9 percent had chemotherapy or no treatment recorded.

Final Comments

With the wider application of exploratory laparotomy for staging and the improvement of objective response rates and survival results now obtainable with radiotherapy and chemotherapy, it is obvious that the future role of surgery will be quite different from the past. The number of cases receiving radical surgical excision alone has diminished to zero at the present time.

Since about 50 percent of our patients with Hodgkin's disease and about 28 percent with other malignant lymphomas had stage I and stage II disease at the time of diagnosis, and if pretherapy exploratory laparotomy is practiced routinely on patients with early malignant lymphomas, it is clear that the proportion of patients having surgical procedures, particularly for staging purposes, will probably be more than 30 percent in the future (pp. 127–128). However, we feel major operations still may be required for the initial diagnosis and therapy in a certain number of patients whose disease is not present in one of the peripheral lymph nodes. At the time of diagnosis in the present EFSCH series, 25 percent of those with Hodgkin's disease had extranodal involvement and 49 percent of those with non-Hodgkin's lymphoma did also (including 8 percent whose viscera lesions appeared to be unifocal).

It is not known whether complications secondary to malignant lymphoma itself will decrease after the current trend of aggressive therapy or not. However, both radiotherapy and chemotherapy have their own complications, and with the prolongation of life, other unrelated conditions and secondary cancers might develop (pp. 384–396). Thus major surgery will always be required for a certain proportion of the patients who present with nodal or extranodal disease internally. Surgery will also continue to be important in the diagnosis and management of new conditions related or unrelated to lymphomas.

SURGICAL TREATMENT OF PERIPHERAL ADENOPATHY

Historical Review

The discovery of x-rays in 1896 by Roentgen was followed by the finding of their effectiveness in treating certain blood and hematopoietic diseases. As early as 1902, Pusey and Senn observed success in the treatment of various lymph node swellings, including Hodgkin's disease (cited by Anglesio 1969). In 1917, Yates and Bunting were the first to champion the surgical removal of localized Hodgkin's disease. They also warned: "If extirpation is not to be complete, it should not be attempted." Apparently, Yates became very skilled in the technique of lymph node excision and had few untoward reactions following wide removal of nodes. Willis (quoted by Guerriero, 1931) related that Yates treated the former's son for Hodgkin's disease by removal of nodes all over the body followed by administration of anti-diphtheroid horse serum in large quantities. The patient recovered completely and had no recurrence at the time of the report, 16 years later.

Since then, the role of surgical therapy for peripheral adenopathy in malignant lymphomas has been a controversial issue. To date there has been no controlled study published that permits comparison of surgical removal with irradiation therapy or with a combination of the two. Thus, when comparative data are quoted here, they come from uncontrolled and heterogeneous series.

Although today surgery alone has no place in the treatment of malignant lymphoma, for historical interest, a review of the pros and cons of this therapeutic modality over the past 30 years is given below.

In 1940, Baker and Mann reported two cases of cervical Hodgkin's disease in which the patients had been free of disease for periods of 10 and 12 years after radical removal and postoperative irradiation. Sugarbaker and Craver (1940) reported a series of 196 cases with either reticulum cell sarcoma or lymphosarcoma. Twenty-five patients had some extirpative procedure plus radiation (12 had nodal dissection, 11 had extranodal lesions removed, and 2 underwent both procedures). The overall 5-year cure rate was 24 percent. In 1942, Slaughter and Craver questioned the concept that Hodgkin's disease was inevitably fatal when they found four long-term survivors who were free of disease and who were accidentally treated with surgery because of a mistaken diagnosis.

Gall and Mallory (1942) found that about 10 percent of cases of malignant lymphoma had localized lesions accessible for surgical excision at the time of autopsy. In a series of 618 cases, 77 were treated with surgery. Excluding 44 patients who had diseases extending beyond the limits of eradication at the time of operation and 10 who died postoperatively, the remaining 23 patients survived an average of 7 years after the onset of their disease. Gall (1943) reported on 48 patients with malignant lymphoma who had radical surgical excision; 21 patients also had prophylactic irradiation in amounts varying from 600 to 1800 rads. Seventeen patients had node dissection and 31 had surgery for extranodal and visceral diseases. Despite 5 postoperative deaths, the 5-year survival rate was 45 percent. For the 11 cases of Hodgkin's disease treated surgically, the median survival was 5.4 years after surgery and 3.2 years after x-ray therapy.

In 1947, Jackson and Parker stated that there were no valid grounds for assuming that malignant lymphoma represented a systemic disease at its onset; and surgical excision of localized lymphoma, when possible, seemed to result in the longest survivors and some apparent cures. Hellwig (1947) reported a series of 130 cases of malignant lymphoma. Surgical therapy was initially employed in 67 cases with the intention of effecting a cure. Of the 21 patients who had no postoperative x-ray therapy, 12 (57 percent) survived 5 years or longer free of disease. Of the 40 patients who had adequate postoperative radiation, 18 patients survived. He felt radical surgery alone offered an excellent choice of cure in selected cases. On the other hand, Stout (1947) found in 119 cases of non-Hodgkin's lymphomas that 15 (12.7 percent) lived more than 10 years. Seven patients were treated by radiotherapy alone, 3 by surgery, and 5 by surgery followed by radiotherapy. He felt there was no evidence that surgery with or without postoperative radiotherapy resulted in more cures or longer survival than radiotherapy alone.

Williams et al (1951) reported 35 major operations performed on 31 patients among the 240 hospitalized for Hodgkin's disease. One patient was treated with radical neck dissection; he was free of disease 8.5 years later. In 1951, Craver commented on the therapy of Hodgkin's disease: "If the disease is detected while still apparently restricted to one site, and if this early focus is accessible for surgical removal, one may always consider radical surgery as the primary treatment." It was known that those patients with disease clinically localized to one lymph node group and without systemic symptoms had the best long-term prognosis among all the patients.

Hall and Olsen (1956) pointed out that patients with Hodgkin's disease apparently might be free of disease for periods of up to 25 years after a biopsy with or without subsequent roentgenotherapy, and then have recurrences. On the other hand, they felt that patients with lymphosarcoma are less likely to have long, asymptomatic remissions. And a 5- to 10-year remission without evidence of disease is more likely to represent eradication of the disease in a patient with lymphosarcoma than in one with Hodgkin's disease. However, others (Slaughter 1965; Catlin 1966) felt that Hodgkin's disease could remain localized longer than other types of lymphoma, and that the results of surgical treatment were more favorable.

In 1958, Slaughter et al reported 18 patients with localized Hodgkin's disease treated surgically; 10 had postoperative radiotherapy of less than 1200 rads. Seven of the 11 patients who were disease-free for 6 to 14 years had only surgical treatment. He commented that if radical surgery were equally effective as radical radiotherapy, then surgery should be preferable in the young to middle-age groups because "The effects of radiation are both permanent and progressive, whereas the effect of surgery is only permanent." In the same paper, while reporting that localized Hodgkin's disease can be treated surgically with good result, they reported no 5-year arrest in 22 reticulum cell sarcoma and lymphosarcoma patients who had radical neck dissections. However, Kremen, in discussion of Slaughter's paper, reported four 5-year non-Hodgkin's cures, including 3 cases of neck and

1 case of groin lesions treated by radical node dissections. Rosenberg et al (1958) studied lymphosarcoma in childhood and commented that they believed any child with lymphosarcoma in an apparent localized site, whether nodal or extranodal, deserves every attempt at surgical and radiological eradication of the disease. Dargeon (1961) noted that 15 of 75 children seen with lymphosarcoma between 1926 and 1959 were alive for more than 5 years; 9 were treated primarily by operative means, 3 had operation and radiation therapy, and 1, operation and chemotherapy.

In 1958, Diamond pointed out various guidelines in selecting patients with Hodgkin's disease for radical surgery: "When the sole evidence of disease is on one side of the neck, radical neck dissection should be undertaken only when such disease is superior to an imaginary line bisecting the neck horizontally at the midpoint of another imaginary line drawn from the mastoid eminence of the temporal bone to the midportion of the clavicle. If the mass is at or inferior to this axis point, surgery should not be selected. In the axilla, the disease should be confined to the lower portion of the axilla and not up near or in the apex. In the groin, radical groin dissection is elected only for clinical class I cases with palpable femoral nodes or a femoral mass but no enlarged inguinal nodes."

Craver (1964) believed that when adenopathy of Hodgkin's disease first appeared in the axilla or groin there should be suspicion of disease within the thoracic cavity or the abdomen respectively. He also speculated that when the first enlarged nodes appear at the base of the left side of the neck, the disease may have started internally, having been carried through the thoracic duct (Slaughter and Craver 1942).

However, Slaughter (1965) disagreed with this dictum that nodal involvement in the low neck precluded surgery, because several of his 5- to 20-year survivals had retroclavicular disease removed by neck dissection. Unfortunately, his reports did not specify whether the adenopathy was located in the right or left side. Pack and Molander (1966) commented that it seemed strange that Diamond, an internist, should attempt to instruct surgeons concerning the limitations in selecting patients for radical surgery by proposing two imaginary lines in the neck.

Smith and Klopp (1961) and Klopp (1968) reported a series of 54 patients with localized lymphomas. The 5-year survival rates of those treated by surgery alone, by surgery plus irradiation, and by irradiation alone were 75 percent, 50 percent, and 10 percent, respectively. For the 31 patients with Hodgkin's disease the 5-year cure rate was 56 percent for the surgical group as contrasted to 9 percent for the irradiated group. For lymphoma of the peripheral lymph node, there was a 90 percent 5-year survival rate in patients treated surgically as contrasted to 19 percent for those treated by x-ray.

Lacher (1963) compared survival rates in 11 Hodgkin's patients treated surgically, 8 also had postoperative radiotherapy, with the total 93 stage

I patients and found the 5-year survival rates were similar (63.6 percent versus 65.6 percent). He emphasized that the argument in favor of radical surgery in Hodgkin's disease remained equivocal and the advantages seemed obscure. Molander (1969) pointed out that some of the non-surgical patients of Lacher had other types of therapy as well, and the findings reported were the work of a heterogeneous group of surgeons. However, Molander did agree with Lacher "That if surgery is elected, it should be combined with postoperative irradiation," using the same dosage factors as for primary irradiation of Hodgkin's disease.

Holloway (1965) reported that 7 of 30 patients with malignant lymphoma seen from 1955 to 1959 underwent operation for the purpose of cure. The 5-year survival rate of the 7 patients was 85 percent, whereas the mean survival of 23 patients not operated upon was 2 years and all were dead within 5 years. Of the 6 long-term survivors, 2 patients with Hodgkin's disease had radical node dissection for lesions of the axilla and neck. Two of the 4 patients with non-Hodgkin's lymphoma had resection of the stomach, 1 had right colectomy and pneumectomy, another had resection of a large retroperitoneal mass.

In 1965, Slaughter reiterated his criteria for confirming the "localized" or "unicentric" lymphomatous involvement as normal chest film, no clinical enlargement of the spleen, normal blood counts without eosinophilia, lack of fever or generalized pruritus, and normal lymphangiogram of the femoral to retroperitoneal nodes. He reported that 10 of the original 11 patients reported in 1958 stayed well for 12–20 years (ond died 11 years postoperatively of multiple sclerosis). In addition, 16 more patients achieved 5-year survival status after radical neck dissection. The percentage of disease-free survival remained the same (60 percent) and only half of the patients received postoperative radiotherapy.

Molander and Pack (1963, 1965) reported that the best survival of patients with malignant lymphoma was found in the few patients who were eligible for an initial radical surgical approach followed by postoperative radiotherapy of 3000 to 3600 rads. The results of Hodgkin's disease and non-Hodgkin's lymphomas were quite similar: Of 12 patients with Hodgkin's disease, 66.6 percent survived 5 years; of 42 patients with other lymphomas (23 were for excision of visceral lesions) 62 percent survived 5 years. The corresponding figures for patients treated initially with irradiation were 37.5 percent and 35 percent, respectively. The 10-year survival rate of the 12 patients with Hodgkin's disease was 60 percent, while 62 patients unsuitable for surgical therapy and treated with x-ray alone had a rate of 10 percent. There were no recurrences in the operated group (Pack and Molander 1966).

Molander and Pack commented that the proportion of patients with Hodgkin's disease suitable for surgical treatment was small (12/316 = 4 percent). But out of the 316 patients, 159 asserted that the initial manifestation of the disease was an enlarged lymph node in one of the 3 superficial regional groups (neck, axilla, and groin). They believed that if peripheral node biopsy was done immediately, cases suitable for radical node dissection could be increased by 1000 percent. Favorable prognostic factors pointed out by them included normal peripheral blood and marrow cell counts; absence of leukocytosis, leukopenia, eosinophilia, and thrombocytopenia; early surgical intervention for stage I disease or unicentric bulky growth; and the histologic type of nodular sclerosis. Factors contraindicating curative surgical efforts were primary abdominal disease; fever; splenomegaly; multiple regions of nodal involvement; severe pruritus; and antecedent acute infection.

Catlin (1966) reported that 36.5 percent of 249 patients with head and neck lymphoma had surgery. Out of the 91 patients who had some definitive surgery, 48 percent survived 5 years. Out of 49 neck dissections, 23 patients were free of recurrence for over 5 years (10 Hodgkin's disease, 7 lymphosarcoma, and 6 reticulum cell sarcoma). He listed 5 of the more common and important indications for surgical intervention: (1) bulky lymph nodes in only one side of the upper neck; (2) many localized thyroid and parotid gland tumors; (3) infection and/or obstruction in tumors involving the nasal cavity and paranasal sinuses; (4) residual lymphoma which failed to respond to x-ray treatment; and (5) inability to establish accurate diagnosis, despite several preoperative biopsies.

Schamaun (1967) mentioned 8 patients who had radical excision of cervical, axillary, supraclavicular, or mediastinal nodes for Hodgkin's disease. All patients had other manifestations of the disease subsequently despite postoperative irradiation or chemotherapy. Four patients died 2, 3, 5, and 5.5 years after surgery. Four patients were still living at 5, 6, 7, and 7.5 years after surgery.

The current role of surgery in treating peripheral adenopathy of malignant lymphoma appears to be rather limited. Bonadonna (1971) commented that, although the reported results of surgical therapy were satisfactory (the 5-year survival rate being in the range of 75 percent–80 percent), "At the present time, with high-energy radiation equipment available, the surgical treatment of stage I cases has been practically abandoned because intensive irradiation of the upper or lower trunk lymphoid regions can yield equivalent results, and has the advantage of allowing a precautionary irradiation of the adjacent areas." Kaplan (1972) agreed with such a view, but he said that in isolated instances, recurrences after tumoricidal radiotherapy might sometimes be controlled by limited excisional surgery. Patterson (1973) emphasized that the surgeon and the radiotherapist must be allies, and for the present, there is no good case for purposing a radical dissection of stage I Hodgkin's disease in the neck, axilla, or groin.

Scope of Surgical Excision of Peripheral Adenopathy

The scope of surgical exenteration of localized Hodgkin's disease in the lymph nodes of the neck, axilla, and groin as described by Pack and Molander (1966) are as follows: "The radical neck dissection includes the removal of the sternocleidomastoid, omohyoid, and platysma muscles, the internal jugular vein, the adventitial coat of the carotid artery and all of the lymphoid and areolar tissues in the neck, including the unilateral triangles. In dissecting the involved axilla, the pectoralis major and minor muscles are removed and the axilla freed of all lymph nodes from the apical region down to and including the subscapular nodes, sparing only the long thoracic and subscapular nerves. In groin dissections, a liberal ellipse of skin is sacrificed, the skin flaps dissected widely back, the inguinal ligament temporarily detached from the anterior superior iliac spine, the retroperitoneum entered, and all lymph nodes from the bifurcation of the aorta dissected downward to include the iliac, obturator, inguinal, and femoral groups. In some instances postirradiation dissection is indicated for the removal of nodes that have become resistant to irradiation."

On the conservative side, Smith and Klopp (1961) pointed out that radical surgical therapy did not appear to be better than complete total excision of all localized lymphoma, especially for cases of giant follicular lymphomas. There are many cases recorded that were controlled by excisnal biopsy. Among a series of 65 patients with Hodgkin's disease reported by Hall and Olson (1956), one patient with Hodgkin's paragranuloma was free of disease 146 months after a biopsy and another case, also in remission, was treated with roentgenotherapy for a recurrence 8 years after the initial local excision. Dawson and Harrison (1961) reported 44 cases of so-called "benign Hodgkin's disease," which was characterized histologically by the presence of Reed-Sternberg cells in a background of mature lymphocytes intermingled with a small number of reticulum cells. The prognosis was good: 93 percent of the patients survived 5 years and 85 percent 10 years. Local excision was the only form of initial therapy in 14 patients and 1 patient had radical node dissection. In 11 of these, the disease recurred at the same site after intervals varying from 1 to 13 years, and the remainder of the patients were free from disease 1, 4, 4, and 20 years later.

Craver (1964, 1968) said Hodgkin's disease was known to relapse after an interval of 15 to 17 years of apparent remission. Thus, something more in the order of a 20-year disease-free interval should be demanded as an approximation of a measure of cure for Hodgkin's disease.

Non-Hodgkin's lymphoma could have long-term cure with either limited or radical operations too. Catlin (1966) reported an 11-year-old boy who had simple excision of 2 solitary nodes of lymphosarcoma in both sides of the upper neck. He was well 13 years later without further treatment. Another remarkable case was that of a 33-year-old man who had an ulcerative tumor in the right tonsil with neck adenopathy. Preoperative of the biopsy mass suggested anaplastic carcinoma. An uncomplicated right tonsillectomy and "commando" operation were done. The final diagnosis was reticulum cell sarcoma of the tonsil and neck nodes. Postoperative x-ray therapy was discussed, but never given. Two months after the operation, enlarged nodes appeared in the left side of the neck, and a dissection was done for metastatic sarcoma. The patient was well 13 years later without any additional therapy.

Results of Surgical Treatment of Peripheral Adenopathy

All of the patients that had radical surgical treatment of peripheral adenopathy as published in the English literature were reviewed. Those series that gave enough description of the anatomical location and pathological classification of the adenopathies are summarized in Tables 5-7 and 5-8. In these selected patients, the overall 5-year survival rate for patients with Hodgkin's disease was 76 percent, and for those with non-Hodgkin's lymphoma, 69 percent. In reference to Craver's warning (1964) that disease appearing in the axilla or groin meant possible disease within the thoracic cavity or the abdomen, it is interesting that Gall (1943), Hellwig (1947), Slaughter et al (1958), Holloway (1965), Molander and Pack (1965), and Pack and Molander (1966) all reported long-term success with surgical therapy of axillary and inguinal nodes with or without postoperative radiotherapy. Werf-Messing (1968) reported a series of 343 patients with reticulum cell sarcoma and lymphosarcoma treated by local radiotherapy. Among the 142 patients with early disease (stage I), 11 patients presented with inguinal adenopathy. During follow-up, none of these 11 patients developed regional extension, and only one developed distant spread to the hilar region. This suggested that non-Hodgkin's lymphoma presented in the groin could be controlled very effectively with local therapy too.

Among the present EFSCH series, there were 7 patients who had radical node dissection as the initial step in establishing diagnosis and controlling of the disease. Two additional patients had nodal dissections after radiotherapy. Their clinicopathological characteristics are summarized in Table 5-9. In the 2 patients with Hodgkin's disease who had radical node dissection, one was done because of a wrong preoperative diagnosis of inguinal hernia. The other had axillary adenopathy 1 year after having had a simple mastectomy for papilloma of the breast. Both died within 2 years despite radiotherapy. In the 7 patients with other lymphomas, 2 had radical neck dissection as treatment for separate but coexisting neoplasms (lip and pyriform sinus cancers). Of these 7 patients, 4 developed distant disease 2–10 months later and 1 patient had local recurrence 21 months later, despite radiotherapy of 3000 rads. Only 2 patients were free of disease: one over 3 years after inadequate radiotherapy to the groin (550 rads) and another patient died of heart disease 8 years after radical neck dissection for a submandibular mass.

Table 5-7
Radical Dissection for Peripheral Lymphadenopathy of Hodgkin's Disease of Specific Regions

Year	Author	No. of patients	Neck No*	Neck Yes*	Axilla No*	Axilla Yes*	Groin No*	Groin Yes*	Disease-free (years)	Survival (years)
1940	Baker and Mann	2	2						12, 10	12, 10
1942	Slaughter and Craver	5		5					11, 11, 10, 8, 4	33, 11, 10, 8, 5
1943	Gall	9	3	4		1			15, 6, 3 / 6, ?, 2, 0 / 5	15, 10, 3 / 10, 5, 2, 0.5 / 5
1947	Hellwig	3	2				1		14, ? / 9	14, 10 / 9
1951	Williams, et al.	1	1						8	8
1958	Slaughter, et al.	18	8	9		1			10, 9, 9, ?, 7, 6, 2, ? / 13, 12, ?, 9, 7, 6, ?, 0, 0 / 5	10, 9, 9, 7, 7, 6, 2, 2 / 13, 12, 11, 9, 7, 6, 2, 1, 1 / 5
1963	Lacher	11	3	7	1	1		1	2, 6, 2 / 12, 10, 10, 3, 3, 1, 1 / 1	6, 6, 4 / 12, 10, 10, 10, 7, 4, 3 / 2
1965	Holloway	2	1		1				5, 7	7, 7
1966	Pack and Molander	11		3		3		5	12, 10, ? / 11, 10, ? / 11, 11, 10, 7, ?	12, 10, 3 / 11, 10, 2 / 11, 11, 10, 7, 3
	Overall	62	18	30	7	7	1	6	39/62 5-year or more (63%)	47/62 5-year or more (76%)

*Postoperative radiation therapy.

Table 5-8
Radical Peripheral Dissection of Lymphadenopathy of Non-Hodgkin's Lymphoma

Year	Author	No. of patients	Site of adenopathy						Disease-free (years)	Survival (years)
			Neck		Axilla		Groin			
			No*	Yes*	No*	Yes*	No*	Yes*		
1940	Sugarbaker and Craver	12		12						3 (24%) survived 5 years
1943	Gall	8	5	1			2		2, 0, 7, 0, 0 5 8, 4	11, 9, 7, 3, 2 5 8, 4
1947	Hellwig	12	9		1			2	15, 12, 9, 8, 7, ?, 5, ?, ? 8 8, 5	15, 12, 9, 8, 7, 7, 5, 5, 5 8 8, 5
1947	Stout	3		1	1		1		10 13.5 ?	10 13.5 10
1958	Kremen (Slaughter)	4	3				1		All well over 5 years	
1965	Molander and Pack	19		5		3		11	none recurred	3 (60%) survived 5 years 2 (67%) survived 5 years 8 (73%) survived 5 years
	Overall	58	17	19	2	3	4	13	31/46 5-years or more (67%)	40/58 5-years or more (69%)

*Postoperative radiation therapy.

Table 5-9
Radical Node Dissection for Malignant Lymphoma (EFSCH series)

Patient No.	Age	Sex	Date	Indication	Operation	Pathology diagnosis	Positive node	Postoperative Radiotherapy (rads)	Chemotherapy	Subsequent Lesion Local	Elsewhere	Interval	Survival months (* = alive)	Lymphoma at follow-up
Hodgkin's disease														
08968	16	M	9-46	R-axillary mass	Axillary dissection	LP	+	2000	–	–	L-axilla, mediastinum	3M	26M	+
40360	34	M	9-71	R-groin mass	Radical groin dissection	NS	+	6000	–	–	Para-aortic (by staging laparotomy)	2M	6M	? pneumonia
Non-Hodgkin's Lymphoma														
06371	56	M	5-44	L-upper and lower neck nodes	Radical neck dissection	LPD	10/54	2500	–	–	Aortic	10M	12M	+
18935	57	M	3-54	Submandibular node (lip cancer)	Radical neck dissection	LWN	1/37	–	–	35M	Mesentery	7M	91M	+
22308	63	F	9-57	Submandibular mass	Suprahyoid dissection	HWN	+	–	–	–	–	–	98M	– heart attack
31826	60	M	9-63	R-neck mass (pyriform sinus cancer)	Laryngectomy and radical neck dissection	MC	+	–	–	5M	L-neck	2M	9M	+
25160	75	F	10-63	L-post. neck node. 3.5 yr after RT	Radical neck dissection	LWD	20/34	–	+	–	CNS	8M	53M*	+
30125	66	M	3-64	Inguinal hernia, 2 yr after RT to leg nodules	Radical groin dissection	HPD	0/17	3000	+	21M	–	–	92M*	+
36951	63	M	2-68	Groin mass	Superficial groin dissection	HPD	+	550	–	–	–	–	39M*	–

In addition, there were 4 patients who had radical mastectomy (Table 5-10). One patient with Hodgkin's disease had radical mastectomy because biopsy of the axillary mass was read as unclassified malignant tumor. Among the 364 patients with non-Hodgkin's lymphomas, 3 patients had radical mastectomy. In one patient (No. 36548) the lymphoma was coexisting with breast cancer. Another patient (No. 01590) who had radical mastectomy for breast and axillary mass was free of disease for 7.5 years without any other therapy.

During the study of 163 EFSCH patients with Hodgkin's disease, we have excluded 10 other patients because the diagnosis was made elsewhere and the tissue slides could not be reviewed. One patient (No. 30024), a 22-year-old white female, had a right lower neck dissection in continuity with a mediastinal node dissection through a sternal splitting incision. Multiple nodes containing Hodgkin's disease typical of nodular sclerosis type were found and postoperative radiotherapy was given (3000 rads to the neck, 2400 rads each to anterior and posterior mediastinum). The patient has had 3 subsequent pregnancies and has been well and free of disease for more than 13 years. Another patient, a brother of one of the 163 patients, also treated elsewhere, had a radical neck dissection for right midneck mass. Surgical specimen showed that numerous nodes were involved with Hodgkin's disease of the lymphocyte predominance type. The patient was given intravenous nitrogen mustard, 18 mg daily, for 14 days. No other therapy was given and the patient has been free of disease for over 10 years.

In the EFSCH series, wide but local excision of adenopathy was done in 6 of the 364 patients with non-Hodgkin's lymphoma as shown in Table 5-11. Three of these patients had axillary mass excised and 5 received no other therapy. Excluding the 1 patient who died postoperatively, it is interesting to note that 3 patients are still free of disease 4, 10, and 12 years after the operation, 1 patient died with recurrence 10 years later, and another patient is free of disease 16 years after 3 separate excisions of lesions of the thigh, neck, and axilla. We present these unusual cases not to propose surgery as the treatment of choice, but to emphasize our ignorance in understanding the natural history of these diseases. In very selected cases, surgery, perhaps by removing the bulk of the tumor might tip the balance in favor of the host immunity against the tumor and achieve the phenomenon of tumor dormancy (Fisher and Fisher 1962) or even spontaneous regression (Everson and Cole 1966).

SUMMARY

Surgery as treatment of malignant lymphoma has never been practiced widely. Historically, Yates and Bunting (1917) were the first to champion the surgical removal of localized Hodgkin's disease. This approach became

Table 5-10
Radical Mastectomy for Malignant Lymphoma (EFSCH series)

Patient No.	Age	Sex	Date	Indication	Pathological diagnosis	No. positive nodes	Postoperative		Subsequent lesion		Interval (months)	Survival (months)	Lymphoma at follow-up
							Radiotherapy (rads)	Chemotherapy	Local	Elsewhere			
Hodgkin's Disease													
13154	64	M	1-50	L-axilla mass	MC	+	2450	+	–	neck, R-axilla	3	20	+
Non-Hodgkin's Disease													
01590	67	M	4-43	Breast and axilla mass	Und	0/15	–	–	–	–	–	87	–(pneumonia)
10347	68	F	10-47	Axilla mass	Und	11/25	2600	–	–	viscera	3	4	+
36548	71	F	6-66	Breast ca. and axilla mass	Breast: ductal ca. Node: lymphoma	4/15	–	–	–	liver	1	2	+

Table 5-11
Excision as Treatment of Non-Hodgkin's Lymphoma (EFSCH series)

Patient No.	Age	Sex	Date	Indication	Pathological diagnosis	Radiotherapy (rads)	Chemotherapy	Local recurrence	Survival months (* = alive)	Lymphoma at follow-up
04376	72	F	11-42	Post-RT axillary mass	HPD	4000	–	–	1	+
17335	58	M	10-54	L-thigh mass	LPD	–	–	–	204*	–
			6-55	R-neck mass	LPD					
			8-55	R-axilla mass	LPD					
24516	25	M	11-57	L-low neck mass	MC	(abdomen only)	–	10 years	120	+
27310	72	F	10-59	R-low neck mass	UC	–	–	–	145*	–
29423	75	F	6-62	Axillary mass	LWN	–	–	–	110*	–
31976	66	F	4-68	Submandibular mass	LPN	–	–	–	44*	–

an obsolete issue when Patterson (1972) stressed the current concept as no radical surgery for Hodgkin's disease. The overall 5-year survival rates for patients who were selected to have surgical excision of peripheral lymphadenopathy, with or without post-operative radiotherapy, were 76 percent for Hodgkin's disease and 69 percent for non-Hodgkin's lymphoma.

Since radiotherapy has proved to be more effective in treating nodal disease and combination chemotherapy in disseminated lesions, surgery should no longer be used as the definitive treatment of malignant lymphoma. Before the days of utilizing pretreatment staging laparotomy and splenectomy, in the EFSCH series about 1 out of every 5 patients with Hodgkin's disease and 1 out of every 3 with other lymphomas had various major surgical procedures for diagnosis, therapy, and complications of malignant or non-malignant origin.

Presently, staging laparotomy and splenectomy seem to overshadow the other roles of surgery in the management of patients with malignant lymphoma. However, major operations still may be required for the initial diagnosis in certain number of patients whose disease is not present in one of the peripheral lymph nodes. Both radiotherapy and chemotherapy have their own complications, and with the prolongation of life other unrelated conditions and additional cancers might develop. Thus, major surgery will always be required for a certain proportion of the patients who have nodal or extranodal disease internally. And surgery will also continue to be important in the diagnosis and management of new conditions related or unrelated to lymphomas.

REFERENCES

Anglesio E: The Treatment of Hodgkin's Disease. New York, Springer, 1969

Baker C, Mann WN: Hodgkin's disease. Lancet 1:25–25, 1940

Banfi A, Bonadonna G, Carnevali G, et al: Malignant lymphomas: Further studies on their preferential sites of involvement and possible mode of spread. Lymphology 2:130–138, 1968a

Banfi A, Bonadonna G, Carnevali G, et al: Preferential sites of involvement and spread in malignant lymphomas. Eur J Cancer 4:319–324, 1968b

Bonadonna G: Present position of radical and palliative treatment of malignant lymphomas, in Chiappa R, Musumeci R, Uslenghi C (eds): Endolymphatic Radiotherapy in Malignant Lymphomas. New York, Springer, 1971, pp 1–22

Catlin D: Surgery for head and neck lymphomas. Surgery 60:1160–1166, 1966

Craver LF: Etiology and pathogenesis, in Molander DW, Pack GT (eds): Hodgkin's Disease. Springfield, Ill, Thomas, 1968, pp 3–19

Craver LF: Hodgkin's disease, in Tice F (ed): Practice of Medicine, vol 5. Hagerstown, Md., Prior, 1951, pp 107–152

Craver LF: Treatment of Hodgkin's disease, in Ariel IM, Pack GT (eds): Treatment of Cancer and Allied Diseases (ed 2). New York, Hoeber, 1964, pp 168–191

Dargeon HW: Lymphosarcoma in childhood. Am J Roentgenol Radium Ther Nucl Med 85:729–732, 1961

Dawson PJ, Harrison CV: A clinicopathological study of benign Hodgkin's disease. J Clin Pathol 14:219–231, 1961

Diamond HD: The Medical Management of Cancer. New York, Grune and Stratton, 1958

Everson TC, Cole WH: Spontaneous Regression of Cancer. Philadelphia, Saunders, 1966

Fisher B, Fisher ER: Host factors influencing the development of metastases. Surg Clin North Am 42:335–351, 1962

Freeman C, Berg JW, Cutler SJ: Occurrence and prognosis of extranodal lymphomas. Cancer 29:252–260, 1972

Fridman M, Ezdinli EZ: New trends in lymphoma management. NY State J Med 71:2661–2664, 1971

Gall EA: The surgical treatment of malignant lymphomas. Ann Surg 118:1064–1071, 1943

Gall EA, Mallory TB: Malignant lymphoma; Clinico-pathologic survey of 618 cases. Am J Pathol 18:381–429, 1942

Glatstein E, Guernsey JM, Rosenberg SA, et al: The value of laparotomy and splenectomy in the staging of Hodgkin's disease. Cancer 24:709–718, 1969

Guerriero HE: Four cases of Hodgkin's disease treated with radium. New Orleans Med & Surg J 83:698–705, 1931

Hall CA, Olson KB: Prognosis of the malignant lymphomas. Ann Intern Med 44:687–706, 1956

Hanks GE, Terry LN, Bryan JA, et al: Contribution of diagnostic laparotomy to staging non-Hodgkin's lymphoma. Cancer 29:41–43, 1972

Hass AC, Brunk SF, Gulesserian HP, et al: The value of exploratory laparotomy in malignant lymphoma. Radiology 101:157–1971

Hellwig CA: Malignant lymphoma: The value of radical surgery in selected cases. Surg Gynecol Obstet 84:950–958, 1947

Holloway JB Jr: Definitive surgery for malignant lymphomas. Am Surg 31:349–353, 1965

Jackson H Jr, Parker F Jr: Hodgkin's Disease and Allied Disorders. New York, Oxford University Press, 1947

Jenkin RD, Sonley MJ, Stephens CA, et al: Primary gastrointestinal tract lymphoma in childhood. Radiology 92:763–767, 1969

Kaplan HS: Hodgkin's Disease. Cambridge, Mass., Harvard University Press, 1972

Klopp CT: Surgical treatment of primary lymphoma. Cancer Management: A Special Graduate Course on Cancer. Sponsored by American Cancer Society. Philadelphia, Lippincott, 1968, pp 393–397

Lacher MJ: Role of surgery in Hodgkin's disease. N Engl J Med 268:289–292, 1963

Lee BJ, Nelson JH, Schwarz G: Evaluation of lymphangiography: Inferior venacavography and intravenous pyelography in the clinical staging and management of Hodgkin's disease and lymphosarcoma. N Engl J Med 271:327–337, 1964

Molander DW: When to hospitalize for Hodgkin's disease. Hospital Practice 4:57–67, Sept 1969

Molander DW, Pack GT: Lymphosarcoma: Choice of treatment and end-results in 567 patients: Role of surgical treatment for cure and palliation. Rev Surg 20:3–31, 1963

Molander DW, Pack GT: Management and survival of 883 patients with malignant lymphoma. Am J Roentgenol Radium Ther Nucl Med 93:154–159, 1965

Newall J, Friedman M: Reticulum-cell sarcoma. Part III. Prognosis. Radiology 97:99–102, 1970

Newall J, Friedman M, Narvaez, F de: Extra-lymph-node reticulum-cell sarcoma. Radiology 91:708–712, 1968

Pack GT, Molander DW: The surgical treatment of Hodgkin's disease. Cancer Res 26:1254–1263, 1966

Patterson WB: Current concepts in cancer. 39. Updated Hodgkin's Disease, no radical surgery. JAMA 223:64–65, 1973

Peters MV: Current concepts in cancer. 2. Hodgkin's Disease: Radiation therapy. JAMA 191:28–29, 1965

Peters MV: Radiotherapy, in Molander DW, Pack GT (eds): Hodgkin's Disease. Springfield, Ill., Thomas, 1968, pp 78–115

Peters MV: Hasselback R, Brown TC: The natural history of the lymphomas related to the clinical classification, in Zarafonetis CJ (ed): Proceedings of the International Conference on Leukemia-Lymphoma. Philadelphia, Lea & Febiger, 1968, pp 357–371

Röentgen WC: On a new kind of rays. Science 3:227–231, 1896

Rosenberg SA, Diamond HD, Craver LF: Lymphosarcoma: Survival and the effects of therapy. Am J Roentgenol Radium Ther Nucl Med 85:521–532, 1961

Rosenberg SA, Diamond HD, Dargeon HW, et al: Lymphosarcoma in childhood. N Engl J Med 259:505–512, 1958

Schamaun M: Surgical treatment in Hodgkin's disease, in Rüttimann A (ed): Progress in Lymphology, vol 1. Stuttgart, Thieme, 1967, pp 125–217

Slaughter DP: Current concepts in cancer. 2. Hodgkin's Disease: Radical surgery. JAMA 191:26–27, 1965

Slaughter DP, Economou SG, Southwick HW: Surgical management of Hodgkin's disease. Ann Surg 148:705–710, 1958

Slaughter DP, Craver LF: Hodgkin's disease; five year survival rate; value of early surgical treatment; notes on 4 cases of long duration. Am J Roentgenol Radium Nucl Ther Med 47:596–606, 1942

Smith DF, Klopp CT: The value of surgical removal of localized lymphomas. Surgery 49:469–476, 1961

Stout AP: Lymphosarcoma and Hodgkin's disease. RI Med J 32:436–439, 1949

Stout AP: The results of treatment of lymphosarcoma. NY State J Med 47:158–164, 1947

Sugarbaker ED, Craver LF: Lymphosarcoma: Study of 196 cases with biopsy. JAMA 115:17–23, 112–117, 1940

Werf-Messing B van der: Reticulum cell sarcoma and lymphosarcoma: A retrospective study of potential survival in locoregional disease. Eur J Cancer 4:549–557, 1968

Williams RD, Andrews NC, Zanes RP Jr: Major surgery in Hodgkin's disease. Surg Gynecol Obstet 93:636–640, 1951

Yates JL, Bunting CH: Results of treatment of Hodgkin's disease. JAMA 68:747–751, 1917

6

Staging Laparotomy and Splenectomy

The advent of megavoltage radiotherapeutic equipment made it possible to deliver tumoricidal doses of radiation to large volumes. To carry out curative radiation therapy of Hodgkin's disease, precise knowledge of the extent of involvement is essential. Although lymphangiography has proved to be an important advance in the macroscopic diagnosis of disease of the para-aortic and iliac lymph nodes, there are practical situations in which the clinician is still uncertain of the meaning of palpable spleen and liver, abnormal laboratory tests or scans, equivocal lymphangiograms, or suspicious gastrointestinal x-rays. Thus, diagnostic laparotomy with splenectomy, biopsy of liver, lymph nodes, and other tissues was introduced.

The main value of staging laparotomy lies in finding focal and minute visceral and nodal diseases not detectable by nonoperative means. When liver involvement is found, systemic chemotherapy rather than radiation therapy is the preferred treatment. Splenectomy facilitates the administration of radiation therapy, decreases the complication of radiation pneumonitis and nephritis, and possibly also increases patients' tolerance to radical radiotherapy as well as intensive chemotherapy. The additional bonus of staging laparotomy includes preserving ovarian function for the young female patient and gaining knowledge of the patterns of spread of malignant lymphomas. Presently, it is still too soon to know whether surgical staging will help alter the natural course of the disease and/or improve prognosis or not.

INDICATIONS FOR HODGKIN'S DISEASE

In an effort to delineate more precisely the extent of involvement below the diaphragm in patients with Hodgkin's disease, Glatstein et al (1969) from Stanford University performed laparotomy, splenectomy, and liver and para-aortic lymph node biopsies. Their first report covered the period from 1960 to November, 1968 and included 37 previously untreated and 28 treated patients; all patients were under the age of 65. The indications for laparotomy included splenomegaly, hypersplenism, equivocal lymphangiogram, hepatomegaly, or abnormal liver function tests. Their results showed that all of the methods of nonoperative evaluation of involvement of the spleen, liver and nodes had serious limitations. A general correlation was observed between the occurrence of systemic symptoms and the extent of disease below the diaphragm. There was no liver involvement without concomitant splenic involvement. In conclusion, they suggested that this operative procedure was a valuable supplement to the diagnostic evaluation of selected patients. Knowledge of presence or absence of intraabdominal involvement is important for the delivery of extended-field megavoltage radiation therapy with curative intent.

Two subsequent reports from Stanford University appeared shortly (Enright et al 1970; Glatstein et al 1970). Needle biopsy of the bone marrow was done preoperatively and additional open bone marrow biopsy was performed during the staging laparotomy. There were 50 consecutive new patients operated upon from August, 1968 to April, 1969. During the same period, 7 patients were excluded because of massive obesity, positive needle biopsy of the bone marrow, or previously performed celiotomy for diagnosis. Approximately 30 percent of those patients whose preoperative work-up was negative or inconclusive proved to have unsuspected abdominal Hodgkin's disease, primarily in the spleen and lymph nodes of the splenic hilum. Left supraclavicular adenopathy appeared to correlate with the presence of intraabdominal disease. On the other hand, abdominal tumor was found in 34 percent of those with mediastinal involvement and in 67 percent of those without.

Allen et al (1969), from the University of Chicago, and Lowenbraun et al (1970), from the Baltimore Cancer Research Center, reported 38 additional patients who had diagnostic laparotomy and splenectomy for Hodgkin's disease. They also expressed great enthusiasm for this procedure: "The low operative morbidity and worthwhile results in these initial patients led to the performance of laparotomy in all except stage IV patients." Nuland (1970) of Yale University even conducted laparotomy in patients with stage IV disease prior to the commencement of chemotherapy. The only patients who were not operated upon were those too ill to withstand surgery, either because of Hodgkin's disease or an intercurrent medical condition.

However, words of caution were raised by others such as Jelliffe et al (1970) from England; they pointed out the greater risk of thromboembolic complications in patients who developed thrombocytosis after splenectomy. Jelliffe commented that exploratory staging should not be regarded as a routine method of investigation if the patient was in poor general condition, had a history of thrombotic episodes, had severe varicose veins, or was taking estrogen or contraceptive pills.

Peters (1970) commented that she would not advise laparotomy for patients over 50 years of age, because the older patients usually had more disease than suspected and such a discovery at laparotomy might result in more radical treatment than often was advisable. But for young patients, especially those under 30 years of age, it often is vital to verify the extent of disease before prescribing radical radiation to sites which might entail distressing complications in the future.

Aisenberg et al (1971), from the Massachusetts General Hospital, published their more rigid indications for laparotomy in Hodgkin's disease. They selected patients below the age of 50 with fever, sweats, or chills; a palpable spleen or a positive lymphangiogram; or any 2 of the following minor indications: equivocal lymphangiogram, splenomegaly by x-ray; palpable liver, elevated bromosulfophthalein or alkaline phosphatase levels, unfavorable histology of mixed cellularity or lymphocyte depletion type. Their data showed that the spleen was the initial abdominal organ involved, and from there the disease spread to the celiac and para-aortic lymph nodes. However, they had a particular attitude toward cases who had positive lymphangiograms but negative biopsy of abdominal nodes. They would stage the patients as though the lymphangiogram were in error, but treat them to include the possibility of retroperitoneal lymphoma by irradiating the para-aortic nodes. They felt this approach was particularly appropriate for individuals with systemic symptoms since such patients did better after extensive radiotherapy.

Kadin et al (1971), from Stanford, published another report covering the period from 1964 through 1969. Abdominal involvement was present in 51 of the 117 previously untreated patients. Among the 51 patients, it was clinically unsuspected in 11 (21 percent) and equivocal in 10 (20 percent). Although lesions of the mixed cellularity type showed the highest risk of abdominal involvement (63 percent), a high frequency of abdominal disease was also seen in those with lymphocyte predominance (46 percent) and nodular sclerosis (39 percent). The incidence of abdominal involvement by the last type was higher when the initial biopsy showed a cellular pattern. Twenty-five patients had mesenteric node biopsies; only one, who was diagnosed at the time of cholecystectomy, had a positive result, and the histological pattern was that of lymphocyte predominance. Enlarged spleens of more than 400 g were usually involved, although 15 spleens weighing less than 200 g also contained disease. Occult abdominal lesions of splenic hilar nodes alone were found in 4 patients. Another 4 had positive disease of the marrow diagnosed by the open iliac crest biopsy, despite negative preoperative biopsies taken with the Jensen-Westerman needle.

Allen et al (1971) pointed out the importance of removing even apparently normal spleens, since 4 of the 6 patients with splenic involvement were not suspected at the time of laparotomy. In 3 patients, only a single nodule (one less than 5 mm in size) was present in the spleen. Farrer-Brown et al (1971) reported that 22 out of 44 untreated patients had splenic involvement. In 2 spleens, single nodules of 2 and 3 mm, respectively, were present. Three additional spleens contained only 2 to 5 small foci of up to 7 mm in diameter.

Zarembok et al (1972) found that 40 percent of normal sized spleens were involved. If gross examination of spleen, lymph node, or liver biopsies were normal, the specimens were fixed overnight in formalin, and all of the tissues were cut into 3 mm slices and submitted for sectioning. One of the 15 positive spleens had a lesion of only 2 mm in diameter; 4 had solitary nodules of less than 1 cm. Spleenic involvement appears to begin in the periarteriolar area in the periphery of the Malpighian bodies (Farrer-Brown et al 1972).

Schwartz (1971) mentioned the removal of 2 spleens which showed no lesions grossly but were positive for Hodgkin's disease microscopically. Gutterman et al (1972) reported 2 spleens which contained only a single microscopic focus of Hodgkin's disease. But Rosenberg (1972) said that of more than 200 splenectomies in his series, none had involvement of the spleen detected only under the microscope without lesions grossly evident.

Hass et al (1971) found that even normal-sized abdominal nodes could contain focal lesions. In addition, they found involved nodes together with uninvolved nodes in 33 percent of the patients in whom 2 or more lymph node areas were sampled at laparotomy. One patient had positive lesions in splenic hilar nodes without demonstration of disease in the spleen, abdominal or retroperitoneal lymph nodes. Perlin et al (1971) performed staging laparotomy on 30 patients. In 2 patients, minute foci of disease were found only in nodes about the celiac axis and peripancreatic area. In another patient, a node adjacent to the common bile duct was involved, requiring a lateral enlargement of the standard port for extended-field radiotherapy.

Hanks et al (1971), of North Carolina, selected patients for celiotomy only after both bone marrow and needle biopsy of the liver were interpreted as negative or not diagnostic for malignancy. But even a needle biopsy of the liver could miss pathological lesions. Perlin et al (1972) reported that 2 of their 3 patients who had Hodgkin's disease of the liver by biopsy taken at laparotomy showed only nonspecific hepatitis in the needle biopsy specimen obtained preoperatively. Zarembok et al (1972) mentioned that even open liver biopsy had its limitation of sampling errors. One of their patients died of an acute myocardial infarction 3 months after staging laparotomy. Although the liver biopsy taken at operation was negative, hepatic involvement was found at autopsy.

Givler et al (1971), from Iowa City, reported that clinical evaluation of the liver was in disagreement with biopsy findings in about one-third of the patients. Alkaline phosphatase was the most sensitive parameter and liver scan the least. In cases of questionable hepatic infiltrations without Reed-Sternberg cells, the liver was considered to be involved if the splenectomy specimen showed definite involvement. If splenic involvement was not demonstrated, the questionable hepatic lesions were considered negative.

The practice of staging laparotomy was gaining popularity when Johnson (1971) raised the question of whether staging laparotomy is routinely indicated in Hodgkin's disease. For Hodgkin's disease clinically limited to lymph nodes above the diaphragm (stages I and II) as is commonly the initial presentation, he felt that surgical exploration of the abdomen rarely contributed to treatment decision-making and was not routinely justified. His reasoning was as follows: (1) Random sampling of abdominal lymph nodes has a high false negative rate and is unlikely to detect all the minute microscopic lesions. Thus, it cannot help determine the need for prophylactic abdominal irradiation. (2) Splenectomy for the purpose of facilitating radiotherapy is not sound because with proper field localization, prophylactic irradiation of a normal-sized spleen is without complication and effective in controlling occult disease in this organ. (3) Unsuspected disease in sites outside the standard prophylactic treatment fields (i.e., lymph nodes in the porta hepatis or mesentery) is extremely uncommon. He conducted a retrospective study of 164 consecutive cases in which radiotherapy was delivered to different areas of the lymphoid system. When relapse was suspected in the abdomen, repeated meticulous diagnostic evaluation including exploratory laparotomy was done (Johnson et al 1970). In 124 patients without splenomegaly and with negative lymphangiogram, none had disease outside the standard radiation ports. Only 2 patients had extension of their disease to the liver. However, he felt that for patients with positive lymphangiogram and or splenomegaly (stage III), the chance of having unrecognized disease in the abdominal viscera or nodes was high and routine exploratory laparotomy seemed indicated (Browde 1971).

In response to Johnson's question, Lokich (1972) said that routine laparotomy was needed in staging Hodgkin's disease. Other than the usual reasons of detecting hepatic and splenic disease and gaining information useful for adjusting the field of irradiation, he commented that "the scientific data from laparotomy provide an understanding of the mode of spread of the disease, increase understanding of the host response to Hodgkin's disease, and aid in estimating prognosis." For patients with no retroperitoneal disease, irradiation was given only down to the aortic bifurcation and the pelvic areas were spared. Ultmann (1972) summarized experiences reported in the literature and also said that: (1) Laparotomy improves assessment of the extent of disease beyond what is possible by clinical, biochemical, and radiological studies alone; (2) The incidence of atypically located adenopathy is not extremely small, since 7.5 percent of 145 patients had nodes in the porta hepatis, mesentery, or splenic hilum. In his own institution, among 81 Hodgkin's patients, 12 had involvement of a single node: 7 were portal and 3 splenic lymph nodes (Ferguson et al 1973). (3) When the spleen is not palpable, there is a 5 percent chance of liver involvement; when the spleen is palpable, liver involvement can be predicted in over 50 percent of the cases. Thus, staging laparotomy can detect those patients who really need chemotherapy or radiotherapy to all the lymphoid tissues and can help avoid giving prophylactic abdominal irradiation to all.

This last point is debatable, because treatment fields for the abdomen used by different radiotherapists vary from total abdominal field, to para-aortic field only, to the "inverted Y" field. Most physicians would consider liver involvement as an indication for chemotherapy since fatal complication of radiation hepatitis resulted when tumoricidal doses of approximately 4000 rads were delivered to the entire liver (Ingold et al 1965). However, Hass et al (1971) did not commit such patients to chemotherapy alone but still treated them with external radiation therapy in dosages of 2000 to 2500 rads with or without combined chemotherapy. Kaplan (1973) treated several patients with biopsy-proven liver disease with external megavoltage x-rays and radioactive gold (Au 198). Two patients have had no relapse at 6 and 7 years after treatment, and a third, who died of an acute myocardial infarction 3 years after treatment, was found to have no evidence of Hodgkin's disease at autopsy.

Johnson et al (1971) reported on the results of a randomized study of assigning patients with stages I, II, and III lesions to limited versus intensive prophylactic irradiation. For patients without symptoms, the rate of developing relapse in extranodal sites was less than 5 percent for those with the histology of nodular sclerosis and lymphocyte predominance. For patients with symptoms and the histologic subtype of mixed cellularity and lymphocyte depletion, the relapse rate for extranodal sites was over 46 percent. The use of total nodal irradiation in the latter group decreased incidence of relapse and improved survival. Thus, they maintained that "exploratory laparotomy for all patients would have infrequently provided information essential for treatment planning and would not have improved the results of radiotherapy. But patients who might benefit from exploration could be identified prospectively either by clinicohistological factors or by the observation of vascular invasion on the original peripheral node biopsy."

As an alternative to full abdominal exploration but still capable of accomplishing a good tissue biopsy of the liver, DeVita et al (1971b), performed peritoneoscopy in 38 previously untreated patients. In most cases, 4 deep biopsies were taken with needles, 2 in each lobe of the liver. If lesions were visualized, additional forcep biopsies were performed as indicated. In 16 percent of the patients who had no evidence of disease on the basis of liver function tests and liver size, the biopsy specimen contained tumor.

And, hepatomegaly, the presence of symptoms and the Lukes histological classification of lesions did not help in predicting positive biopsies (Bagley et al 1973). There was no mortality nor significant morbidity resulting from this procedure. The reported mortality of peritoneoscopy in 11 large series of 1455 examinations was only 0.1 percent. Limitations of this procedure included inability to visualize the retroperitoneal area and the removal of the spleen. Their yield of positive biopsies is similar to the result reported from Stanford, using staging laparotomy. In both series the patients at higher risk of having liver involvement are those with preoperative evidence of disease below the diaphragm. The Committee on Hodgkin's Disease Staging Procedures at the Ann Arbor Conference suggested peritoneoscopy as a suitable alternative to celiotomy in patients with the highest risk of liver involvement, those with apparent involvement of the para-aortic nodes and spleen, or those with marked splenomegaly (Rosenberg et al 1971).

Prosnitz et al (1972b), from Yale University, reported their experience with laparotomy and splenectomy in 40 untreated patients. Surgery was carried out in a little more than half of the patients before any radiation therapy was given, and in the remainder, the operation was done between irradiation given to the mantle field and to the abdominal area. They felt that splenectomy performed after the mantle field irradiation might improve the hematologic tolerance to a greater extent than if the splenectomy were performed before any radiotherapy. Two of the 25 patients, who had the operation before any treatment, required interruption of radiotherapy to the abdominal field because of platelet depression, whereas none of the 15 who had surgery between chest and abdominal field irradiation did so. In their series, about 25 percent of the patients who were felt to have no disease below the diaphragm had abdominal disease on surgical exploration. In their institution, if disease is found in the nodes and spleen below the diaphragm, all of the abdominal nodes are treated with the "inverted Y" field. If the lymphangiogram is equivocal or positive and the exploration is negative, the treatment is the same. If the lymphangiogram and exploration are both negative, the para-aortic, but not the pelvic lymph nodes are treated prophylactically (Prosnitz et al 1972b).

Mitchell et al (1972) from Toronto, Canada, reported 29 untreated and 16 treated patients. In 19 of the untreated patients, diseases suspected in the abdomen were not confirmed, and the additional trauma of abdominal irradiation was avoided. Twenty patients had intraabdominal disease, 18 had involvement of the spleen, including 2 with only splenic disease. In 4 patients, the celiac nodes were involved; in 2, nodes along the superior border of the pancreas were also involved. Lymph nodes in the mesentery were involved on 3 occasions. Except one patient with iliac node and one with celiac node, all patients with para-aortic lymph node disease also had positive spleens. Contrary to the findings of Glatstein et al (1969), who reported that a spleen which weighed 400 g or more was always involved with Hodgkin's disease, they found 3 out of 7 such spleens did not have lesions.

Rosenberg (1971b) emphasized: "The major value and utility of exploratory laparotomy and splenectomy are to determine the extent of the disease, and then, only if the identification of abdominal disease would alter the therapeutic program planned." He explained further: "If the therapeutic plan is to use radiotherapy only to known sites of disease, or to limit the use of radiotherapy to those patients with stages I or II disease above the diaphragm either as a general rule, or for particular patients, then the exploratory laparotomy and splenectomy are indispensable for adequate staging and therapeutic decisions. If the therapeutic plan is to treat so-called total lymphoid fields as a general rule, or for particular patients, even in the absence of identified abdominal disease, then the surgical procedure has only the limited value of identifying the few patients with liver involvement and the facilitation of treatment to some extent. If young women wish to preserve ovarian function and pelvic irradiation is planned, surgical oophoropexy is recommended and then the full exploration and splenectomy would seem to be justified at the time of operation."

Trueblood et al (1972) attempted to suggest some guidelines that will avoid the two extremes of total irradiation to all and exploratory laparotomy for all. They felt that patients with a positive lymphangiogram, which had an accuracy rate of 80 percent, could be treated with extensive abdominal fields without laparotomy and splenectomy. For the remaining patients, about two-thirds of the patients in any large series, laparotomy would be carried out. They listed four criteria which suggested significantly increased risk of intraabdominal diseases: (1) systemic symptoms, (2) equivocal lymphangiograms, (3) large spleen, and (4) enlarged liver with abnormal liver function tests. However, they were not ready to use these four criteria in the selection of patients for staging laparotomy because they felt after applying the above four criteria and excluding those with positive lymphangiogram, about 6 percent of the patients were left with undiagnosed abdominal involvement. They felt that this 6 percent of the entire series with untreated disease was unacceptable since this exceeded the morbidity of laparotomy and splenectomy combined with abdominal irradiation. This last point is debatable since mortalities have been reported and several recent reports (see below) have shown that the morbidity of staging laparotomy could be as high as 30 percent.

Similar to Johnson's view, Smith et al (1973) felt that laparotomy is not necessary in patients who had stage I or II Hodgkin's disease above the diaphragm, if extended field and splenic irradiation is administered routinely. Of 19 preoperative stage I and II cases, 2 became stage III and none became stage IV. One of the cases which were advanced to stage III had involvement of the spleen; and the other, the celiac node. On the other hand, 4 of the 10 patients who were thought to have stage III disease became stage II because of false-positive lymphangiogram; and one became stage IV because of a positive liver biopsy. Two of the 4 patients who were classified as having stage IV disease became stage III after a negative liver biopsy. Thus, they felt that only patients whose disease is initially staged as III or IV should have a laparotomy.

For the present, the value of pretreatment staging laparotomy in the detection of occult abdominal malignant lymphoma is well documented. In fact, this concept has been applied to other conditions, and several institutions are conducting exploratory laparotomy as part of the routine initial investigations in cancer of the uterine cervix (Averette et al 1972; Buchsbaum 1972; Ucmakli and Bonney 1972). Similar to the results with Hodgkin's disease, it was found that clinical staging was inaccurate in over one-third of the cases. And unsuspected metastases in bowel, liver, and coexistent ovarian carcinomas were discovered.

In any case, exploratory laparotomy with splenectomy and tissue biopsy is a major surgical procedure requiring general anesthesia and should not be undertaken lightly. It is hoped that "with increasing experience, it may become possible to further define the indications for laparotomy and splenectomy with respect to such variables as age, sex, sites of peripheral adenopathy, presence of constitutional symptoms, histological type, abnormal tests, and to predict those parameters for which the highest expectation of diagnostic yield would obtain" (Kaplan 1972a).

In a Forum (1973), Dr. Stutzman, of Roswell Park Memorial Institute, said: "The complexities, expense, and delay in institution of therapy imposed by the ever-increasing number of staging tests have led to the deletion of isotope scanning, lymphangiography, gastrointestinal studies, bone marrow biopsy, and pyelography in patients being staged by laparotomy and surgical marrow biopsy in our institution." However, other experts in the Forum had different opinions. But they seem to agree on the recommendation that staging laparotomy be undertaken in all patients, *except:* (1) those who have biopsy-proven stage IV disease, (2) those who have localized supradiaphragmatic disease (especially stage IA or IIA nodular sclerosis lesions), an unequivocally negative lymphangiogram, negative liver–spleen scan, normal liver function tests, and normal bone core biopsy, (3) those over 65 years of age because of a significant immediate postoperative risk, (4) those younger than 15, especially under 5, years of age because of the long-term risk of fulminant infection after splenectomy, and (5) those who have medical contraindications to surgery. Dr. Meeker added a relative contraindication of secondary hypersplenism due to Hodgkin's disease, since mortality occurred in such circumstance.

OPERATIVE TECHNIQUE

Since staging laparotomy and splenectomy is a relatively new operation, many versions with slightly different details of how the biopsy specimens were taken have been described. Even in the same medical center, the technique may still be undergoing modification and evolution. Thus, it seems interesting to compare the technical aspects reported in the literature here.

Lowenbraun et al (1970) described exploration through a left paramedian or subcostal incision, with careful examination of the liver, porta hepatis, spleen, gastrointestinal tract, mesentery, kidneys, and retroperitoneal space. Splenectomy was performed and a wedge biopsy of the liver was taken. Splenic hilar, mesenteric, and abnormal retroperitoneal nodes were biopsied. If no grossly involved nodes were detected, left para-aortic nodes were biopsied. Metal clips were placed at the site of removed nodes, splenic pedicle and, if present, the lateral boundary of retroperitoneal disease. Later, Zarembok et al (1972) said that in most cases, the iliac and mesenteric nodes were biopsied routinely.

Enright et al (1970) described the use of a midline incision, extending below the umbilicus for female patients who needed oophoropexy. Liver biopsy was done with both the removal of a wedge biopsy and the use of a Vim-Silverman needle to sample the deeper hepatic parenchyma. In instances in which the para-aortic lymph nodes were not remarkable, the left para-aortic nodes from below the left renal vein to the inferior mesenteric artery were resected as a chain. The area was approached by reflecting the transverse colon superiorly and the small intestine to the right; a vertical incision was made in the base of the colonic mesentery between the fourth portion of the duodenum and the inferior mesenteric vein. Mesenteric nodes were biopsied routinely (Kadin et al 1971). A 1-cm core of bone and marrow was removed from the lateral aspect of the iliac crest by means of a cutting cylinder activated by a Stricker saw mechanism. Hass et al (1971) and Ferguson et al (1973) took a thin wedge of bone 1.5 to 2 cm wide with a sharp chisel, since the use of a hollow drill did not always provide the minimal area of undistorted marrow (one sq cm) needed to find focal disease.

Nuland (1970) described removal of suspicious nodes through short, separate incisions in the posterior peritoneum. If there were no suspicious tissues, sample nodes were removed from both sides of the aorta at approximately L2 position. He also made an opening in the gastrocolic omentum to palpate the celiac axis and the entire length of the splenic artery. The celiac node was biopsied and the proximal splenic artery was dissected out of the superior surface of the pancreas for about 2 to 3 in. lateral to the celiac axis, ligated, and marked with metal clips. Mitchell et al (1972) ligated the splenic artery close to the celiac axis before splenectomy.

Schwartz (1971) described transection of the ligament of treitz and mobilization of the duodenum and jejunum medially to biopsy the celiac node and to dissect the para-aortic nodes in continuity downward to the iliac region. Mitchell et al (1972) would commence the random dissection of the nodes along the iliac arteries and proceed along the aorta toward the diaphragm. Ferguson et al (1973) excised iliac nodes through separate 2 cm incisions in each groin.

Allen et al (1971) said they routinely biopsy nodes from the porta hepatis. They pointed out that the surgeon should obtain the largest nodes for biopsy, not just the most accessible ones. Even normal looking spleen and lymph nodes should be removed. Also, the pathologist should use the semiserial section technique for whole organs to detect minute foci of disease.

Hanks et al (1971) included taking radiographs during the operative procedure to locate specific suspicious lymph nodes. They also emphasized that accessory splenic tissue should be searched and removed. Hass et al (1971) reported 6 patients with accessory spleens among 75 staging splenectomy operations. These were involved with lymphoma when the main spleens were involved. Ferguson et al (1973) found accessory spleens in 18 percent of the cases, of which 20 percent contained tumor.

Statistically, one-third of the patients could have accessory spleens. Curtis and Movitz (1946) encountered 131 accessory spleens in 56 patients among a series of 174 consecutive splenectomies. Of these, 54 percent were located in the hilum; 25 percent in the pedicle; 12 percent in the omentum, especially along greater curvature of the stomach; 6 percent, retroperitoneum; 3 percent, splenocolic ligament and mesentery. The left pelvic adnexa in females, or left scrotum in males, should be examined because of the embryonic contiguity of the splenic anlagen to the genital ridge. In both sexes, the hollow of the sacrum could be a possible site for accessory spleen (Schwartz 1971).

In grossly normal livers, Givler et al (1971) suggested taking the wedge biopsy at 10 cm left of the falciform ligament. In contrast, Exelby (1971) described taking a biopsy from the midportion of the right lobe in pediatric patients. Perlin et al (1972) only took one liver biopsy by wedge resection. Trueblood et al (1972) said that the liver biopsy should be the first step during laparotomy in order to keep round cell infiltration in the biopsy specimen to a minimum. Schwartz and Cooper (1972) explained that prolonged application of the retractor rapidly resulted in cellular infiltration.

Bilateral oophoropexy is usually performed by attaching the ovaries to the front or back of the uterus as low as possible and marked with braided wire suture tags (Trueblood et al 1970). Exelby (1971) and Nahhas et al (1971) did oophoropexy differently. They transposed the ovaries upward and lateral to the iliopsoas muscles and sutured them to the parietal peritoneum just below the iliac crest. Metal clips are used to mark the lateral and medial borders of the ovary, and the ovarian pedicle is sutured to the posterior peritoneum to prevent herniation and strangulation of bowel.

Paglia et al (1973) believed that moving ovaries to the anterior iliac crest region offered more protection from radiation therapy and, on occasion, patients who had midline ovaries complained of pelvic pain during sexual intercourse. In addition, they did appendectomy routinely, since patients with Hodgkin's disease might on occasion develop gastrointestinal involvement and abdominal pain. Also this avoids the confusion between Mittelschmerz pain from a transposed ovary and appendicitis.

Prosnitz et al (1972b) reported that their attending radiotherapists were present in the operating room at almost all of the 40 staging operations. All of their operations were carried out through a left rectus-splitting incision from the costal margin to a point just superior to the umbilicus (Nuland 1970). In cases where oophoropexy was desired, it was done through a separate small suprapubic abdominal incision. However, "when grossly benign-looking tissue proved to be microscopically involved or when unsuspected disease was found in the abdomen, a second operation was performed to remove the ovaries." It is not known why they wanted to do oophorectomy, unless they felt the ovary might harbor disease and become the focus for later dissemination.

Ferguson et al (1973) routinely take at least 8 lymph node specimens from the following areas: portal, celiac (aorta at level of T-12 and L-1), splenic, para-aortic on both sides below and behind the duodenum (level of L-2 to L-4), external iliac on both sides, and superior mesenteric. Each of these sites was found to be involved in at least 10 percent of the patients with Hodgkin's disease, and much oftener in those with other lymphomas. Seven of their 81 patients with Hodgkin's disease and 1 of the 37 patients with other lymphomas had involvement of the portal nodes without other abdominal lymphadenopathy.

CLINICOPATHOLOGICAL CORRELATIONS

Staging laparotomy was initially undertaken as a clinical investigation to find out if it would increase the precision of diagnostic tests, better define the extent of disease, promote more effective therapy and clarify the natural history of Hodgkin's disease. So far, staging laparotomy has demonstrated its value in all of these aspects. What remains to be shown, which requires many more years of careful follow-up, is that there is better control of the disease and increased survival of such patients.

The accumulated data up to the present time showed that splenectomy specimens revealed evidence of Hodgkin's disease in 36 percent of the spleens thought to be uninvolved by clinical and/or radioisotopic examinations; and in 64 percent of the clinically positive spleens (Table 6-1). The result of open liver biopsy also pointed to a high false positive rate

Table 6-1

Clinical Impressions versus Results of Liver Biopsy and Splenectomy in Hodgkin's Disease

	Spleen				Liver			
	Clinical (−)		Clinical (+)		Clinical (−)		Clinical (+)	
	Patient No.	Biopsy (+)	Patient No.	Biopsy (+)	Patient No.	Biopsy (+)	Patient No.	Biopsy (+)
Jelliffe et al (1970)	12	7	10	5	12	1	10	1
Lowenbraun et al (1970)[a]	7	1	5	4	7	0	5	3
Aisenberg et al (1971)	19	9	6	4			16	9
Hass et al (1971)[a]	38	14	12	11	34	4	26	6
Kadin et al (1971)	90	29	27	15	91	3	4	1
Hanks et al (1972)	8	2	6	4	10	1	12	4
Meeker et al (1972)	18	8	10	7	18	1	13	7
Mitchell et al (1972)[a]	21	6	24	11	32	2		
Parker et al (1972)	12	2	8	8			9	4
Perlin et al (1972)	20	8	10	6	21	0		
Prosnitz et al (1972b)	38	14	2	1	40	0		
Ultmann (1972)	23	8	7	4	20	1	12	0
Zarembok et al (1972)	23	9	7	6	20	0	10	1
EFSCH[a]	9	5	3	2	7	0	5	1
Total	338	122 (36%)	137	88 (64%)	312	13 (4%)	122	37 (30%)

[a] Series includes patients who had previous therapy.

of 70 percent among abnormal livers checked by physical examinations, laboratory tests, and radioisotopic scans. And about 4 percent of clinically normal livers had positive biopsy of Hodgkin's disease.

The poor reliability of lymphangiogram in diagnosing involvement of retroperitoneal and abdominal lymph nodes was also clearly defined by results of multiple nodal biopsies during staging laparotomy (Table 6-2). In those patients who had normal lymphangiograms, 12 percent had positive retroperitoneal nodes confirmed by biopsy; and for those who had a definitely abnormal lymphangiogram, only 72 percent had positive nodes. The limitation of lymphangiogram in outling abnormal nodes of the upper abdomen and of atypically located nodes in the porta hepatis, mesentery, or splenic hilum was also well demonstrated. Ultmann (1972) said the incidence of involvement of such unusual nodes was about 7.5 percent. But Zarembok et al (1972) found involvement of nodes outside the para-aortic chain in 5 of 30 consecutive untreated patients.

In the accumulated surgical experiences reported in the literature (Table 6-3), only 61 percent of the patients had no change in their clinical stage designations before and after laparotomy. About 24 percent of the patients had their stages advanced, mainly from stages I and II to III, and III to IV. About 15 percent had their stages decreased, especially stage III dropping to II, reflecting the high false positive rate of lymphangiogram (28 percent) and clinical impression of involvement of spleen (36 percent). In patients with negative lymphangiograms, 40 percent of those with symptoms (stages IB and IIB) and 20 percent without (stage IA and IIA) are found to have lymphoma below the diaphragm (Aisenberg 1973).

In 100 cases admitted with Hodgkin's disease, Rosenberg (1971c) reported that the initial distribution of stages I to IV was 13 percent, 67 percent, 10 percent, and 10 percent, respectively. After lung tomogram, lymphangiogram, and needle biopsy of the bone marrow, the distribution changed to 11 percent, 36 percent, 29 percent, and 24 percent. After laparotomy and splenectomy, the relative distribution became 10 percent, 30 percent, 32 percent, and 28 percent. In 54 patients, Piro et al (1972) showed that preoperative disease staging was changed in 18 patients (31 percent) and 37 percent required alteration of preoperative plans of therapy as a consequence of the procedure. Specifically, 10 patients received less nodal irradiation and 2 were given more than planned. Two patients had nodal irradiation rather than chemotherapy and 4 received cytotoxic drugs instead of x-ray therapy.

Findings of staging laparotomy have improved our understanding of the natural pattern of involvement and the possible mode of spread of Hodgkin's disease. Patients without mediastinal disease had a higher frequency of having subdiaphragmatic disease than those with mediastinal disease 2/3 versus 1/3 (Glatstein, et al 1970; Zarembok et al 1972). And abdominal involvement was found in 17 percent of the patients with only right cervical

Table 6-2

Correlation of Lymphangiographic Appearance versus Involvement of Retroperitoneal Nodes in Hodgkin's Disease

	Negative		Equivocal		Positive	
	Patient No.	Biopsy (−)	Patient No.	Biopsy (−)	Patient No.	Biopsy (−)
Jelliffe et al (1970)	11	1	4	2	6	6
Lowenbraun et al (1970)[a]	4	0			8	4
Aisenberg et al (1971)	7	1	5	0	13	8
Hass et al (1971)[a]	27	0			16	15
Kadin et al (1971)	60	8	25	5	30	24
Hanks et al (1972)	9	1			5	5
Mitchell et al (1972)[a]	19	4	2	0	22	12
Perlin et al (1972)	6	1	2	1	6	4
Prosnitz et al (1972b)	14	4	11	2	14	13
Ultmann (1972)	13	2	4	2	12	6
Zarembok et al (1972)	12	0	3	0	15	9
Total	182	22 (12%)	56	12 (21%)	147	106 (72%)

[a] Series includes patients who had previous therapy.

adenopathy versus 54 percent with left or bilateral neck nodes (Dorfman 1971). In addition, there is a correlation of mediastinal involvement with side of cervical adenopathy, i.e., 86 percent of those with right neck lesions had mediastinal disease versus 50 percent of those with only left-side lesions or 66 percent of those with bilateral neck lesions (Rosenberg 1971a). This is explained by the known lymphatic drainage of the mediastinum predominately to the right supraclavicular area (Smithers 1970). Kaplan (1968–69) explained that the reason for the seemingly noncontiguous distribution of disease in the lower neck and abdomen, but not the mediastinum (the so-called "mediastinal skip"), was retrograde extension of the disease by way of the thoracic duct from the upper abdominal nodes. He believed this was retrograde specifically because there were cases where lesions in the neck appeared more than 4 years before the involvement of para-aortic nodes, which made antegrade spread unlikely.

However, Prosnitz et al (1972b) found no distinct pattern of cervical or mediastinal involvement which correlated with a higher frequency of abdominal disease, and in about 50 percent of the cases, abdominal disease failed to have a contiguous pattern of spread. Ibrahim et al (1972) reported that Hodgkin's disease of the spleen was found in 2 of 5 patients with presentations in the right side of the neck and in 2 of 7 patients with lesions in the left side of the neck. Meeker et al (1972) found abdominal involvement in 8 of 10 patients with right, 5 of 9 with left, and 1 of 3 patients with bilateral cervical adenopathy, as well as 2 of 2 patients with inguinal adenopathy. Zarembok et al (1972) and Gutterman et al (1972) also found no correlation between laterality of cervical adenopathy and the frequency of abdominal involvement.

Peters et al (1973) analyzed their data of 63 patients who had laparotomy in a slightly different fashion. They divided the patients into 3 groups and found a strong correlation between patterns of presentation and frequency of intraabdominal disease. Twenty-one patients had adenopathy of a single peripheral region, excluding supraclavicular area, and none had disease below the diaphragm. Thirty-one had involvement of the mediastinum and a peripheral nodal region, 42 percent of this group had positive abdominal lesions. Of the 12 patients with adenopathy of 2 or more peripheral regions but without lesions of the mediastinum, 100 percent had abdominal diseases on exploration.

It was shown that about two-thirds of the patients with splenic involvement had retroperitoneal disease, and almost all of those who had nodal lesions in splenic pedicle also had positive spleens (Zarembok et al 1972). In about 8 percent of the patients, the only documented site of Hodgkin's disease below the diaphragm might be the spleen (Rosenberg 1972). This data seemed to confirm the suggestion of Aisenberg et al (1971) that the spleen was the initial abdominal organ involved and from there the disease spread to the celiac and para-aortic lymph nodes. However, Kadin et al

Table 6-3
Overall Stage Changes After Staging Laparotomy and Splenectomy in Hodgkin's Disease

	Total	Same	Advanced				Declined		
	Patient No.	Patient No.	Patient No.	I,II–IV	II–IV	III–IV	Patient No.	III–I,II	IV–I,II,III
Glatstein et al (1970	50	29	11	8		3	10	6	4
Jelliffe et al (1970)	22	8	9	7		2	5	5	
Lowenbraun et al (1970)[a]	12	9	1	1			2	2	
Aisenberg et al (1971)	25	13	7	3		3	5	5	
Hanks et al (1972)	14	10	2	1	1		2		
Meeker et al (1972)	26	10	14	10	1	4	2	2	2
Parker et al (1972)	20	11	2				7		
Perlin et al (1972)	30	22	5	3		2	3	3	
Prosnitz et al (1972b)	40	33	7	7		0			
EFSCH[a]	12	9	2	1			1		
Total	251	154 (61%)	60 (24%)	41[b]	3[b]	14[b]	37 (15%)	23[b]	7[b]

[a] Series includes patients who had previous therapy.
[b] Incomplete data.

(1971) reported 4 patients and Hass et al (1971) had 1 patient in whom positive splenic hilar nodes were the only site of intraabdominal disease. Perlin et al (1971) and Mitchell et al (1972) had 4 patients whose only positive nodes were located in the celic axis and peripancreatic area. Dettman and Storaasli (1972) and Ferguson et al (1973) had 8 patients whose only disease was found in a porta hepatis node.

In Kaplan's experience, clinical and/or radiographic finding of splenomegaly has almost invariably been accompanied or preceded in time by lymphangiographic evidence of involvement of the upper lumbar para-aortic nodes (Kaplan 1968–69). Thus, he felt the evidences strongly indicated that the pattern of progression of Hodgkin's disease in the abdomen was from the upper para-aortic nodes to the lymph nodes of the splenic pedicle and hilus and thence into the substance of the spleen itself. Involvement of the spleen in turn posed the threat of hepatic parenchymal involvement. And bone marrow involvement in patients with previously untreated disease came only after involvement of the para-aortic nodes, and possibly also the spleen, via hematogenous spread (Kaplan 1972a).

Massive involvement of the spleen is accompanied by biopsy evidence of liver involvement in over 50 percent of cases, whereas positive liver biopsies are seldom obtained when spleens shown to contain Hodgkin's disease are still within or near the normal limits of size. Furthermore, spread of disease to the liver occurred subsequently in 15 of 34 cases in which prior splenic involvement had been documented (Kaplan 1968–69). Ferguson et al (1973) found that the correlation of massive splenomegaly with hepatic involvement is not absolute. Seventeen patients had malignant lymphoma of the liver on biopsy; in 7, the diseased spleen weighed less than 300 grams.

Almost all of the patients who had Hodgkin's disease of the liver also had involvement of the spleen. The only exception was that reported by Schwartz and Cooper (1972) who said 1 of their 30 patients had hepatic involvement without accompanying splenic or abdominal lymphatic lesions. They also pointed out that the spleen has no lymphatic supply, thus Hodgkin's disease probably reaches it via the blood stream, although the alternative explanation of retrograde lymphatic spread is not ruled out by present knowledge. Reed-Sternberg cells have been observed to circulate in the peripheral blood of 37 percent of patients with advanced Hodgkin's disease (Bouroncle 1966); and similar cells have been found in the lymph of the thoracic duct (Engeset et al 1969). Thus it is possible that lymphoid tumor cells may be continuously circulated in the blood stream and the lymph channels, suggesting that the vascular and lymphatic systems are not independent but intimately interrelated (Fisher and Fisher 1967).

In the accumulated surgical experience with staging laparotomy (Table 6-4), about 48 percent of the patients had some intraabdominal involvement (nodal involvement in 44 percent, spleen in 43 percent, and the liver in

Table 6-4
Distribution of Overall Intraabdominal Involvement in Hodgkin's Disease

	Total Patient No.	Node(+) Patient No.	Spleen(+) Patient No.	Liver(+) Patient No.	Any one(+) Patient No.
Jelliffe et al (1970)	22	9	11	4	15
Aisenberg et al (1971)	25	9	13	4	13
Dorfman (1971)	185	86	78	15	86
Ibrahim et al (1972)	27	2	6		6
Mitchell et al (1972)[a]	45	18	17	9	20
Prosnitz et al (1972b)	40	19	15	4	22
Zarembok et al (1972)	30	9	15	1	16
EFSCH[a]	12	8	7	1	8
Total	386	170 (44%)	162 (43%)	38 (11%)	186 (48%)

[a] Includes patients who had previous therapy.

11 percent). Apparently the degree of exceptions to the usual pattern of involvement is related to the different histological types. Trueblood et al (1972) summarized their experience at Stanford. About 46 percent of 185 patients had intraabdominal disease. When the figure was analyzed by subtypes, it was 62 percent for the mixed cellularity type, 46 percent for the lymphocyte predominance, and 42 percent for the nodular sclerosis (only 3 patients had lymphocyte depletion). When there was intraabdominal disease, the spleen was the single most commonly involved organ: in about 100 percent of patients with mixed cellularity, in 92 percent of those with the nodular sclerosis and in 50 percent of those with the lymphocyte predominance. Liver involvement also showed a similar distribution: mixed cellularity had the highest incidence (28 percent), lymphocyte predominance the next (15 percent), and nodular sclerosis the lowest (12 percent). It was surprising that nodular sclerosis, which had the highest predilection for mediastinal involvement also had a high incidence of extranodal and extrasplenic involvement. Among 137 patients, there were 16 lung, 7 liver, 6 bone marrow, 5 rib or pelvic bone, 4 vertebra, 3 pericardium, and 2 subcutaneous tissue lesions.

Meeker et al (1972) summarized the interrelationship of histological subtypes and sites of involvement in 30 patients who had staging laparotomy. Twenty-five patients had cervical adenopathy and 2 patients had primary intra abdominal Hodgkin's disease. Nodular sclerosis showed an almost equal distribution between peripheral lymph nodes, abdominal nodes, and spleen, while lymphocyte predominance occurred most often in peripheral and abdominal nodes. Lymphocyte depletion was seen most often with liver and spleen lesions, while mixed cellularity was most prevalent in peripheral lymph nodes.

Several old and new tests were found to have value in selecting patients who might have a higher chance of having abdominal Hodgkin's disease. Ratkin et al (in press) found the presence of unexplained anemia correlated with infradiaphragmatic involvement. In 41 patients with Hodgkin's disease, 53 percent of anemic patients had positive spleens and 37 percent had involved abdominal lymph nodes, contrasted with 18 percent and 5 percent, respectively, for nonanemic patients. Najean et al (1967) showed that anemia of Hodgkin's disease resembled iron deficiency anemia but iron stores were not depleted and iron administration did not correct the anemia. Using radioactive labeled hemoglobin, they demonstrated that the incorporation of iron into erythrocytes was smaller and slower than normal in patients with active disease, but not in those whose disease was inactive. Lanaro et al (1971) studied red blood cell survivals in a series of 22 consecutive patients with Hodgkin's disease. Seventy-three percent of the patients had values within the normal limits established in their laboratory tests (half-life 36.6 ± 4.3 days). They found patients with early disease had normal survival values, whereas half of the cases in advanced stages had decreased erythrocyte survival. The exact cause of this abnormality is not known.

Aisenberg (1962) and Brown et al (1967) conducted delayed hypersensitivity studies in patients with Hodgkin's disease, and they found those with advanced disease were more likely to be anergic. Gutterman et al (1972) evaluated skin-test reactivity in 11 patients prior to staging laparotomy. They could not correlate the results of delayed hypersensitivity with the presence or absence of intraabdominal disease. They also reviewed 6 reports in the literature and believed that the histological type as well as the presence or absence of systemic symptoms should not be given major consideration in selecting patients for laparotomy and splenectomy. Schwartz (Meeker et al 1972) mentioned he had 2 patients back-to-back who had clinically stage IA unicentric cervical disease who had hepatic involvement on open biopsy.

Other than the significance of splenomegaly which means a higher chance of lymphomatous involvement, Halie et al (1972a) described two types of abnormal cells in the peripheral blood which correlated highly with Hodgkin's lesion in the spleen. They believed this finding supported the thesis of hematogenous spread or a multicentric origin of the disease. Using the finding of this blood test and examination of the spleen removed at surgery, they found all 5 "localized" cases were in remission after total nodal irradiation, whereas only 1 of 12 patients with "disseminated" disease reached remission and all others had recurrences (Halie et al 1972b).

Presently, clinical manifestations, similar to the findings of laboratory tests, x-ray or radioisotopic studies have not been useful in excluding patients who would not be benefited from exploratory laparotomy. The distribution of histological subtypes of Hodgkin's disease in patients who underwent staging laparotomy is different from the overall distribution of 12 clinical series as summarized before (Table 6-5). The percentage of patients with nodular sclerosis is definitely higher among the operative series (60 percent versus 18–53 percent); and the percentage of lymphocyte depletion is certainly lower (3 percent versus 4–25 percent). With the knowledge that the

Table 6-5

Distribution of Histological Types Among Hodgkin's Patients Who Had Laparotomy

	Total Patient No.	Histology			
		LP	NS	MC	LD
Jelliffe et al (1970)	22	1	17	4	
Aisenberg et al (1970)	25	1	16	8	
Dorfman (1971)	185	13	137	32	3
Farrer-Brown et al (1971)	44	7	23	14	
Hass et al (1971)	50	10	27	12	1
Ibrahim et al (1972)	27	9	8	9	1
Mitchell et al (1972)	45	6	23	15	1
Prosintz et al (1972b)	40	2	21	14	3
Zarembok et al (1972)	30	3	19	4	4
Ratkin et al (in press)	40	7	18	13	2
EFSCH	12	4	5	2	1
Total	520	63	314	127	18
Percentage		12%	60%	25%	3%
12 Clinical Series (p. 41)		10–26%	18–53%	20–35%	4–25%

different histological subtypes might have different findings at exploration, we have summarized the results reported in the literature in Table 6-6. It appears that nodular sclerosis has a relatively low incidence (7 percent) of liver involvement, but 39 percent had splenic and/or abdominal node disease. Patients with lymphocyte predominance had a higher rate of liver involvement (15 percent). And the other 2 histological subtypes (mixed cellularity and lymphocyte depletion) had the highest rate of positive findings in the liver (18 percent), spleen and lymph node (51–72 percent).

These data supported Rosenberg's contention that: "no matter what the histology, in patients where there was a totally negative clinical evaluation, even in lymphocyte predominance or nodular sclerosis type and, even in the presence of a negative lymphangiogram, there still were patients who had disease below the diaphragm. Even in the absence of systemic symptoms, where there was a negative or an equivocal lymphangiogram, there were still 5 patients out of 16 with unsuspected disease. Young patients have the lowest risk of all the selected groups, but there are examples of various patients under 30 in whom the laparotomy was of value" (Tubiana 1971). Trueblood et al (1972) also concluded that the recognition of histological patterns is not a reliable indication of the extent of disease. However, Kaplan (1972b) once reported that "had we performed a splenectomy in all women with Hodgkin's disease in stage I with lymphocyte predominance or nodular sclerosis or in all men in stage I with lymphocyte predominance over the past 7 years, all would have been done unnecessarily judged by the fact that there has so far been no recurrence of disease since treatment in any of the 3 groups." Thus his treatment plan for patients with stage

Table 6-6
Histology of Hodgkin's Disease versus Sites of Involvement*

	Total patient No.	Abdominal node(+)				Mediastinum(+)				Spleen(+)				Liver(+)			
		LP	NS	MC	LD	LP	NS	MC	LD	LP	NS	MC	LD	LP	NS	MC	LD
Jelliffe et al (1970)	22					-/-	8/17	0/4		0/1	9/17	2/4	-/-	0/1	2/17	2/4	0/3
Aisenberg et al (1971)	25					-/-	4/16	4/8		-/-	7/16	5/8	-/-	-/-	3/16	0/8	-/-
Dorfman (1971)	185	0/13	98/137	11/32	1/3	6/13	58/137	20/32	2/3	3/13	53/137	20/32	2/3	1/13	7/137	7/32	0/3
Mitchell et al (1972)	45	0/6	17/23	5/15	-/-	3/6	7/23	7/15	-/-	2/6	7/23	7/15	-/-	2/6	5/23	1/15	-/-
Prosnitz et al (1972b)	40	0/2	10/20	4/15	2/3	0/2	11/20	7/15	1/3	0/2	7/20	7/15	1/3	0/2	0/20	4/15	0/3
Zarembok et al (1972)	30	1/3	17/19	4/4	2/4	1/3	3/19	2/4	3/4	1/3	7/19	3/4	4/4	0/3	0/19	0/4	1/4
Total	347	1/24	142/199	24/66	6/11	12/26	91/232	40/78	7/11	7/26	90/232	44/78	8/11	4/26	17/232	14/78	2/11
Percentage of each		4%	71%	36%	55%	46%	39%	51%	64%	27%	39%	56%	72%	15%	7%	18%	18%
Overall Percentage		$\frac{165}{300} = 55\%$				$\frac{150}{347} = 44\%$				$\frac{149}{347} = 43\%$				$\frac{37}{347} = 11\%$			

*Number of patients with positive lesions/total number of patients with the particular histology subtype.

209

IA, and IIA of the upper half of the body with histological subtypes of lymphocyte predominance and nodular sclerosis was to give supervoltage irradiation to the mantle field without prior staging laparotomy.

ADDITIONAL BENEFITS

Exploratory laparotomy not only determines for certain whether or not the intraabdominal lymph nodes or organs are involved, but presents additional benefits important for the clinical management of the patient. Glatstein et al (1969) pointed out that with the spleen removed and the splenic pedicle marked radiographically by a silver clip, it became possible to irradiate the nodes along the splenic pedicle without causing damage to the left lower lobe of the lung, pleura, diaphragm, heart, and the upper half of the left kidney. In the past these areas had to be included in the treatment field due to splenic movement with respiration. In addition, the reduced size of the upper abdominal field made it possible in some patients to treat the pelvic fields simultaneously and thereby reduce the total treatment time.

It was also felt that splenectomized patients seemed to have fewer and less severe episodes of thrombocytopenia, leukopenia, and related complications during radiation therapy. Salzman and Kaplan (1971) did a comparative study of hematologic changes during total lymphoid radiotherapy of 50 patients who had splenectomy (group A) and 50 patients who retained their spleens (group B). Group A maintained higher counts throughout treatment, and the differences between the 2 groups were statistically significant for platelets in all fields of treatment and for white blood cells during the mantle and pelvic fields, but not the para-aortic field. During the follow-up period, group A recovered toward pretreatment levels faster and more completely than group B. Treatment interruptions were required in 7 group A patients and 16 group B patients. All group A patients had completion of therapy after an average of 25 weeks of treatment whereas 16 of the group B patients were not able to resume original planned therapy because of persisted low blood counts.

Marks et al (1971) also felt that splenectomy played a role in the success of extended mantle therapy for patients with Hodgkin's disease and other malignant lymphomas. "Theoretically, the spleen removes functionally competent red and white cells and platelets with minor morphological aberrations; hence when the spleen is not present to filter out these functional components of the peripheral blood, radiotherapist and chemotherapist alike can apply more vigorous therapy."

Rosenthal (1948) first used splenectomy to elevate the white blood cell count and to enhance patients' tolerance to nitrogen mustard therapy. Nies and Creger (1967) reported 11 patients (including 4 with Hodgkin's disease,

3 each of lymphosarcoma and reticulum cell sarcoma) who had splenectomy for leukopenia or thrombocytopenia which prevented necessary chemotherapy. White cell counts rose to at least 5000 in all 8 patients who previously had had leukopenia, and platelet counts rose to at least 140,000 in 9 of the 11 patients who had thrombocytopenia. In two-thirds of the patients whose peripheral counts responded to splenectomy, at least a moderate dose of chemotherapy could be given without severe depression of the white cell and platelet counts for 2 months or longer.

Lowenbraun et al (1970) reported that 5 of the 12 Hodgkin's patients who did not have extensive radiotherapy had excellent tolerance of combination chemotherapy (MOPP) after laparotomy and splenectomy. Even in 10 patients with advanced Hodgkin's disease (9 with stage IVB and one stage IIIA), 8 of whom had bone or marrow involvement and poor tolerance to myelosuppressive drugs, Lowenbraun et al (1971) reported good amelioration of the cytopenia after splenectomy and excellent tolerance to chemotherapy.

Prosnitz et al (1972a) commented that bone marrow depression during the course of therapy of stage III patients was common in those who had not had splenectomy. Splenectomized patients, in contrast, had little difficulty. Fuller and Gamble (1973) utilized combined chemotherapy and radiotherapy in 33 patients with stage III Hodgkin's disease. They said some difficulty was encountered in patients treated with two courses of MOPP therapy who did not have a splenectomy performed.

However, De Vita (1971a) commented that the efficacy of splenectomy as part of the initial treatment of Hodgkin's disease remained largely unproven. In some 140 patients treated with the MOPP protocol, 12 presented with pancytopenia and their blood counts invariably improved rather than worsened on a full dose of drugs. Viola et al (1973) reported a Hodgkin's patient who had extensive myelofibrosis, pancytopenia and abnormal cells in the peripheral blood. Following four courses of MOPP therapy, the patient had a normal peripheral blood picture and a normal bone marrow biopsy. Panettiere and Coltman (1973) reported that patients with Hodgkin's disease received more chemotherapeutic agents in a shorter period of time when they had undergone prior splenectomy, because they had higher circulating platelet and lymphocyte counts prior to chemotherapy. However, after 4 courses of chemotherapy, there was a proportionately greater fall in the white blood cell and platelet counts in the asplenic group. Preliminary data suggest that there may be enhanced response rate in the asplenic group.

It is interesting to note that Woods et al (1971) conducted a retrospective study of 53 consecutive patients who had renal allograft transplants and found that the incidence of Imuran-induced leukopenia in nonsplenectomized patients was significantly higher than in patients who had splenectomy prior to transplantation. They reported 2 patients who had marked increase in tolerance to immunosuppressive chemotherapy when splenectomy was performed. Hartley et al (1971) also reported 4 patients who were on regular hemodialysis therapy and who were incapacitated by anemia probably secondary to excess splenic activity. After splenectomy, all patients had diamatic and sustained symptomatic relief without further transfusions.

One important aspect of conducting a pretreatment staging operation is to perform oophoropexy to avoid sterilization in young female patients. When ovaries are placed in the midline, they can be shielded with a lead block during radiotherapy to the external iliac, obturator, and hypogastric nodes. The dose of radiation received by such ovaries, calculated as immediately beneath the middle of the 10-cm lead block, was 9 percent of the incident dose (Ray et al 1970). Primary transmission accounts for only 0.5 percent of this, the remainder being due to scattered radiation. The midline ovaries received a minimal dose of 263 rads and a maximal of 4400 rads. Thus, it is not surprising that Trueblood et al (1970) reported that 12 of 23 patients (52 percent) had preservation of normal menstrual periods following radiotherapy, 1 other patient resumed spontaneous menstruation after 22 months of sustained amenorrhea. One patient became pregnant after radiotherapy and gave birth to a normal infant. Baker et al (1972) used an 8-cm lead block and found that the maximal dose received by the midline ovaries was about 13 percent of the doses given to the pelvic nodes, about 500 rads over a period of 4 weeks. Three of their 8 patients had normal menstruation. Another patient, who had stage IIIA disease, resumed menstruation after 2 years of amenorrhea and gave birth to a normal baby 6 years after irradiation.

In laterally transposed ovaries, which are located about 5 cm from the edge of the "inverted Y" radiation field, Nahhas et al (1971) found that the dose received was 8 percent or less of the incident dose. Of this, about 3 percent was transmitted through the lead block and 5 percent scattered. Menstruation was normal in 3 of the 4 patients who had pelvic irradiation. All 12 patients who had radiotherapy to the second lumbar area were menstruating normally. It is obvious that not all female patients are so fortunate. Schwartz et al (1971) commented that "in actual practice, few radiotherapists are able to deliver adequate doses of radiotherapy without damage or sterilization of the ovaries even after oophoropexy."

INDICATIONS FOR NON-HODGKIN'S LYMPHOMA

Rosenberg (1971) mentioned that studies using routine laparotomy and bone marrow biopsies are in progress, and hopefully, applying the newer histopathological classification of Rappaport (1966), it might be possible to identify the patterns of intraabdominal involvement of non-Hodgkin's disease.

Later, Jones et al (1973) of Stanford reported that the Rappaport classification did segregate the non-Hodgkin cases into two very distinct groups which exhibited marked differences in behavior after radiotherapy. Patients with localized *diffuse* histiocytic lymphoma suffered a relapse very rapidly after conventional therapy, with 95 percent of the relapse occurring within 13 months after admission; the median survival was only 13 months. Patients with localized *nodular* mixed cell or lymphocytic poorly differentiated lymphomas had a median survival of 80 months, but they continued to have a significant high and relatively constant risk of relapse several years (11 percent at 5 years) after initial radiotherapy. Starting in July, 1971, they conducted a new clinical trial including all untreated patients with biopsy-proven non-Hodgkin's lymphoma, age ranges 10 to 70 years. Routine exploratory laparotomy was performed on the first 69 patients, (stage I to IV). This disclosed involvement of para-aortic lymph nodes in 42 percent of the patients, splenic lymphoma in 32 percent, and hepatic involvement in 16 percent. In particular, mesenteric lymph nodes were affected by lymphoma in 61 percent of the 31 patients who underwent mesenteric node biopsies. Approximately 30 percent of the patients had their clinical stages changed as a result of the laparotomy findings.

Hanks et al (1971) presented a series of 24 patients who had staging laparotomy and 10 of these had non-Hodgkin's lymphoma. They mentioned that these 10 patients came from 46 patients seen during the same time period. Elias and Mittelman (1971) included 8 patients of non-Hodgkin's lymphoma in the 27 patients who had exploratory laparotomy. Hass et al (1971) presented a series of 75 patients operated on after June, 1969; 25 of them had stages I to IV non-Hodgkin's disease (13 patients were untreated and 12 had prior therapy).

Hass et al (1971) showed that in their hands, the lymphangiographic evaluation of non-Hodgkin's lymphoma was 100 percent accurate, but clinical and radioisotopic scanning evaluation of the spleen was reliable in about 60 percent of the cases. About half of the patients with splenic tumors also had liver involvement. When the liver was clinically abnormal, 33 percent had histologic lymphoma; and when it was felt to be normal, 20 percent had disease. Hepatic involvement by lymphoma was typically limited to nodules in the triads or capsule. In untreated patients, the liver was involved only in stage IIIB patients; in previously treated patients, the liver was involved in 1 out of 7 IIIA patients. Two patients, both of poorly differentiated lymphocytic type, were found to have bowel involvement with extensive diseases in the retroperitoneal region and mesentery.

Brunk et al (1970) reported about 16 percent of non-Hodgkin's patients had their stage changed as a result of exploratory laparotomy. None of the 12 patients with stage I or II disease had hepatic or splenic involvement. In stage III, 18 of 28 had involvement of the spleen and 7 of 28, the liver. In stage IV, 1 of 2 had involvement of both organs. They seemed to feel that in patients with stage III disease, exploratory laparotomy provided most valuable information about areas of involvement and permitted more carefully planned radiation therapy.

Gutterman et al (1972) felt that staging laparotomy and splenectomy appeared to be justified in patients with non-Hodgkin's lymphoma, since 2 of their 5 patients had their stages changed. Hanks et al (1972) showed that preoperative clinic stages of 7 of the 15 untreated patients with non-Hodgkin's lymphoma were in error as a result of laparotomy, (2 of 9 stage I and II patients were advanced to III, 1 to IV; 4 of 6 stage III patients were changed, 1 improved to I, 3 to IV). Three of 15 patients with normal liver tests, scans, and needle biopsies proved to have hepatic involvement by open biopsy. All also had splenic disease histologically. The spleen was normal in 3 of the 7 patients with positive mesenteric nodes, illustrating the contrasting sites of abdominal extension in non-Hodgkin's lymphoma as compared to Hodgkin's disease, which rarely involves mesenteric lymph nodes. When mesenteric nodes were involved they delivered 2000 rads in 2 to 3 weeks to the entire abdomen and an additional 2000 rads in 2 weeks to the retroperitoneal area and any surgically delineated involved nodes.

Thus, staging laparotomy appears to achieve the same purposes in non-Hodgkin's lymphoma as in Hodgkin's disease. These are: (1) to detect and confirm intraabdominal visceral involvement, especially liver or gastrointestinal disease; (2) to detect errors in clinical staging by biopsy of nodal areas not defined by lymphangiogram such as the region around and above the cisterna chyli, the splenic hilus, and the mesenteric lymph nodes; (3) to direct radiotherapy with greater accuracy after surgical definition of the extent of intraabdominal involvement. However, Aisenberg (1973) felt it is difficult to justify routine laparotomy for patients with non-Hodgkin's lymphoma because in such cases a choice between curative therapies does not exist. Rosenberg also expressed his opinion in a Forum (1973): "Until the results of several of the ongoing studies are known, and unless the patient in question is part of an appropriate clinical investigation, it would be wise for physicians to limit surgical staging to patients with Hodgkin's disease and not use the procedure for other lymphomas."

Bagley et al (1973) reported on the value of peritoneoscopy and multiple liver biopsies in detecting hepatic involvement in 46 patients with untreated non-Hodgkin's lymphomas as compared with percutaneous liver biopsies. Among patients with lymphocytic or mixed cell lymphoma, positive percutaneous liver biopsies were found in 50 percent of patients with hepatomegaly, but in only 11 percent of those without hepatomegaly (p < 0.025). Of the patients who had negative percutaneous biopsy, peritoneoscopy specimen was positive in about 27 percent, but 50 percent of patients with negative peritoneoscopy had diagnosable hepatic lymphoma by wedge biopsy at laparotomy. Thus, it appears that peritoneoscopy was unreliable in patients with non-Hodgkin's lymphomas. However, if the sole purpose of laparotomy were to determine the status of the liver involvement, then approximately one third of patients with negative percutaneous biopsies would have been spared a laparotomy by the finding of positive liver biopsies on peritoneoscopy.

COMPLICATIONS AND MORTALITIES

The complication rates of splenectomies in Hodgkin's patients who had either massive splenomegaly or significant hypersplenism were high. In the first series of 65 patients who had staging laparotomies, there were no wound infections, dehiscence, or subphrenic abscess (Glatstein et al 1969). Approximately 1 out of every 3 patients did have postoperative fever and basilar atelectasis. There were 28 patients who had previous therapy and, in a footnote, the authors cited postoperative death of a patient who had a laparotomy 18 months after mantle radiotherapy. Preoperatively, he had splenomegaly, pancytopenia, and abnormal liver function tests. At autopsy, sepsis, left subphrenic abscesses, and disseminated Hodgkin's disease were found.

In the second series of patients reported from Stanford University, Enright et al (1970) listed a complication rate of 9 percent in 68 previously untreated patients. These included 3 wound infections; and 1 each of pneumonia, mild pancreatitis, and urinary tract infection. In another report, Glatstein et al (1970) mentioned one serious complication of a colonocutaneous fistula which healed after approximately 2 weeks of conservative management.

In the 22 patients reported by Jelliffe et al (1970) 1 suffered 2 pulmonary emboli from which he recovered completely. It was pointed out that all patients showed a rise in the platelet count which usually reached its highest level 10 to 14 days after surgery. In 2 patients, it rose to just under 900,000/mm^3. Among 12 patients reported by Lowenbraun et al (1970), 1 developed a platelet count of greater than 1,000,000/mm^3 that decreased after therapy. Abrahamsen (1972) presented data to show that there appeared to be a considerable pooling of platelets in the spleens of patients with untreated Hodgkin's disease. After the splenectomy, the degree of thrombocytosis correlated with the weight of the removed spleen and might, to a large extent, have been due to removal of the splenic platelet pool.

In the 21 patients undergoing staging laparotomies reported by Allen et al (1971) 1 had acute gastrointestinal bleeding on the fourth postoperative day due to a reactivation of peptic gastritis. Nahhas et al (1971) reported that among 18 young women who had lateral ovarian transpositions, 1 required a second laparotomy 3 months later and a pelvic hematoma was found. Among the 18 patients reported by Zarembok et al (1972) 1 developed small bowel obstruction 6 months after the laparotomy. He had received abdominal radiotherapy during this period, and multiple adhesions were found at surgery.

Ferguson (Meeker et al 1972) reported a 5.3 percent complication rate in 151 staging laparotomy operations (including 50 non-Hodgkin's lymphomas and 7 mycosis fungoids). A serious gastric hemorrhage and subphrenic abscess occurred in a patient who had a gastrectomy, and a pancreatic fistula in a patient who had chronic pancreatitis. The others were wound complications, 3 of which occurred in patients with mycosis fungoids. It is important to note that the author performed additional procedures during the laparotomy: 2 gastrectomies, 1 jejunal resection for lymphomas, and 6 incidental cholecystectomies. In the small series operated upon at EFSCH (Table 6-7), 3 of the 15 staging operations had additional procedures: appendectomy and resection of ileum, cholecystectomy, thoracotomy and lung biopsy. There was no complication. But 1 of the other 12 patients had a minor complication which consisted of a tear of the diaphragm during the splenectomy; this was treated with short-term thoracostomy.

Prior to early 1972, there were approximately 600 cases who had staging laparotomies for untreated Hodgkin's disease which were recorded in the literature, and no mortality was reported. Jewell et al (1972), of the University of Kentucky, described the first death occurring in a healthy 19-year old male. The patient, who had asymptomatic mediastinal and right supraclavicular adenopathy, died of irreversible bronchospasm following a laparotomy and splenectomy. Whether the bronchospasm was related to the presence of Hodgkin's disease is not known, but a possible explanation, relating to an excess of bradykinin which can cause bronchospasm, is offered. Eilam et al (1968) found patients with Hodgkin's disease had significantly lower levels of plasma bradykininogen than either normal subjects or those with inactive Hodgkin's disease. The finding was compatible with increased release of bradykinin, a substance thought to be a chemical mediator of inflammation. The spleen has cathepsins which inactivate bradykinin (Greenbaum and Yamafuji 1966); removal of the spleen may thus indirectly result in excess bradykinin.

Mitchell et al (1972) reported another death among 45 patients. They specifically mentioned that this patient was the last of their series, all operated upon by one surgeon. (Later, a larger series of 64 patients was reported from the same institution by Peters et al 1973.) The patient developed a rapidly advancing thrombophlebitis on the 11 postoperative day. Pulmonary embolism resulted and the patient died of hemorrhagic diathesis and gastrointestinal hemorrhage. Two obese patients with body weights over 200 pounds had wound dehiscence (1 also had a subphrenic abscess). A third patient developed partial small bowel obstruction relieved by conservative measures.

Meeker et al (1972), also of the University of Kentucky, reviewed 30 patients operated upon at the University Medical Center and at community hospitals. A second mortality occurred in a 26-year old patient with clinical stage III disease. He developed a postoperative massive gastrointestinal hemorrhage which necessitated a subtotal gastrectomy. Unfortunately, this

Table 6-7
Exploratory Laparotomy and Splenectomy for Malignant Lymphoma (EFSCH series)

Patient No.	Age	Sex	Date	Histology	Neck	Supraclavicular	Axilla	Groin	Mediastinum	Marrow	Lymphography	Clinical liver	Clinical spleen	Liver scan	Stage	Marrow	Para-aortic	Splenic hilum	Spleen (g)	Liver	Other	Stage	Radiotherapy	Chemotherapy	Survival (months) * = alive
					Lymphadenopathy							Preoperative impression				Operative findings						Postoperative			
Hodgkin's disease																									
37933	40	M	1/69	LP	R,L	−	R,L	R,L	−	−	0	+	+	+	IVA (ileum)	0	−	+	+(735)	−	Ileum (+) mesenteric (−)	IVA	−	+	10
38097	59	M	4/69	LP	R,L	R,L	R,L	−	+	−	+	−	−	0	IIIB	0	0	+	− (0)	0	−	IIIB	+	+	34*
38375	39	M	[1]4/69	MC	−	R	−	−	+	−	+	+	+	0	IIIB	0	0	+	+(520)	0	−	IIIB	+	+	4
37306	23	F	7/69	NS	−	R,L	−	−	+	−	0	+	−	+[2]	I₂B	0	0	+	+(212)	+	−	IVB	−	+	27*
38712	22	F	12/69	NS	−	R,L	R,L	−	+	−	0	+	−	+	IVB (liver)	−	+	+	+(221)	−	Peripancreatic(+)	IVB	+	+	30*
38821	42	M	[1]2/70	NS	−	R	L	−	+	0	0	+	−	0	IVB (lung)	−	+	+	+(320)	−	Mesenteric(+) lung(+)	IVB	−	+	25*
22169	75	M	3/70	LD	R	−	R,L	R,L	−	−	0	−	+	−	IIIB	0	−	−	−(245)	−	Mesocolon(−) iliac(−)	IIIB	+	+	3
38901	38	M	[1]3/70	LP	−	L	R	R,L	+	−	0	−	−	+[2]	IIIA	−	+	−	+(195)	−	−	IIIA	−	+	25*
39607	28	F	1/71	LP	L	L	−	−	+	0	0	−	−	0	IIA	0	−	−	+(120)	−	−	IIA	+	−	15
39906	23	M	4/71	NS	R,L	R,L	−	−	+	−	0	−	−	−	IIA	−	−	+	+(415)	−	−	IIIA	+	+	12
40360	35	M	9/71	MC	R,L	R	−	R,L	−	0	0	−	−	−	IIB	0	+	−	−(330)	−	−	IIB	+	−	6
40471	20	F	11/71	NS	R,L	R	−	−	−	+	0	−	−	−	I₂A	−	−	−	(84)	−	mesenteric(−)	IA	+	−	7*
Non-Hodgkin's lymphoma																									
38101	47	M	8/70	Und	−	−	−	−	−	0	−	+	−	+	IVA (liver)	0	+	0	−	−	mesenteric(−)	IIIA	−	+	18
39711	49	M	2/71	LPD	−	L	−	R,L	−	−	0	−	+	−	IIIA	0	+	−	−(144)	+	mesenteric(−)	IIIA	−	−	14
39644	43	M	2/71	LWN	R,L	−	L	R,L	+	+	0	−	+	−	IVA (marrow)	+	+	+	+(1687)	+	mesenteric(+)	IVA	−	−	9

0 = Test not done.
1 = Patients who had previous therapy.
2 = Abnormal scan suggested lesion at porta hepatis.

217

was followed by wound dehiscence and culminated in his death with liver failure thought to be secondary to severe hepatitis. In the discussion of the paper, Ferguson said there was 1 death among the 94 consecutive staging operations for Hodgkin's disease, all supervised by one surgeon. The 52-year-old patient, who had had a cholecystectomy shortly before the staging exploration, died 11 days after an uneventful operation from a pulmonary embolism (Ferguson et al 1973).

Prior to September, 1972, there were reports from 22 institutions in the English literature concerning the experience of over 1000 patients (about 10 percent had previous therapy) who had staging laparotomies for Hodgkin's disease. With the 5 deaths reported, the overall operative and postoperative mortality rate was about 0.5 percent. However, the true incidence of deaths associated with staging laparotomies must be higher, since many surgical complications are not reported. For instance, Kaplan (1972a) mentioned one fatal instance which occurred in one of his affiliated teaching hospitals. There was no death in the 185 patients with untreated Hodgkin's disease who had diagnostic laparotomies performed at Stanford University (Kadin et al 1971; Dorfman 1971).

Since 1972, the incidence of postlaparotomy complications reported in the literature also became higher. Perlin et al (1972) reported that 4 out of their 30 patients developed postoperative complications: one had bleeding from the splenic bed; another had a subdiaphragmatic abscess secondary to gastric perforation; in a third, paroxysmal atrial tachycardia occurred during anesthesia, followed by transient encephalopathy; a fourth had a bacteroides septicemia, thought to be directly related to his stage IV Hodgkin's disease. All patients had thrombocytosis, but only 3 were treated with heparin because the platelet count was over $1,000,000/mm^3$.

Terz et al (1972) encountered 3 patients with significant complications among 20 patients who had surgical staging procedures. One developed mechanical intestinal obstruction on the fifth postoperative day. Another, with a history of pulmonary embolism, developed a similar episode after the operation, despite partial occlusion of the inferior vena cava with a clip at the time of the laparotomy. A third patient required re-exploration a few hours after surgery for bleeding from a lumbar artery at the site of removal of a para-aortic node. Among the 40 patients reported by Prosnitz et al (1970a) there were 2 wound infections and 1 wound dehiscence. Two patients developed intestinal obstruction (2 and 18 months after surgery); both required exploration and lysis of adhesions in the left upper quadrant. In another patient, the hepatic artery was ligated at the celiac axis. This was recognized and corrected at the time. Postoperatively, while on anticoagulants, the patient developed a bleeding stress ulcer. He underwent a vagotomy and gastroenterostomy and eventually recovered. In 13 patients (5 with non-Hodgkin's lymphomas) who had staging laparotomies reported by Gutterman et al (1972), 4 had postoperative complications: pneumonia, wound infection, hematoma, and upper gastrointestinal bleeding.

Meeker et al (1972) reported a high complication rate of 27 percent (8 of 30) within 30 days of surgery. There was unexplained high fever (102°F), bronchospasm, massive gastrointestinal hemorrhage, pneumonia, and generalized herpes. They also studied other factors such as duration of the operation, amount of blood loss, and fluid replacement; but they did not say whether or not these factors correlated with the frequency of post-operative complication. The amount of estimated blood loss recorded had a range of 50–1400 ml. Five of 25 patients required blood transfusions of 500–1000 ml. Fluid replacemement had a range of 700–3700 ml. The average operation lasted for 114 minutes, with a range of 55–205 minutes. In the discussion of this paper, Beattie said a careful laparotomy in his hospital usually took about 4 hours.

Ratkin et al (in press) reported their experience of staging laparotomies of 41 patients with Hodgkin's disease and 11 with other lymphomas. Nine of these 52 patients (17 percent) had severe complications, defined as life-threatening or delaying antineoplastic therapy, within 3 weeks after surgery. There were 6 staphylococcal infections (2 subdiaphragmatic abscesses and 4 chronic deep wound infections), 1 upper gastrointestinal hemorrhage, 2 pulmonary emboli, and 1 hepatitis. One patient died from a cerebrovascular accident. Eight other patients had minor complications of atelectasis and urinary tract infections. The development of complications was not associated with the presence or absence of anemia nor with the histologic type of disease, although the complication rate was higher for those with non-Hodgkin's lymphomas and for those who had received previous therapy. Older patients generally had a higher frequency of severe complications. It was emphasized that thromboembolic phenomenon should be carefully watched for even after the patient is discharged from the hospital. They also recommended that individual institutions monitor their experiences carefully to determine if their patient populations are subject to higher morbidity from staging laparotomies.

Another serious and often fatal complication, recently reported by several authors, is septicemia or severe infection after splenectomy. This problem was thought not to be important in patients with untreated Hodgkin's disease, although it had been well studied and documented, especially in children. In 1952, King and Shumacker suggested that splenectomy might predispose to infection. Lowdon et al (1962) showed that the risk, although present at all ages, was probably greatest if the operation was performed in infancy. About 80 percent of the infections occurred within 2 years after surgery, and they had a tendency towards recurrent episodes (Horan and Colebatch 1962). Pneumococcal infections appeared to play a major role. Hemophilus influenza, neisseria meningitidis, and other cocci were found less frequently. It was recommended that splenectomized patients, especially children, be placed on prophylactic penicillin therapy for 2 years after the operation.

Eraklis et al (1967) studied the hazard of overwhelming infection after splenectomies in 467 pediatric patients. They found the most important variable in determining the risk of infection was the presence or absence of certain underlying or primary disease. There was no infection if a normal spleen was removed because of accidental injury; the risk was high (over 33 percent) in patients who had serious primary disease such as Cooley's anemia, Wiscott-Aldrich syndrome, or other immunologic deficiency states. Erickson et al (1968) showed that the frequency of meningitis and sepsis following a splenectomy before the age of 1 year was abnormally high. The frequency of postsplenectomy infection among older children did not appear to be significantly higher than normal, but the mortality from these infections which did occur was devastating (78 percent).

In 40 persons (only 3 were children), Pedersen and Videbaek (1966) also found that splenectomy for traumatic rupture of the spleen had no lasting sequal of any severity. But Whitaker (1969) reported that 8 of 77 patients who had severe pneumococcal infections had splenectomy (including 3 for traumatized spleens), whereas only one postsplenectomy infection existed among 523 patients with nonpneumococcal infections. Overwhelming bacterial infections (usually pneumonia, septicemia, or meningitis) or hemostatic defects, especially disseminated intravascular coagulation, and the Waterhouse-Friderichsen syndrome of adrenal collapse in adults undergoing splenectomies were also reported (Lowdon et al 1966; Bisno and Freeman 1970).

Rosenberg (1971b) mentioned a 10-year-old patient who had fatal hemophilus bacteremia and meningitis 2 years after the splenectomy for staging of Hodgkin's disease, although he did receive total lymphoid irradiation followed by combination chemotherapy. Later, more reports of late complications from splenectomies in patients with Hodgkin's disease appear in the literature. Stiver et al (1972) reported a 41-year-old man died of pneumococcal sepsis and disseminated intravascular coagulation without Hodgkin's disease 16 months after a staging laparotomy and splenectomy. Ravry et al (1972) reported 2 pediatric patients (ages 6 and 13) who developed life-threatening meningitis caused by pneumococci in one and hemophilus in the other within one year after the splenectomy. The second patient also suffered another episode of sepsis and peritonitis caused by pneumococci. Fortunately, both survived. Nixon and Aisenberg (1972) reported a fatal infection by hemophilus influenza in a 13-year-old girl 18 months after the staging splenectomy without residual Hodgkin's disease. Desser and Ultmann (1972) commented that 2 of the 4 cases described above had combination chemotherapy (MOPP). Moore et al (1972) also mentioned 2 other patients who developed septicemia after combination chemotherapy.

Donaldson et al (1972), from Stanford University, reviewed 494 patients seen from 1968 through 1971 for the occurrence of postsplenectomy bacteremia. There were 238 patients with Hodgkin's disease and 31 with non-

Hodgkin's lymphomas who had laparotomies and splenectomies as part of their initial evaluation procedure. The incidence of bacteremia in patients with lymphomas (4.5 percent) was no higher than that of the non-lymphoma group (9.3 percent). When bacteremia did develop, the mortality rate did not differ among patients with or without lymphomas. However, 5 of the 33 episodes of bacteremia which were due to pneumococcus occurred in patients with lymphomas (ages 14, 19, 21, 21, and 48 years). They mentioned that 4 of 27 patients with lymphomas seen during a 10-year period prior to this particular study did develop pneumococcal infections. But, unfortunately, a concurrent group of patients with lymphomas and without splenectomies was not available in their institution to do a comparable study. Only 1 of the 5 patients with pneumococcal bacteria died; he also had widespread lymphoma. They mentioned an 11-year-old child who died after the cutoff point of their study. He had fulminant pneumococcal pneumonia 9 months after the splenectomy. Assuming 10 percent of the 269 patients with lymphomas belonged to the pediatric age group, this means that mortality due to delayed septicemia is close to 7 percent (2 of 27).

Another possible, but unconfirmed, complication related to the splenectomy could be an increased incidence of viral infections. Goffinet et al (1972) found herpes zoster-varicella infections occurring in 11.4 percent of 1130 patients with malignant lymphomas. In 592 patients with Hodgkin's disease, the figure was higher (15.4 percent), especially in patients with advanced disease who received multiple chemotherapy after radiotherapy. They also noted a significantly increased incidence of viral infections in patients seen during 1969 (32 percent). Since both splenectomies and combination chemotherapy (MOPP) were aggressively utilized after 1968, it was not possible to say which contributed the most to this high rate of infection. Ravry et al (1972) noted that 5 of their 13 pediatric patients who had staging laparotomies had herpes zoster infections within 1 year after the splenectomy. However, Schimpff et al (1972) found the incidence of zoster in Hodgkin's patients was similar whether or not a splenectomy had been done (25 percent).

Desser and Ultmann (1972) conducted a preliminary survey of 12 institutions in this country (including the 269 cases reported by Donaldson et al 1972). Among a total of 1170 splenectomies carried out during staging laparotomies (934 were for Hodgkin's disease and 236 for non-Hodgkin's lymphomas), the incidence of severe bacterial infection was 1.4 percent and the mortality rate was 0.5 percent. They felt that these figures were substantially less than those reported for infections after splenectomies for other causes. They were unable to calculate age-adjusted rates, especially for children. However, they commented that the clustering of cases in the younger age patients indicated that this group deserved special consideration. They felt that patients under 15 years old, with nodular sclerosis and disease clinically restricted to the high neck or to the mediastinum alone, who had negative lymphangiograms, and who would be treated with extended mantle or total lymphoid radiotherapy, would probably be the least likely to derive additional benefit from laparotomies and splenectomies. Trueblood et al (1972) also commented that one cannot ignore the syndrome of pneumococcal septicemia and meningitis as being totally unrelated to the splenectomy.

Hays et al (1973) reported a series of 23 pediatric patients, ages 2 to 15 years, who had staging laparotomy for Hodgkin's disease from 1967 to 1972. The findings are similar to those of the adults; the clinical stage was altered by laparotomy in 11 of 23 patients (10 had stages advanced from I-II to III-IV), resulting in major changes of management. There was no intraoperative or postoperative complication; although one 22 month old patient died two months after the operation, probably caused by the hyperacute infection related to his asplenic state, and another died 18 months later of extensive pulmonary infiltration unrelated to the staging laparotomy. They commented that total nodal radiation therapy would produce distortion of skeletal growth in all infants and young children, and the effect of prolonged combination chemotherapy (COPP or MOPP) in early childhood were unknown. Because of these factors it would appear that laparotomy is probably of greater value in the child than in the adult with Hodgkin's disease.

SUMMARY

In an effort to more precisely delineate the extent of involvement of Hodgkin's disease below the diaphragm, exploratory laparotomy, splenectomy, biopsy of liver and abdominal lymph nodes were introduced. Later open biopsy of the bone marrow was added and ovaries of young female patients were transposed to areas outside the field of irradiation. It was emphasized that even the grossly normal spleen and lymph node should be removed for tissue diagnosis because they can harbor Hodgkin's disease.

Results of staging laparotomy showed that all the methods of nonoperative evaluation of spleen, liver and lymph nodes had serious limitations. Specifically, the spleen was involved in one-third of the cases thought to be uninvolved, and in two-thirds of those who had splenomegaly or abnormal radioisotopic scan. Liver biopsy was positive only in 30 percent of the patients who had hepatomegaly, abnormal scan or blood tests. About 4 percent of clinically normal livers had Hodgkin's disease by open biopsy. In the face of a normal lymphangiogram, 12 percent of the cases had lesions in retroperitoneal nodes by biopsy. Another 7 percent or so had positive nodes in the atypical locations of the porta hepatis, mesentery, or splenic hilum. And for those who had a definitely abnormal lymphangiogram, only 72 percent had positive nodes confirmed. In general, about 24 percent of the patients had their clinical stages advanced after staging laparotomy, and 15 percent had their stages decreased.

Findings of staging laparotomy have also improved our understanding of the natural pattern of involvement and the possible mode of spread of Hodgkin's disease. The different histological subtypes do have somewhat different natural histories. Splenectomy facilitates the administration of radiotherapy, decreases the complication of radiation pneumonitis and nephritis, and possibly also increases the patient's tolerance to radical radiotherapy as well as intensive chemotherapy. An additional bonus of performing laparotomy includes preservation of ovarian functions for the young female patients.

The practice of conducting pretreatment exploratory laparotomy has been extended to patients with non-Hodgkin's lymphoma and carcinoma of the uterine cervix. Involvement of mesenteric nodes and other viscera occurred more often in patients with non-Hodgkin's lymphoma, and staging laparotomy appears to achieve the same purposes as it does in Hodgkin's disease.

From the first report of Glatstein et al (1969) until early 1972, there were approximately 600 patients recorded in the literature who had staging laparotomy for untreated Hodgkin's disease. The postoperative complication rate was about 5 percent and no mortality was reported. Jewell et al (1972) reported the first operative death of a healthy 19-year-old man. Subsequently other reports appeared, and the overall mortality associated with staging laparotomy and splenectomy was about 0.5 percent. After 1972, the incidence of postoperative complications reported in the literature also became higher—as high as 30 percent. Case reports of severe postsplenectomy infections, which were thought not to be important in patients with early Hodgkin's disease, also appeared.

Presently, the major value and benefit of exploratory laparotomy and examination of tissues are to determine the extent of the disease, and then only if the identification of abdominal lesions would alter the therapeutic program planned preoperatively. Although certain correlations have been found between some of the clinicopathological factors and a higher incidence of abdominal involvement, none of these factors has been useful in excluding patients who would not have positive intraabdominal lesions. However, staging laparotomy and splenectomy is a major surgical procedure and should not be undertaken lightly. Moreover, it remains to be proven whether surgical staging will help alter the natural course of the disease and improve prognosis.

REFERENCES

Abrahamsen AF: Effects of an enlarged splenic platelet pool in Hodgkin's disease. Scand J Haematol 9:153–158, 1972

Aisenberg AC: Studies on delayed hypersensitivity in Hodgkin's disease. J Clin Invest 41:1964–1970, 1962

Aisenberg AC: Malignant lymphoma. N Engl J Med 288:883–890, 935–941, 1973

Aisenberg AC, Goldman JM, Raker JW: Spleen involvement at the onset of Hodgkin's disease. Ann Intern Med 74:544–547, 1971

Allen LW, Strum SB, Ultmann JE, et al : The staging of lymphoma, in Ultmann JE, Griem ML, Kirsten WH, et al (eds): Current Concepts in the Management of Leukemia and Lymphoma. New York, Springer, 1971, pp 13–46

Allen LW, Ultmann JE, Ferguson DJ, et al: Laparotomy and splenectomy in the staging of Hodgkin's disease. J Lab Clin Med 74:845, 1969

Averette HE, Dudan RC, Ford JH Jr: Exploratory celiotomy for surgical staging of cervical cancer. Am J Obstet Gynecol 113:1090–1096, 1972

Bagley CM Jr, Thomas LB, Johnson RE, et al: Diagnosis of liver involvement by lymphoma: Results in 96 consecutive peritoneoscopies. Cancer 31:840–847, 1973

Baker JW, Morgan RL, Peckham MJ, et al: Preservation of ovarian function in patients requiring radiotherapy for para-aortic and pelvic Hodgkin's disease. Lancet 1:1307–1308, 1972

Bisno AL, Freeman JC: The syndrome of asplenia, pneumococcal sepsis, and disseminated intravascular coagulation. Ann Intern Med 72:389–393, 1970

Bouroncle BA: Sternberg-Reed cells in the peripheral blood of patients with Hodgkin's disease. Blood 27:544–556, 1966

Browde S: Current concepts in the approach to Hodgkin's disease. South African Cancer Bull 15:137–147, 1971

Brown RS, Haynes HA, Foley HT, et al: Hodgkin's disease: Immunologic, clinical, and histologic features of 50 untreated patients. Ann Intern Med 67:291–302, 1967

Brunk SF, Gulesserian HP, Hass AC, et al: Exploratory laparotomy and splenectomy in staging lymphomas. Clin Res 18:470, 1970

Buchsbaum HJ: Para-aortic lymph node involvement in cervical carcinoma. Am J Obstet Gynecol 113:942–947, 1972

Curtis GM, Movitz D: The surgical significance of the accessory spleen. Ann Surg 123:276–298, 1946

Desser RK, Ultmann JE: Risk of severe infection in patients with Hodgkin's disease or lymphoma after diagnostic laparotomy and splenectomy. Ann Intern Med 77:143–146, 1972

Dettman PM, Storaasli JP: The status of Hodgkin's disease. Am J Med Sci 263:347–356, 1972

DeVita VT: Hodgkin's disease. Lancet 2:46–47, 1971a

DeVita VT Jr, Bagley CM Jr, Goodell B, et al: Peritoneoscopy in the staging of Hodgkin's disease. Cancer Res 31:1746–1750, 1971b

Donaldson SS, Moore MR, Rosenberg SA, et al: Characterization of postsplenectomy bacteremia among patients with and without lymphoma. N Engl J Med 287:69–71, 1972

Dorfman RF: Relationship of histology to site in Hodgkin's disease. Cancer Res 31:1786–1793, 1971

Eilam N, Johnson PK, Johnson NL, et al: Bradykininogen levels in Hodgkin's disease. Cancer 22:631–634, 1968

Elias EG, Mittelman A: The role of surgery in malignant lymphoma. Exhibit presented at the 57th Annual Clinical Congress, Am Coll Surg Meeting, Atlantic City, Oct 1971

Engeset A, Höeg K, Höst H, et al: Thoracic duct lymph cytology in Hodgkin's disease. Internatl J Cancer 4:735–742, 1969

Enright LP, Trueblood HW, Nelsen TS: The surgical diagnosis of abdominal Hodgkin's disease. Surg Gynecol Obstet 130:853–858, 1970

Eraklis AJ, Kevy SV, Diamond LK, et al: Hazard of overwhelming infection after splenectomy in childhood. N Engl J Med 276:1225–1229, 1967

Erickson WD, Burgert EO Jr, Lynn HB: The hazard of infection following splenectomy in children. Am J Dis Child 116:1–12, 1968

Exelby PR: Method of evaluating children with Hodgkin's disease. CA 21:95–101, 1971

Farrer-Brown G, Bennett MH, Harrison CV, et al: The diagnosis of Hodgkin's disease in surgically excised spleens. J Clin Pathol 25:294–300, 1972

Farrer-Brown G, Bennett MH, Harrison CV, et al: The pathological findings following laparotomy in Hodgkin's disease. Br J Cancer 25:449–457, 1971

Ferguson DJ, Allen LW, Griem ML, et al: Surgical experience with staging laparotomy in 125 patients with lymphoma. Arch Intern Med 131:356–361, 1973

Fisher ER, Fisher B: Recent observations on concepts of metastasis. Arch Pathol 83: 321–324, 1967

Forum on "Surgical staging of Hodgkin's disease: advantage or risk?" Participants: Perlin E, Stutzman L, Ultmann JE, Brunk SF, Rosenberg SA, Meeker WR. Mod Med 41(6):86–90, March 19, 1973

Fuller LM, Gamble JF: Current concepts in cancer. 40. Updated Hodgkin's Disease, combined chemotherapy-radiotherapy program. JAMA 223:168–169, 1973

Givler RL, Brunk SF, Hass CA, et al: Problems of interpretation of liver biopsy in Hodgkin's disease. Cancer 28:1335–1342, 1971

Glatstein E, Guernsey JM, Rosenberg SA, et al: The value of laparotomy and splenectomy in the staging of Hodgkin's disease. Cancer 24:709–718, 1969

Glatstein E, Trueblood HW, Enright LP, et al: Surgical staging of abdominal involvement in unselected patients with Hodgkin's disease. Radiology 97:425–432, 1970

Goffinet DR, Castellino RA, Kim H, et al: Staging laparotomies in unselected previously untreated patients with non-Hodgkin's Lymphomas. Cancer 32:672–681, 1973

Goffinet DR, Glatstein EJ, Merigan TC: Herpes zostervaricella infections and lymphoma. Ann Intern Med 76:235–240, 1972

Goldman JM: Laparotomy for staging of Hodgkin's disease. Lancet 1:125–127, 1971

Greenbaum LM, Yamafuji K: The in vitro inactivation and formation of plasma kinins by spleen cathepsins. Br J Pharmacol 27:230–238, 1966

Gutterman JU, Rodriguez V, McClure JB: Staging of malignant lymphoma by laparotomy and splenectomy: Review of the literature. Milit Med 137:251–254, 1972

Halie MR, Eibergen R, Nieweg HO: Observations on abnormal cells in the peripheral blood and spleen in Hodgkin's disease. Br Med J 2:609–611, 1972a

Halie MR, Seldenrath JJ, Stam HC, et al: Curative radiotherapy in Hodgkin's disease: Significance of haematogenous dissemination established by examination of peripheral blood and spleen. Br Med J 2:611–613, 1972b

Hanks GE, Newsome JF, Terry LN Jr: The value of laparotomy in staging lymphomas. South Med J 64:585–588, 1971

Hanks GE, Terry LN Jr, Bryan J, et al: Contribution of diagnostic laparotomy to staging non-Hodgkin's lymphoma. Cancer 29:41–43, 1972

Hartley LC, Innis MD, Morgan TO, et al: Splenectomy for anemia in patients on regular hemodialysis. Lancet 2:1343–1345, 1971

Hass AC, Brunk SF, Gulesserian HP, et al: The value of exploratory laparotomy in malignant lymphoma. Radiology 101:157–165, 1971

Hays DM, Karon M, Issacs H, et al: Hodgkin's disease: Technique and results of staging laparotomy in childhood. Arch Surg 106:507–512, 1973

Horan M, Colebatch JH: Relation between splenectomy and subsequent infection: A clinical study. Arch Dis Child 37:398–414, 1962

Ibrahim E, Fuller LM, Gamble JF, et al: Stage I Hodgkin's disease: Comparison of surgical staging with incidence of new manifestations in lymphogram- and prelymphogram-studied patients. Radiology 104:145–151, 1972

Ingold JA, Reed GB, Kaplan HS, et al: Radiation hepatitis. Am J Roentgenol Radium Ther Nucl Med 93:200–208, 1965

Jelliffe AM, Millet YL, Marston JA, et al: Laparotomy and splenectomy as routine investigations in the staging of Hodgkin's disease before treatment. Clin Radiol 21:439–445, 1970

Jewell WR, Furman R, Hasbrouck JD: Irreversible bronchospasm in Hodgkin's disease: An operative death. Surgery 71: 419–422, 1972

Johnson RE: Is staging laparotomy routinely indicated in Hodgkin's disease? Ann Intern Med 75:459–462, 1971

Johnson RE, Glover MK, Marshall SK: Results of radiation therapy and implications for the clinical staging of Hodgkin's disease. Cancer Res 31:1834–1837, 1971

Johnson RE, Thomas LB, Schneiderman M, et al: Preliminary experience with total nodal irradiation in Hodgkin's disease. Radiology 96:603–608, 1970

Jones SE, Fuks A, Kaplan HS, et al: Non-Hodgkin's lymphomas. V. Results of Radiotherapy. Cancer 32:682–691, 1973

Jones SE, Kaplan HS, Rosenberg S A: Non-Hodgkin's lymphomas. III. Preliminary results of radiotherapy and a proposal for new clinical trials. Radiology 103:657–662, 1972

Kadin ME, Glatstein E, Dorfman RF: Clinicopathologic studies of 117 untreated patients subjected to laparotomy for the staging of Hodgkin's disease. Cancer 27:1277–1294, 1971

Kaplan HS: Current concepts in Cancer. 39. Updated Hodgkin's Disease radiother-, apy of advanced Hodgkin's disease with curative intent. J A M A 223:50–53, 1973

Kaplan HS: Hodgkin's Disease. Cambridge, Mass, Harvard University Press, 1972a

Kaplan HS: Hodgkin's disease: Prognosis as related to pathology, staging and treatment. Proc R Soc Med 65:62–64, 1972b

Kaplan HS: On the natural history, treatment, and prognosis of Hodgkin's disease. Harvey Lect 64:215–259, 1968–69

King H, Shumacker HB Jr: Splenic studies. I. Susceptibility to infection after splenectomy performed in infancy. Ann Surg 136:239–242, 1952

Lanaro AE, Bosch A, Frias Z: Red blood cell survival in patients with Hodgkin's disease. Cancer 28:658–661, 1971

Lokich JJ: Staging laparotomy. Ann Intern Med 76:143–144, 1972

Lowdon AG, Stewart RH, Walker W: Risk of serious infection following splenectomy. Br Med J 1:446–450, 1966

Lowdon AG, Walker JH, Walker W: Infection following splenectomy in childhood. Lancet 1:449–504, 1962

Lowenbraun S, Ramsey H, Serpeck AA: Splenectomy in Hodgkin's disease for splenomegaly, cytopenias, and intolerance to myelosuppresive chemotherapy. Am J Med 50:49–55, 1971

Lowenbraun S, Ramsey H, Sutherland J, et al: Diagnostic laparotomy and splenectomy for staging Hodgkin's disease. Ann Intern Med 72:655–663, 1970

Marks JE, Pinsky SM, Griem ML: The extended mantle field in the radiotherapeutic treatment of malignant lymphoma. Radiology 100:423–425, 1971

Meeker WR Jr, Richardson JD, West WO, et al: Critical evaluation of laparotomy and splenectomy in Hodgkin's disease. Arch Surg 105:222–229, 1972

Mitchell RI, Peters MV, Brown TC, et al: Laparotomy for Hodgkin's disease: Some surgical observations. Surgery 71:694–703, 1972

Moore MR, Bull JM, Jones SE, et al: Sequential radiotherapy and chemotherapy in the treatment of Hodgkin's disease. Ann Intern Med 77:1–9, 1972

Nahhas WA, Nisce LZ, D'Angio GJ, et al: Lateral ovarian transposition. Obstet Gynecol 38:785–788, 1971

Najean Y, Dresch C, Ardaillou N: Trouble de l'utilisation due fer hemoglobinique au cours des maladies de Hodgkin evolutives. Nouv rev Fr hematol 7:739–754, 1967

Nies BA, Creger WP: Tolerance of chemotherapy following splenectomy for leukopenia or thrombocytopenia in patients with malignant lymphomas. Cancer 20:558–562, 1967

Nixon DW, Aisenberg AC: Fatal *hemophilus influenzae* sepsis in an asymptomatic splenectomized Hodgkin's disease patient. Ann Intern Med 77:69–71, 1972

Nuland SB: Splenectomy as an adjunct to the treatment of Hodgkin's disease. Conn Med 34:851–855, 1970

Paglia MA, Lacher MJ, Hertz RE, et al: Surgical aspects and results of laparotomy and splenectomy in Hodgkin's disease. Am J Roentgenol Radium Ther Nucl Med 117:12–18, 1973

Panettiere F, Coltman CA, Jr.: Splenectomy effects on chemotherapy in Hodgkin's disease. Arch Intern Med 131:362–366, 1973

Parker JC Jr, Richards JD, Meeker WR Jr: Histopathologic revelations of the staging of abdominal exploration in Hodgkin's disease-combined morphologic types. Am J Pathol 66:76a–77a, 1972 (Abstr)

Pedersen B, Videbaek A: On the late effects of removal of the normal spleen: A follow-up study of 40 persons. Acta Chir Scand [Suppl] 131:89–98, 1966

Perlin E, Ryan TF, Ebersole JH, et al: Diagnostic laparotomy and splenectomy in the clinical staging of Hodgkin's disease. Milit Med 137:97–102, 1972

Perlin E, Ryan TF, Moquin RB: Laparotomy for staging of Hodgkin's disease. Lancet 1:494, 1971

Peters MV: Changing concepts in radiotherapy for the lymphomas. Leukemia-Lymphoma. Chicago, Year Book, 1970, pp 261–274

Peters MV, Brown TC, Rideout DF: Current concepts in cancer. 39. Updated Hodgkin's Disease prognostic influences and radiation therapy according to pattern of disease. JAMA 223:53–59, 1973

Piro AJ, Hellman S, Moloney WC: The influence of laparotomy on management decisions in Hodgkin's disease. Arch Intern Med 130:844–848, 1972

Prosnitz LR, Fischer JJ, Vera R, et al: Hodgkin's disease treated with radiation therapy: Follow-up data and the value of laparotomy. Am J Roentgenol Radium Ther Nucl Med 114:583–590, 1972a

Prosnitz LR, Nuland SB, Kligerman MM: Role of laparotomy and splenectomy in the management of Hodgkin's disease. Cancer 29:44–50, 1972b

Rappaport H: Tumors of the hematopoietic system, Atlas of Tumor Pathology. Section III, Fascicle 8. Armed Forces Institute of Pathology, 1966

Ratkin GA, Present CA, Weinerman B: Correlation of anemia with infradiaphragmatic involvement in Hodgkin's disease and other malignant lymphomas. (in press)

Ravry M, Maldonado N, Velez-Garciá E, et al: Serious infection after splenectomy for the staging of Hodgkin's disease. Ann Intern Med 77:11–14, 1972

Ray GR, Trueblood HW, Enright LP, et al: Oophoropexy: A means of preserving ovarian function following pelvic megavoltage radiotherapy for Hodgkin's disease. Radiology 96:175–180, 1970

Rosenberg SA: The clinical evaluation and staging of patients with malignant lymphoma, in Ultmann JE, Griem ML, Kirsten WH, et al (eds): Current Concepts in the Management of Leukemia and Lymphoma. New York, Springer, 1971a, pp 32–42

Rosenberg SA: A critique of the value of laparotomy and splenectomy in the evaluation of patients with Hodgkin's disease. Cancer Res 31:1737–1740, 1971b

Rosenberg SA: Current concepts in Cancer. 36. Updated Hodgkin's Disease place of splenectomy in evaluation and management. JAMA 222:1296–1298, 1972

Rosenberg SA: Radiotherapy for Lymphoma, in Clark RL, Cumley RW, McCay JE, et al (eds): Oncology 1970, vol 4. Chicago, Year Book, 1971c, pp 518–525

Rosenberg SA, Boiron M, DeVita VT Jr, et al: Report of the Committee on Hodgkin's Disease Staging Procedures. Cancer Res 31:1862–1863, 1971

Rosenthal E: Nitrogen mustard therapy combined with splenectomy; preliminary communication. Lancet 1:408, 1948

Salzman JR, Kaplan HS: Effect of prior splenectomy on hematologic tolerance during total lymphoid radiotherapy of patients with Hodgkin's disease. Cancer 27:471–478, 1971

Schimpff S, Serpick A, Stoler B, et al: Varicella-zoster infection in patients with cancer. Ann Intern Med 76:241–254, 1972

Schwartz SI: Operative staging of Hodgkin's disease. Presented at the 57th Annual Clinical Congress, Am Coll Surg Meeting, Atlantic City, Oct 1971

Schwartz SI, Adams JT, Bauman AW: Splenectomy for hematologic disorders. Curr Probl Surg pp 1–57, May 1971

Schwartz SI, Cooper RA Jr: Surgery in the diagnosis and treatment of Hodgkin's disease. Adv Surg 6:175–203, 1972

Smith J, Pasmantier MW, Silver RT, et al: The staging of Hodgkin's disease: Selective vs routine laparotomy. JAMA 224:1026–1028, 1973

Smithers DW: Spread of Hodgkin's disease. Lancet 1:1262–1267, 1970

Stiver G, Sharrar R, Kendrick M, et al: Bacterial risk in staging splenectomy. Ann Intern Med 76:670, 1972

Terz JJ, King RE, Lawrence W Jr: The role of exploratory laparotomy in the staging of Hodgkin's disease. Va Med Mon 99:418–426, 1972

Trueblood HW, Enright LP, Ray GR, et al: Preservation of ovarian function in pelvic radiation for Hodgkin's disease. Arch Surg 100:236–237, 1970

Trueblood HW, Guernsey JM, Cohn R: Hodgkin's disease and non-Hodgkin's lymphoma—the surgeon's role in therapy. Curr Probl Surg pp 2–36, Aug 1972

Tubiana M: Summary of informal discussion on staging procedures in Hodgkin's disease. Cancer Res 31:1751–1754, 1971

Ucmakli A, Bonney WA Jr: Exploratory laparotomy as routine pre-treatment investigation in cancer of the cervix. Radiology 104:371–377, 1972

Ultmann JE: Hodgkin's disease: Laparotomy or not? Ann Intern Med 76:330–331, 1972

Viola MV, Kovi J, Nukhopadhyay M: Reversal of myelofibrosis in Hodgkin disease. JAMA 223:1145–1146, 1973

Whitaker AN: Infection and the spleen: Association between hyposplenism, pneumococcal sepsis and disseminated intravascular coagulation. Med J Aust 1: 1213–1219, 1969

Woods JE, DeWeerd JH, Johnson WJ, et al: Splenectomy in renal transplantation: Influence on azathioprine sensitivity. JAMA 218:1430–1431, 1971

Zarembok I, Ramsey HE, Sutherland J, et al: Laparotomy and splenectomy in the staging of untreated patients with Hodgkin's disease. Radiology 102:673–678, 1972

7
Gastrointestinal Malignant Lymphomas

Lymphomas of the gastrointestinal tract are more inclined to be localized than are similar lesions affecting other anatomical areas (Warren 1959; Azzopardi and Menzies 1960). Berg (1969) showed that primary gastrointestinal lymphoma tended to have mucosal and submucosal growth, and there were foci of early change in separate mucosal nodules. These findings left little doubt that these lymphomas did arise in the gut wall and did not invade it from any adjacent node. He commented that these small separate mucosal growths could be similar to separate lesions of carcinoma in situ found in the epithelium around invasive squamous cancer or adenocarcinomas. Review of the literature showed that half of the patients with gastric lymphomas and 20 percent of those with intestinal lymphoma who were operable and who survived the postoperative period could be cured. Rather than arguing whether certain lesions are primary or not, he suggested that the challenge for the clinicians and pathologists alike should be the identification of localized and reasonably curable lesions.

Thus, for all practical purposes, malignant lymphoma of the gastrointestinal tract could be divided into two groups: (1) the primary lesions which appear to originate from lymphoid cells in the gastrointestinal tract and are clinically confined to the bowel and adjacent mesenteric nodes; (2) secondary lesions which involve the gastrointestinal tract as part of the generalized disease. Dawson et al (1961) have established five criteria for the diagnosis of primary lymphoma of the gastrointestinal tract (p. 244). Lesions of the secondary type occurred about 10 times more frequently than the primary type (50 percent of the autopsy cases versus less than 5 percent presented initially). Although there are cases in which it is impossible, even at necropsy, to decide whether the lesions actually represent primary or secondary involvement of the gastrointestinal tract, recognition of a primary gastrointestinal lesion is of special interest and importance for surgeons because its diagnosis and management both require surgical procedures. Malignant lymphoma presented at each specific site of the digestive system appeared to have different natural histories and individual problems; thus, they will be discussed in separate sections below. In selected cases, surgery can achieve cure in primary lesions, whereas the goal is only for palliation in secondary lesions.

PRIMARY LESIONS (OVERALL)

In the 316 patients with Hodgkin's disease reported by Pack and Molander (1966), the gastrointestinal tract was the site of initial involvement in 1.9 percent. In the non-Hodgkin's series of Rosenberg et al (1961), the figure was 4.6 percent for 1269 patients. A higher incidence was reported by Skrimshire (1955) who said that 10 percent of all lymphomas diagnosed in a large teaching hospital arose primarily in the gastrointestinal tract. Bush and Ash (1969) said 5.3 percent of 1555 patients with malignant lymphoma had involvement of the digestive tract, and about half had early or primary lesions.

Looking at the incidence differently, Warren and Lulenski (1942) showed that 1 percent of 3132 gastrointestinal tumors were of lymphomatous origins (13 of the 28 cases were of Hodgkin's disease). Talvalkar (1968) found 38 cases of primary malignant lymphoma of the small and large intestine among a total of 1756 malignant neoplasms recorded (an incidence of 2.2 percent). Loehr et al (1969) reviewed 100 cases of primary lymphoma of the gastrointestinal tract and said this comprised 1.7 percent of all malignant gastrointestinal tumors treated since 1932.

The relative incidence of lymphomatous lesion among all gastrointestinal malignant tumors is very low in the esophagus and rectum, and high in the small intestine. Allen et al (1954) reported that of all malignant tumors seen from 1913 to 1953 at their hospital, 0.1 percent of those of the esophagus and rectum were malignant lymphomas, whereas 39.7 percent of small intestinal tumors were such. The figures for the colon and stomach were 0.5 percent and 2 percent, respectively. Faulkner and Dockerty (1952) found 20 percent of small intestinal tumors were of lymphoid origin, and al-Khateeb (1970) of Iraq reported that all of the malignant lesions of the small bowel were lymphomas.

McNeer and Berg (1959) found that 2.5 percent of 1685 gastric tumors were malignant lymphomas, and Cohen (1961) said lymphoid tumors represented 3.4 percent of 2854 cases of gastric neoplasms. Of those patients who died of lymphosarcoma, 40 percent has gastric involvement (McNeer and Pack 1962). With the decreasing incidence of gastric adenocarcinomas in the last 20 years, malignant lymphoma of the stomach will be seen more frequently in the future. Dunn et al (1971) reported 39 patients with gastric lymphomas recorded from 1947 to 1969, and 23 were diagnosed after 1960.

Among patients with Hodgkin's disease, the gastrointestinal tract was the site of initial involvement in 2 percent; and among those with the non-Hodgkin's lymphomas, the comparable figure was 13 to 25 percent (Peters et al 1968). The latter figures were higher than those reported by Skirmshire (1955) and Rosenberg et al (1961). Approximately half the primary gastrointestinal lymphomas were gastric and half intestinal. Lymphomas of the small intestine are about twice as frequent as those of the colon. The most common site in the small intestine was the ileum; for the large intestine, the cecum and rectum. More than half the intestinal lymphomas occurred in the ileocecal region. Berg (1969) summarized 177 cases of primary intestinal lymphomas reported in the literature. The composite distributions were 6 percent for duodenum, 16 percent jejunum, 40 percent ileum, 18 percent cecum, 8 percent colon, and 12 percent rectum. Secondary involvement of the gastrointestinal tract appeared to follow the same trend.

Marshall and Adamson (1959) pointed out that Hodgkin's disease of the gastrointestinal tract carries a much more serious prognosis than lymphosarcoma or reticulum cell sarcoma. Among 21 patients with primary lymphosarcoma of the stomach, 53 percent survived 5 years; while the rate was 27 percent in 11 patients with Hodgkin's disease. Dawson et al (1961) reviewed 117 cases of primary malignant lymphoma of the stomach and 176 cases of the small intestine. Hodgkin's disease comprised 10 percent of the intestinal cases and 20 percent of the gastric lesions. Excluding giant follicular lymphomas which appeared to have the best prognosis, they also found that lymphosarcomas have a better prognosis than reticulum cell sarcomas or Hodgkin's disease. Regarding specific site, other than gastric lesions, which had the best prognosis because of early symptoms, and the duodenum, which fared the worst because of location, they found no significant difference among the lesions of the large or small intestine.

Ullman and Abeshouse (1932) felt that an annular growth was the most common manifestation of lymphoma of the intestine and that the symptoms and x-ray findings would be predominantly those of obstruction. However, Deeb and Stilson (1954) showed that the roentgen appearance of lymphosarcoma of the small bowel could better be described as resembling motor dysfunction. The characteristics were: destruction and obliteration of the mucous membrane pattern; stiffness of the walls and absence of peristalsis; crescentic indentations secondary to small lymphosarcomatous infiltrates. Dawson et al (1961) described four types of primary intestinal lymphomatous tumors: annular, or plaque-like lesions; bulky and protuberant growths; aneurysmal bowel lesions; and multiple lymphomatous polyps spread over long segments of the intestinal tract. Cupps et al (1969) reviewed the x-ray manifestations of 46 patients with primary malignant lymphoma of the small intestine.

Myriad roentgenographic patterns were present in 65 percent of the cases, and the x-ray pictures were indistinguishable from other neoplastic and non-neoplastic disease. They pointed out that when several types of lesions coexisted in the patients, the examiner should be alert to the possible presence of lymphoma in the bowel.

Rubin and Massey (1954) described the details of gastrointestinal exfoliative cytology of malignant lymphoma. Few other clinicans have found this technique useful. Rösch et al (1971) described the gastroscopic aspects of 13 cases of gastric lymphoma. They emphasized that the gross lesions often appeared benign, i.e., ulcers, giant folds, and multiple erosions. A definitive preoperative diagnosis is possible only by biopsy or cytology under direct vision. However, Naqvi et al (1969) said that in 10 of 20 patients with gastric lymphoma who had gastroscopic examinations, the gastroscopist's diagnosis was carcinoma, and positive biopsies were obtained only in 5. A preoperative diagnosis of gastric malignant tumor was made only in 55 of their 100 patients, and only 15 were diagnosed as gastric lymphoma before operation. It is not known how much improvement in diagnostic accuracy will be possible with the newer fiberoptic gastroscope.

The diagnosis of primary gastrointestinal malignant lymphoma may be difficult even on examination of tissue specimens. In a series of 57 patients, Kahn et al (1972) reported 3 cases in which the distinction between carcinoma and lymphoma could not be made by the pathologists. They commented that "although careful examination of multiple blocks and histochemical stains for mucin in doubtful cases may help differentiate carcinoma from lymphoma, we feel that electron microscopic examination of such tumors may be the only way to establish an unequivocal diagnosis."

Many factors could influence the result of surgical treatment of gastrointestinal lymphoma. Most authors found prognosis is affected by the presence or absence of regional adenopathies; however, Dawson et al (1961) disagreed. The degree of localization of gastrointestinal lymphomas is difficult to assess. In many cases regional node enlargement is noted, but only 40–50 percent of the enlarged nodes contained tumor (Berg 1969). Five of the 20 patients of Allen et al (1954) who survived 5 years after radical resection and radiotherapy had involvement of regional lymph nodes, and 6 had involvement of surgical margins. This suggested that tumors in lymph nodes or resection margins did not preclude a long-term success. Warren (1959) also felt that postoperative irradiation could control inadequate margins and the results did not appreciably differ from those in patients who were free of node involvement and had clear margins.

It should be pointed out that multicentricity of tumors has been reported to be present in 60 percent, and extension into other structures was found in 36 percent of primary gastric lymphomas (McNeer and Berg 1959). The tendency for lateral unobtrusive spread of the primary tumor explained the high involvement of margins of resected specimens of gastrointestinal lymphomas. Lymphoma spreads to lymph nodes as does carcinoma. Because of multicentric origin, the surgeon should search for other gastrointestinal lesions at celiotomy before resection of any particular lymphoma.

Loehr et al (1969) reviewed 100 cases of primary gastrointestinal lymphoma. They found an overall 5-year survival rate of 49 percent. The rate was similar among lesions with different microscopic patterns or sites of origin in the digestive tract. The highest survival (85 percent) was in those patients who had definitive resections of the lesion and postoperative x-ray therapy in a tumor dose of 3000 to 4000 rads. Of 6 patients treated by x-ray alone in tumoricidal doses, only 1 survived for more than 5 years.

Naqvi et al (1969) proposed a staging system for malignant lymphoma of the gastrointestinal tract as follows: a tumor confined to a single focus without node involvement (stage I): with node involvement (stage II); with invasion of adjacent structure (stage III); and with distant metastases (stage IV). They reviewed a total of 162 cases. The corrected 5-year survival rate for stomach lesions was 64 percent for stage I, 42 percent for stage II, and less than 18 percent for stages III and IV. For small intestine, the comparable figures were 75 percent, 50 percent, and 28 percent. Although there was an overall 18 percent operative mortality for both stomach and intestinal lesions, they felt that even in secondary lesions, palliative resection should be performed in conjunction with radiotherapy or chemotherapy since nonresected lesions were prone to develop serious complications.

Bush and Ash (1969) conducted a retrospective study of 1555 patients seen with the diagnosis of malignant lymphoma. Of these, 83 patients (5.3 percent) had involvement of the gastrointestinal tract. Eight of the 83 patients had Hodgkin's disease. They considered 45 patients as early or primary cases and the other 38, late cases. The 2-year recurrence-free rate for the early cases was 51 percent and for the late cases, 16 percent. Both in early and locally advanced late disease, postoperative radiation markedly reduced the risks of intraabdominal recurrence. Thus, they recommend the use of wide-field abdominal irradiation to reach a midline dosage of 2500 rads in 4 to 6 weeks with suitable shielding to protect the kidney.

Fuller (1966) reported on the results of large-volume irradiation in the management of Hodgkin's disease and malignant lymphomas originating in the abdomen. Twenty-six of her 57 patients had disease in the gastrointestinal tract, and 19 of the 26 had additional involvement of the abdominal lymph nodes. Palliative resection was performed in all of the small intestinal lesions, but was feasible only in about 50 percent of those of the stomach. The overall survival rate of limited radiotherapy (tumor dose below 3000 rads) was 20 percent, whereas 43 percent of those treated radically survived 5 years. The recommended treatment is to use the cobalt 60 machine, giving radiotherapy through parallel opposed fields to encompass the entire abdomen, and to administer a tumor dose of 3000 rads.

Among a series of 95 patients with histologically confirmed reticulum cell sarcoma, Newall et al (1968) reported that 69 patients had extranodal disease as sites of first presentation. Among these 69 extranodal sites, 8 originated from the gastrointestinal tract. Newall and Friedman (1970) found that the radiosensitivity of reticulum cell sarcoma, arising from the gastrointestinal tract, was similar to that of the lymph nodes, and these lesions were more radiosensitive than lymphomas originating in bone or connective tissues. Kaplan (1972) also said that in rare cases of apparently primary gastrointestinal Hodgkin's disease, surgical resection followed by radiotherapy appeared to be the treatment of choice.

SECONDARY LESIONS (OVERALL)

Gall and Mallory (1942) found that 13 percent of the lymphomas involved the gastrointestinal tract, especially those with the diagnosis of Hodgkin's sarcoma (24 percent) and reticulum cell sarcoma (27 percent). Craver and Herrmann (1946) found that 52 (12.8 percent) of 406 patients with Hodgkin's disease developed gastrointestinal symptoms. Seven of these patients had specific gastrointestinal lesions at autopsy or gastroscopy, the other 45 had secondary or extrinsic gastrointestinal involvement.

In the autopsy series, 47 percent of the patients who had Hodgkin's sarcoma had gastrointestinal lesions (Jackson and Parker 1947). In the non-Hodgkin's series, Rosenberg et al (1961) found that 39.7 percent of those who had necropsy had such lesions. Among 281 patients dying of malignant lymphoma, Cornes (1967) found the gastrointestinal tract was involved in 20 percent of those with Hodgkin's disease, 36.7 percent with lymphosarcoma, and 40.2 percent with reticulum cell sarcoma. Among another series of 690 patients who had autopsy for malignant lymphoma, Richmond et al (1962) reported that the stomach was involved in 12 percent of those with Hodgkin's disease and in 23–32 percent of those with non-Hodgkin's disease. The comparable figures for the small intestine were 7 percent and 26–28 percent, respectively; for the large intestine, 7.5 percent and 21–26 percent.

Ehrlich et al (1968) reported that 63 percent of 323 patients with malignant lymphoma had gastrointestinal involvement at autopsy. Among these, 33 percent had direct involvement by tumor, 15 percent had nontumor pathological changes (i.e., ulcerations, erosions, fungal and bacterial infestations, radiation and drug effects), and 15 percent had both tumor and nontumor effects. The frequency of involvement was highest in reticulum cell sarcoma (82 percent) and lowest in Hodgkin's disease (48 percent). They found that gastrointestinal bleeding originated more often from the upper gastrointestinal tract and, in most cases, was secondary to a nontumor source, whereas perforation was found to be more frequently due to the tumor itself rather than therapy. Ileocecal intussusception was found in children and in young adults.

Marshall and Brown (1950) and Frazer (1959) believed that it is especially dangerous to use irradiation on patients with massive involvement of the viscera because severe, and often fatal, hemorrhage is a frequent complication. In addition, Naqvi et al (1969) reported that 4 of 48 patients with small intestine lymphoma treated with radiotherapy and chemotherapy perforated during the course of the treatment. Presumably, this resulted from dissolution of radiosensitive tumors. Another serious complication which might occur in patients with leukemia and lymphomas was reported by Wynne and Armstrong (1972). They reviewed 14 patients with advanced neoplastic disease who developed clostridial septicemia; 3 had malignant lymphoma. All episodes except one appeared to originate in the bowel and were usually accompanied by signs of intestinal obstruction. In 6 of the 14 patients, infection closely followed some surgical or diagnostic procedures. They warned that "The treatment of clostridial sepsis, which includes removal of the source when possible as well as high dose penicillin, should be prompt, for all the patients who died, with one exception, did so within 24 hours of the onset of clinical sepsis."

Welborn et al (1965) stated that radical palliative surgery for patients with widespread tumors of a more primitive cell type is not indicated. However, radical palliative gastrectomy, followed by irradiation therapy, could produce relatively good results in patients with lymphosarcoma of the mature cell type. Pack and Molander (1966) reported a 13.4 percent incidence of stomach involvement with Hodgkin's disease in 217 patients who had postmortem examinations. Usually, involvement of the gastrointestinal tract results from invasion via retroperitoneal or mesenteric nodes. They performed subtotal gastrectomies in 2 patients for intractable hemorrhage. One patient survived 17 months; the other, 4.5 years. Intestinal obstruction, partial or complete, was the sign of involvement; chidren might have intussusception. Of 6 patients having laparotomy for intestinal obstruction, 2 were inoperable, 2 had by-pass enteroenterostomy and survived 7 and 10 months, and 2 had resection and anastomosis and survived 6 and 16 months. Among 125 patients with Hodgkin's disease, Cornes (1967) reported 2 had laparotomies for intestinal obstruction, and another 13 died from lesions in the gastrointestinal tract (4 of perforation, 9 of hemorrhage). Thus, he emphasized that about 1 in every 5 patients with Hodgkin's disease had tumor deposits in the digestive tract and 1 in 10 died from gastrointestinal involvement.

MALABSORPTION SYNDROME

Malabsorption is an interesting presenting symptom of lymphomatous involvement of the digestive system. Apparently, Fairley and Mackie (1937) first described the association of steatorrhea and lymphoid tumors of the gastrointestinal tract. They postulated obstruction of the mesenteric lymphatics by the tumor as the cause of malabsorption and Kent (1964) found that massive involvement of the mesenteric nodes was the most frequent finding.

Hoskins (1967) stated 7 cases were recorded where celiac disease was diagnosed and lymphoma of the small gut developed subsequently. Thus, it is suggested that idiopathic steatorrhea should be regarded as a premalignant condition. Cornes (1967) studied 19 patients with this condition (10 reticulum cell sarcoma, 7 Hodgkin's disease, and 2 lymphosarcoma). Five of the 7 patients with Hodgkin's disease had subtotal villous atrophy and 4 had proven celiac disease. He pointed out that "the remarkable features of the association between steatorrhea and malignant lymphoma are: the relatively high incidence of Hodgkin's disease, the apparent primary development of these tumors in the gut wall, the multiplicity of the tumors found, and their unusual situation in the jejunum and proximal ileum. Once a lymphoid tumor has developed in a patient with steatorrhea, the outlook would appear to be hopeless. Despite surgical removal, fresh lesions develop and the patients are dead within a year."

Brunt et al (1969) reviewed 13 patients with malabsorption who had Hodgkin's disease and other types of intestinal lymphoma. Infiltration of the lamina propria and villous atrophy were found in 12 patients. The authors suggested that the possibility of an occult lymphoma should be ruled out in adults presenting with celiac disease. Of incidental interest is the finding that none of 20 patients with cancer of the small intestine or mesenteric lymph nodes suffered from malabsorption.

Marcuse and Stout (1950) noted the presence of lymphoid overactivity in the small intestine with primary lymphoma. Naqvi et al (1969) reported 2 patients who had granulomatous lesions before intestinal lymphomas. One patient had regional ileitis and another had nontropical sprue. Strangely, in patients with concomitant ileitis and lymphoma, the tumor was found in the nonileitis segments of the bowel.

Dutz et al (1971) supplied the pathological evidence that the non-lymphomatous mucosa of 18 of the 20 patients with primary intestinal malignant lymphomas showed severe sprue-like villous atrophy. Thus, they concluded that sprue-like atrophy of the small bowel is definitely a triggering factor for the development of primary intestinal reticulum cell sarcoma or lymphosarcoma.

Malignant lymphomas have proved to have certain geographic features, and primary gastrointestinal lymphomas are relatively common in the Middle East. The disease is also unique in that it affects young adults. Clubbing of the fingers is rather common, and malabsorption is a common primary manifestation (al-Bahrani and Bakir 1971; al-Saleem and al-Bahrani 1973; Eidelman et al 1966). Ramot (1971) emphasized that the syndrome of intestinal lymphoma with malabsorption is relatively common among Arabs and Jews of Eastern and North African origin, but is rare among Jews of European origin.

al-Saleem and al-Bahrani (1973) reported on 30 patients with the Middle East lymphoma of the small intestine. Twelve patients presented with malabsorption syndrome, 9 with intestinal obstruction, 4 with symptoms suggestive of peptic ulcer, and 2 with melena; 2 had peritonitis due to perforation, and 1 patient presented with renal failure secondary to lymphomatous infiltration of both kidneys. Histologically, the lesions are poorly differentiated non-Hodgkin's lesions. Most frequently, the lesion involves the proximal parts of the small bowel in a diffuse form. They pointed out that most patients with sprue syndrome had a short history and only 1 patient had a history of steatorrhea over 4 years.

Novis et al (1971) reported a series of 23 patients with abdominal lymphoma and malabsorption syndrome. Of these, 4 had Hodgkin's disease. Barium enema suggested the diagnosis in one-third of the patients, whereas peroral jejunal biopsies were diagnostic in one-third and suggestive in another third. Kahn et al (1972) reported a series of 57 patients with primary gastrointestinal lymphoma from South Africa (19 stomach, 34 small bowel, and 4 large bowel). Small bowel lymphomas in adults occurred almost exclusively in nonwhite patients, and 33 percent of these patients presented with malabsorption syndromes. Lymphomas of the stomach had a better prognosis than those of the small bowel (29 percent versus 6 percent 5-year survival).

Fu and Perzin (1972) found 1 case of malabsorption in their 26 cases of primary lymphosarcomas of the small intestine and another case among their 12 cases of secondary intestinal lesions. Fu and Stewart (1973) reported the unusual case of a patient who had severe malabsorption and immunoglobulin abnormalities for 7 years and who suffered 2 episodes of perforation of the ileum within 16 days. The resected bowel segment and mesenteric lymph nodes revealed histiocytic lymphoma. In view of the disappointing results with cytotoxic chemotherapy, the patient was treated with aggressive radiation therapy to the whole abdomen. All symptoms cleared and a repeat laparotomy for repair of a incisional hernia 26 months later revealed no evidence of lymphoma. Yamashiro and Gray (1972) also reported that the malabsorption syndrome associated with small intestine lymphomas could be "cured" by radiotherapy. In one patient who had blunted villi on jejunal biopsy, there was clinical improvement, returning of villa, and reduced round cell infiltration after 3525 rads were given to the abdomen.

ESOPHAGUS

The esophagus, and particularly the esophageal mucosa, is not too frequently involved by metastatic invasion from any neoplasm. Chioléro (1935) found 5 cases of lymphoma of the esophagus; in 3 there was widespread disease; in 2 the disease was confined to the esophagus (proven at autopsy). Williams (1935) reported Hodgkin's stricture of the esophagus which persisted after radiotherapy. Severe dysphagia ensued, and a gastrostomy was performed.

Goldman (1940) found that none of his 212 Hodgkin's cases involved the esophagus or produced dysphagia. In a review of 335 cases of Hodgkin's disease, Vieta and Craver (1941) reported 2 cases of esophagomediastinal fistula and 1 case of tracheoesophageal fistula, Jackson and Parker (1947) could find evidence of an esophageal lesion in only 1 of their 174 Hodgkin's cases.

Bichel (1951) reported a patient with Hodgkin's disease involving the esophageal wall who survived 5 years after radiotherapy. He found 15 more cases reported in the literature, and said there was no primary isolated Hodgkin's disease of the esophagus as such. Allen et al (1954) reported 1 case of lymphoblastic lymphoma of the esophagus among 79 cases of solitary gastrointestinal lymphoma treated by radical surgery.

Richmond et al (1962) found the esophagus was involved in 2.5 percent of the patients with Hodgkin's disease and in 7.5 percent of those with non-Hodgkin's lymphoma. Craver (1964) showed a case with Hodgkin's disease where marked upper esophagus obstruction was relieved after local roentgenotherapy. One patient of Schamaun (1967) was operated upon for Hodgkin's disease of the cervical esophagus. He was alive and well 6.5 years after surgery, although he had to be treated several times for other localization of the disease.

Hambly and Blundell (1968) reported 3 patients with Hodgkin's involvement of the esophagus. They pointed out that invasion from adjacent mediastinal lymph nodes accounted for most of the patients and involvement of the esophageal mucosa was the least common. All 3 patients developed this complication more than 7 years after the initial diagnosis and all had enlarged supraclavicular nodes and mediastinal mass when the esophagus was involved. Response to radiotherapy was only temporary in all. Esophagoscopy was unrewarding because the lesions appeared benign. However, others established the correct diagnosis by biopsy of the esophageal lesions (Strauch et al 1971).

Ehrlich et al (1968) studied 323 patients with lymphoma who came to autopsy. In 71 instances, pathological changes were present in the esophagus, but two-thirds of the lesions were nontumorous. Reticulum cell sarcoma was the most common tumor and lymphosarcoma the least common. Two among the 7 patients of Hodgkin's disease had perforation resulting in fistula from the esophagus into the mediastinum. Bush and Ash (1969) reported that only 1 case among their 1555 patients with the diagnosis of malignant lymphoma involved the esophagus. Berg (1969) estimated that primary esophageal lymphoma accounted for only a fraction of 1 percent of primary gastrointestinal lymphomas.

Caruso and Berk (1970) reported a case of lymphosarcoma where a well-differentiated lesion of the esophagus presented radiographically as a diffuse intramural submucosal tumor. They reviewed 10 patients who had radiographic findings reported: 3 as ulcerated masses, 3 perforations, 2 polypoid masses, and 1 each as large ulcer and irreglar stenotic lesion. The disease arose in the submucosal lymphois nodules, took one of several forms depending on whether it remained in the submucosa, and grew inward toward the lumen or outward toward the surface.

Papp and Penner (1970) reported a Hodgkin's patient with esophago-mediastinal fistula and superior vena cava syndrome. The syndrome and fistula completely disappeared after nitrogen mustard therapy and super voltage radiotherapy. These appeared to be the treatments of choice for esophageal malignant lymphoma.

PRIMARY LYMPHOMA OF THE STOMACH

Hodgkin's Disease

Either Schlagenhaufer (1913) or Steindl (1924) reported the first case of primary gastric Hodgkin's disease. It was suggested that malignant lymphoma could not only originate in lymph glands, but also in lymphoid structures of various visceral organs. Singer (1931) reviewed the literature and found 7 cases of primary isolated Hodgkin's disease of the stomach. All cases had gastric resection under a mistaken clinical diagnosis. He added a case which was unique in that painstaking examination at autopsy showed the disease to be limited only to the stomach and the perigastric lymph glands. Avent (1939) reported another case and emphasized that the prognosis should be guarded because "lymphogranulomatosis is a progressive disease of the mesenchymal tissue." Marshall and Brown (1950) reported that 1 out of every 30 gastric malignancies was of lymphoid origin, and 8 of their 23 patients with primary malignant lymphomas of the stomach had Hodgkin's disease.

Atlee et al (1951) performed a subtotal gastrectomy for primary Hodg-kin's disease (the first patient who had free gastric perforation, and the 32nd reported with this lesion). The patient was living and well 8 years later without radiotherapy or chemotherapy. In 1954 Portmann et al found 47 such cases and added 6 of their own. The distribution of sites of gastric lesions among these 53 cases were as follows: 45 percent antrum only; 20 percent entire stomach; 12.5 percent antrum plus pars media; and 7.5 percent each of pars media, cardia only, or both. Allen et al (1954) reported 7 cases of Hodgkin's disease among their 44 cases of solitary gastric lymphomas treated with radical surgery. Warren and Littlefield (1955), as well as Marshall (1955), all from the Lahey clinic, reported 9 instances of primary Hodgkin's disease among 30 cases of lymphoma of the stomach. Two of the 9 patients lived 8 and 9 years, respectively, after subtotal gastrec-tomy.

Jackson (1957) reported 3 cases of primary Hodgkin's disease of the stomach and said 36 cases have been reported in American literature. He pointed out that such patients usually complained of pain of long duration but seldom had cachexia or abdominal mass. The treatment recommended is gastric resection followed by deep x-ray therapy. Azzopardi and Menzies (1960) included 1 patient with Hodgkin's disease among 11 with primary lymphomas of the stomach. He had a partial gastrectomy alone, and autopsy 3 years later showed no evidence of residual disease. Kane (1963) reported a patient with Hodgkin's disease of the stomach survived 10 years after subtotal gastrectomy and radiotherapy.

Hodgkin's disease of the stomach apparently has a poorer prognosis than that of the other lymphomas. The 5-year survival rates were 27 percent and 53 percent respectively (Marshall and Adamson 1959). Dawson et al (1961) established the criteria for diagnosing primary lymphoma of the gastrointestinal tract, and reviewed 117 cases of the stomach. They found 21 Hodgkin's disease patients with a 5-year survival rate of 31 percent. Hoerr (1965) reported that 9 out of 20 patients who had surgical resection of all gross disease of malignant lymphoma of the stomach survived 5 years (45 percent), but only 1 out of 7 patients with Hodgkin's disease survived 8 years without recurrence after radical gastrectomy and radiotherapy. Naqvi et al (1969) reported 162 lymphomas of the gastrointestinal tract, 100 of which involved the stomach. There were 74 patients with primary gastric lesions and only 2 with Hodgkin's disease. Neither survived 5 years.

Cornes (1967) reviewed 43 cases of Hodgkin's disease where laparotomy for primary gastrointestinal disease were performed; 22 were for gastric tumors. However, the incidence of primary Hodgkin's disease of the stomach must be very low because the gastric service at Memorial Hospital in New York did not see 1 case so diagnosed by the pathologist from 1932 to 1955 (Pack and Molander 1966). Schenkin and Burns (1961) are among those who believe that the disease is probably never localized exclusively in the stomach. In 53 patients with malignant lymphoproliferative disorders, Rosch et al (1971) found 22 instances of secondary gastric involvement and 4 of primary gastric lesions. Of the 4, only 1 patient had Hodgkin's disease.

The preoperative diagnosis of gastric lymphoma may be difficult. Salmela (1968) reported 39 patients with lymphomas of the stomach diagnosed between 1953 and 1970. Of these, 3 were Hodgkin's disease. All of the cases of Hodgkin's disease were interpreted as carcinoma roentgenologically. Ben-Asher (1971) reported a patient with Hodgkin's disease localized to the stomach and treated with 80 percent subtotal gastrectomy, total omentectomy, and postoperative chemotherapy. The patient had a 10-year history suggesting peptic ulcer, and the upper gastrointestinal series revealed a round, smooth lesion typical of leiomyosarcoma.

Reviewing the reports to date, it would appear that lymphomas comprise approximately 3 percent of all malignant tumors of the stomach; and among all primary gastric lymphomas of 10 series reported since 1950, about one-sixth (70 of 394) were of the Hodgkin's variety. In suitable cases with early localized lesions, surgical resection with or without postoperative radiotherapy can achieve long-term cures. The 5-year survival rate is about 30 percent.

Non-Hodgkin's Lymphoma

Cruveilheir (1829) apparently reported the first case of gastric lymphoma. Palmer (1950) collected 500 cases of gastric sarcoma, and, of these, the relative incidence of lymphosarcoma was 42 percent; of reticulum cell sarcoma, 8.8 percent; and of Hodgkin's disease, 9 percent. Marshall (1955) found that 3 percent of all gastric tumors were sarcomas. With the decreased incidence of stomach cancer over the years, Cathcart et al (1971) reported that the incidence of gastric sarcoma had increased to 6.1 percent.

Among the 23 primary malignant lymphomas of the stomach reported by Marshall and Brown (1950), 15 were of the non-Hodgkin's variety. Among the 10 cases reported by Skrimshire (1955), there were 8 of reticulum cell sarcoma and 2 of lymphosarcoma. Berg (1969) reviewed several reported series and suggested that the incidence of reticulum cell sarcoma among gastric lymphoma is somewhere nearer 50 percent.

The first apparent cure of lymphosarcoma of the stomach (20-year survival) treated by partial gastric resection was that reported by Jones and Carmody (1935). Crile et al (1952) reported 19 cases of primary lymphocytic lymphosarcoma of the stomach. The 5-year survival rate of patients who had subtotal resection and postoperative irradiation was 68 percent. They commented that there was no evidence in the literature to show that treatment with roentgen therapy alone was as satisfactory as gastric resection with or without radiotherapy. Frazer (1959) reported that 7 out of 9 patients who had curative resection for gastric lymphoma, with or without postoperative radiotherapy, survived more than 5 years; 6 patients who had radiotherapy alone all died within 12 months.

Radical or total gastrectomy apparently did not improve survival rates in patients with gastric lymphomas. With postoperative radiation, Allen et al (1954) achieved a 58 percent 5-year survival rate in 26 patients with radical gastric resection, and Warren and Littlefield (1955) secured a 40 percent 5-year survival rate after subtotal gastrectomy. Among 91 total gastrectomies done from 1940 to 1953 reported by Herter and Auchincloss (1957), 3 cases were lymphosarcoma of the stomach. Marshall and Adamson (1959) reported a 5-year survival rate of 33 percent in patients who had total gastric resection for localized malignant lymphomas and 42 percent in those who had partial gastric resection. Among 567 patients with non-Hodgkin's lymphoma, Molander and Pack (1963) reported 9 with gastric lesions. Five patients had subtotal and 4 had total gastrectomies; the 5-year survival rates were 60 percent and 50 percent, respectively. Hoerr (1965) reported 8 out of 13 patients with non-Hodgkin's lymphoma survived 5 years. Of the 8, 1 had local excision only; 1, biopsy and radiotherapy; 1, esophagogastrectomy; another underwent a simultaneous gastrectomy and colectomy. Schamaun (1967) said one of his patients was free of symptoms about 4 years after total gastrectomy. Shepard et al (1969) believed radiotherapy to be adequate for gastric lymphoma, and the complication rate of total gastrectomy to be too high. He mentioned 1 patient who died of nutritional problems after total gastrectomy without evidence of a residual tumor.

Smith and Helwig (1958) differentiated the benign gastric "pseudolymphoma" from true lymphosarcoma of the stomach. They studied 131 patients and found 42 had in reality a benign lymphoproliferative disorder. The histologic criteria for the diagnosis of such pseudolymphomas included the presence of a mixed inflammatory infiltrate with reactive centers and ubiquitous scar tissue intimately mixed in a lymphoreticular mass. Jacobs (1963) reviewed 27 cases of lymphoreticular proliferative disorders of the stomach and found only 15 genuine malignant lymphomas. All were reticulum cell sarcomas; 1 patient was well 17 years after surgical excision of the neoplasm. Faris and Saltzstein (1964) studied 21 cases of gastric lymphoid hyperplasia and stressed the importance of finding true germinal centers in distinguishing these lesions from gastric lymphoma. The presence of mature lymphocytes and other inflammatory cell types in the interfollicular tissue in hyperplasia was important. Berry and Mathews (1967) studied 12 cases of gastric lymphosarcomas retrospectively and changed the diagnosis of 6 cases to pseudolymphoma. They commented that the more favorable prognosis usually given for gastric lymphosarcoma was largely a misconception based on the failure to distinguish the true lymphosarcomas from those of the non-neoplastic reactive pseudolymphomas.

Joseph and Lattes (1966) compared the clinicopathological characteristics of 65 localized gastric lymphosarcomas and 6 with disseminated disease. They found no obvious gross or histological differences between the 2 groups. The overall survival rate for primary tumors was 58.7 percent for 5 years, and 27.6 percent for 10 years. The majority of cases was treated with surgical resection with or without added x-ray therapy. The best prognosis for primary tumors included the characteristics of small lesions which were confined to the stomach, the presence of at least partial follicles, the absence of lymph node spread, and only a superficial infiltration of the wall. Cytologically, the finding of predominant lymphocytic cell types suggested a better prognosis than did the preponderance of reticulum cells. Saltzstein (1969) summarized 3 series of cases and reported that the 5-year survival rate was 83–100 percent for the lymphocytic type and 36–50 percent for the reticulum cell type; 10-year survival rates were 77 percent and 30 percent, respectively.

Primary lymphoma of the stomach appears to be rare in children, only 3 cases have been reported: Bailey et al (1961) described 2 cases, and Jenkins et al (1969) included 1 case among 39 pediatric patients with primary gastrointestinal lymphoma.

ReMine (1970) said that non-Hodgkin's lymphoma comprised two-thirds of all primary sarcomatous lesions in the stomach. Between 1940 and 1965, 224 patients with malignant lymphoma and 55 with leiomyosarcomas were seen at the Mayo Clinic. He believed that the therapeutic approach to gastric lymphomas should be very aggressive, and that surgical extirpation followed by radiotherapy is the treatment of choice. The overall 5-year survival rate obtained was 65 percent, including patients with huge growths, nodal involvement, and extragastric spread. Lesions that were treated by total gastrectomy had a 5-year survival rate of 50 percent and 10-year rate of 44 percent. He recommended that "resection should be carried out even though residual tumor must be left behind in regional nodes, and a measure of hope should be extended to the patient with unremovable tumors because of the proved efficacy of roentgen therapy." Shepard et al (1969) showed that in the 9 patients with extensive lesions judged nonresectable, 1 survived 8 years following radiation therapy alone, and another patient was living with no radiologically demonstrable gastric lesion 2 years after diagnosis. They believed that postoperative radiation should be given to all patients with malignant lymphomas of the stomach regardless of the presence or absence of lymph node metastasis.

Cathcart et al (1971) reviewed 20 cases of primary sarcoma of the stomach, including 6 cases of lymphosarcoma and 6 of reticulum cell sarcoma. Ten of these 12 patients had symptoms of peptic ulceration with an average duration of 17 months. The therapy of choice appeared to be resection, reserving irradiation for unresected remnants or later recurrence. They mentioned 1 patient who had a huge lymphosarcoma of the stomach. After 1700 rads were given preoperatively, he had an esophagogastrectomy, splenectomy, adrenalectomy, partial left hepatectomy, and a pancreatectomy. Nonresectable lymph node metastases were left about the renal vasculature, but no additional x-ray therapy was given. Thirty months later, he had an operation for cholelithiases and no residual lymphoma was found. They commented that this case demonstrated a tendency to spontaneous regression of residual metastases and a satisfactory outcome from major partial resection.

Lee and Cogbill (1971) presented 10 cases of primary lymphosarcomas of the stomach (4 lymphoblastic and 6 reticulum cell sarcomas). The preferred treatment was also gastric resection, using radiotherapy as an adjunct when it was not possible to accomplish wide and complete excision of all tumors. Two of the 4 patients who had subtotal gastrectomy without radiation survived 10 and 23 years without recurrence. From their own experience and a review of the literature, they found that patients with lymphosarcomas had a 5-year survival rate of 50 percent, whereas those with reticulum cell sarcomas had a survival rate of 33 percent. Patients with lymphosarcomas had shorter durations of abdominal pain (mean, 3 weeks) without palpable mass, while those with reticulum cell sarcomas had longer durations of pain (mean, 7 months) frequently with palpable mass.

PRIMARY LYMPHOMA OF THE SMALL INTESTINE

Hodgkin's Disease

Sherman (1938) reported a case of Hodgkin's disease apparently primary in the small bowel. Gall (1943) reported 1 patient with Hodgkin's disease of the jejunum who was treated with radical surgery. Among 95 patients who had autopsy, Jackson and Parker (1947) found one instance of Hodgkin's disease primarily in the duodenum and one in the remainder of the small bowel.

Faulkner and Dockerty (1952) said about 440 cases of primary lymphoma of the small intestine were reported, and they added 33 surgically treated cases (only 3 were of Hodgkin's type). They pointed out that all patients had abdominal symptoms suggestive of chronic obstruction, and significant weight loss was present in those who had symptoms for more than 2 months. Three growth patterns were seen: polypoid, aneurysmal, and ulcerative. The lesion can extend beyond delineated tumor margin for distances up to 2 cm in 36 percent of the cases and operative mortality was high (12 percent).

In 217 patients with Hodgkin's disease, Portmann et al (1954) found 8 primary lesions of the gastrointestinal tract, including one of the jejunum and one of the ileocecal region. Among 25 solitary lymphomas of the small intestine, Allen et al (1954) reported 3 cases of Hodgkin's disease. Ralston and Wasdahl (1958) reported that a patient died of perforation of the mid-ileum without involvement of the spleen or other lymph nodes. Cohen and Canter (1959) added 5 more patients who had no evidence of generalized Hodgkin's disease at the time of laparotomy or necropsy (one had disease in the bowel wall without lymph node involvement). They said such lesions constituted less than 6 percent of all small bowel tumors coming to surgery or postmortem examination. In contrast to other malignant lymphomas which seem to have a predeliction for the ileum, Hodgkin's disease may involve the upper small intestine as frequently as the ileum, and the lesions are often multiple. Teitelman and Brill (1960) also reported a case of Hodgkin's disease of the distal ileum without metastases in the numerous nodes of mesentery of the 26-in. ileum resected.

Dawson et al (1961) established five criteria for the diagnosis of primary lymphoma of the intestine. These are: (1) absence of palpable superficial lymphadenopathy; (2) normal white blood cell count and differential count; (3) absence of enlargement of mediastinal lymph nodes on chest roentgenograms; (4) no grossly demonstrable involvement at the time of surgical treatment beyond the involved segment of intestine and its regional mesenteric lymph nodes; and (5) normal liver and spleen. These criteria have been well accepted.

Pack and Molander (1966) reported that primary Hodgkin's disease of the small intestine occurred in 2 instances in their series of 316 patients. Cornes (1967) found 38 Hodgkin's cases in the literature and added 5 of his own cases where laparotomy was performed for lesions primarily of the gastrointestinal tract without peripheral adenopathy. Among the 43 cases, 22 were for stomach; 6, ileum; 5, jejunum; 3, jejunum and ileum; 1, duodenum; and 6, colorectum. Six of the intestinal tumors were multiple and most of the tumors were plaque-like masses in the muscular coats and submucosa. He pointed out that Hodgkin's disease that developed in the stomach had a better prognosis than if it arose in the small and large intestine.

Among the 162 cases of lymphomas of the gastrointestinal tract reported by Naqvi et al (1969), 48 cases involved the small intestine; 24 of them were primary lesions. Four of the stage I patients had Hodgkin's disease and 3 survived more than 5 years. Details of the treatment were not given, but the authors favored surgical resection whenever possible.

Non-Hodgkin's Lymphoma

Primary neoplasm of the small intestine is very rare. Spratt (1966) said among 34,000 admissions to EFSCH from 1940 to 1965, there were only 30 cases of primary tumors of the small intestine (an incidence rate of 0.09 percent). Nineteen patients had malignant tumors; 2 of these were lymphosarcomas. Alexander and Altemeier (1968) found only 7 patients with malignant tumors primarily of the small intestine among 9721 consecutive autopsies; all occurred in patients over the age of 50. Of these 7, 4 were lymphomas; 2, carcinomas; and 1, sarcoma. Morioka and Starkloff (1968) reported 16 tumors of the duodenum and jejunum among 300,000 admissions. Only 1 case of reticulum cell sarcoma of the jejunum was seen.

Faulkner and Dockerty (1952) reviewed 31 surgical cases of malignant lymphomas of the small intestine; 28 were of non-Hodgkin's type. Over 70 percent had nodal involvement and the 5-year survival rate was only 21 percent. Deeb and Stilson (1954) reported 2 of their 4 patients with lymphosarcomas of the small intestine were free from symptoms more than 7 years after radiotherapy. Irvine and Johnstone (1955) reported 17 cases of non-Hodgkin's primary lymphomas of the small bowel. In their series, perforation was the first evidence of disease in 8 patients, and this complication occurred three times as often in reticulum cell sarcomas as in lymphosarcomas. They pointed out that when treated appropriately, the prognosis was not so bad: 3 out of 5 patients who had resections survived 5 to 7 years free of disease.

Skrimshire (1955) reported 13 cases of primary lymphoma of the small intestine (8 reticulum cell sarcoma, 4 lymphosarcoma, and 1 follicular lymphoma). The sites of the lesions were: ileum (10), duodenum (2), and jejunum (1). Burman and van Wyk (1956) reported 25 cases (9 ileum, 5 cecum, 4 ileum and cecum, 4 jejunum, 3 duodenum). Intussusception occurred in 20 percent of the cases, but anemia was rare. Coller and Flotte (1957) reported 9 cases (6 ileum, 2 duodenum, 1 jejunum). With resection and postoperative radiotherapy, 4 patients were well 1, 3, 6, and 11 years postoperatively.

Warren (1959) described jaundice in three of the 4 cases of lymphoma of the duodenum. One patient with severe hemorrhage required subtotal gastric resection for control. Because of the location of the lesion, radical surgical excision was not applicable. He said this particular lesion should be treated with gastroenterostomy and subsequent x-ray therapy. He saw 10 other patients: 5 jejunum and 5 ileum. All had obstructive symptoms without palpable mass. Patients whose lesions were resectable had the best prognosis. Frazer (1959) found that non-Hodgkin's lymphoma of the small intestine had a poorer prognosis than lymphoma of the stomach, because only 3 of the 11 patients (all with lesions of the ileum) lived 5 years or longer, whereas 7 of 18 patients with gastric lesions did so.

Following the diagnostic criteria of primary lymphomas of the intestinal tract proposed by Dawson et al (1961), Weaver and Batsakis (1964) found that 10 of the 18 cases of lymphomas in the small intestine were indeed "primary." Nine patients had lymphosarcomas and 1 had giant follicle lymphoma. Two patients had no concomitant regional mesenteric node involvement, but one still died 7 months later of disseminated disease; the other had no recurrence for 17 years. Excluding 2 deaths in the postoperative period, the average survival was 8 years after surgical resection although only 3 patients had postoperative radiotherapy. They also reported on 3 cases of pseudolymphoma of the small intestine (Weaver and Batsakis 1965).

Henderson and Paterson (1968) reported a patient who had perforation of the jejunum by reticulum cell sarcoma during pregnancy. They reviewed a total of 760 cases of non-Hodgkin's lymphomas of the small intestine and found the incidence of perforation was only 6 percent. Among the more than 80 cases of perforation reported, the female-to-male sex ratio was about 1 : 4.

Mestel (1959) reported 13 cases of non-Hodgkin's lymphomas of the small intestine in children (13 years of age or younger) and found 25 cases in the literature. The sites of lesions were the ileum in 11 and the jejunum in 2. The disease is most common in the 3- to 8-year-old group, and 5.5 times more prevalent in males than females. The prognosis is almost always bad with a mean survival of 13.7 months. Jenkin et al (1969) studied 121 children (less than 16 years old) with non-Hodgkin's lymphoma; 39 had primary gastrointestinal lesions. There were 35 lesions involving the lower ileum, and 1 case each of stomach, duodenum, jejunum, and upper ileum. They pointed out that in localized lymphomas, with or without associated mesenteric nodes, 5 out of 6 patients were alive 5 years after being treated with wide surgical excision and postoperative irradiation of the whole abdomen (2500 rads in 4 weeks). In contrast, only 1 out of 12 children survived 5 years with surgery alone.

It has been pointed out that primary intestinal lymphomas are relatively common in the Middle East (p. 236). al-Khateeb (1970) of Iraq reported that 8.7 percent of the gastrointestinal tract cancers were primary malignant lymphomas of the small intestine. All the malignant lesions of the small bowel were malignant lymphoma. All 30 patients had laparotomy for diagnosis; 8 radical and 11 palliative resections, 5 by-pass procedures, and 6 biopsies were done, al-Bahrani and Bakir (1971) reported 45 cases of primary intestinal lymphomas; all were diagnosed at laparotomy for abdominal pain. Forty-one were of the non-Hodgkin's type. The sites of involvement were: jejunum alone in 16; ileum alone in 8; colon in 2; duodenum in 1; multiple sites in 11; the whole small bowel was affected in 7.

Fu and Perzin (1972) reported 26 cases of primary intestinal lymphomas. Regional lymph nodes in one-third of the cases showed marked lymphoid hyperplasia. The overall 5-, 10-, and 15-year survival rates for the 26 cases were 48 percent, 33 percent, and 17 percent, respectively. They believed "the preferred treatment is a wide segmental resection of the lesion and adjacent bowel, as well as resection of the contiguous mesenteric lymph nodes. Radiotherapy is recommended if any of the following unfavorable features are present: lymph node involvement; tumor on the margins of resection; perforation; fistula; and multicentric tumors."

COLON AND RECTUM

Warren and Lulenski (1942) found only 0.3 percent of 2510 colon and rectal cancers was of lymphomatous origin. Gall (1943) reported 1 patient with Hodgkin's disease who had resection for colon lesions. Among 16 patients with lymphosarcoma who survived more than 10 years, Stout (1947) reported 1 patient with giant follicle lymphoma of the rectum who was well 14 years after surgical treatment alone.

Allen et al (1954) included 9 cases of lymphomas of the colorectum among 79 solitary gastrointestinal malignant lymphomas (4 cecum, 3 transverse colon, 1 each of sigmoid and rectum). Only 1 case was Hodgkin's disease. Portmann et al (1954) described 1 case involving the ileocecal region and found 8 other Hodgkin's cases reported: 4 involved cecum, 2 rectum, and 1 each of splenic flexure and site unspecified. Warren and Littlefield (1955) reported 2 cases of cecum and 7 of rectum involvement among their 49 cases of lymphomas of the gastrointestinal tract. One of the patients with a rectal lesion had Hodgkin's disease.

Burman and van Wyk (1956) reported 5 cases of primary lymphoma of the cecum and 4 cases of the cecum and ileum. Warren (1959) pointed out that the prognosis for lymphoma of the cecum was poor because the lesion could be present for years before symptoms appeared. However, Azzopardi and Menzies (1960) said cecal lesions might have a better prognosis than those of the small intestine because 2 of their patients survived 6 and 15 years after resection. Frazer (1959) reported 2 patients with malignant lymphomas localized in the colon. One had a lesion in the cecum; the other had 2 lesions, 1 in the transverse colon and 1 in the cecum, both of which perforated.

Primary lymphoma of the appendix appeared to be rare. Coller and Flotte (1957) included 1 case of lymphoma of the appendix among 36 non-Hodgkin's lymphomas of the gastrointestinal tract. Raiford (1962) said lymphosarcoma of the appendix was more common than sarcoma, probably because of the relatively large amount of lymphoid tissue in and around the appendix. He said about 30 cases were reported up to his time. Wychulis et al (1966) reported one appendiceal lymphoma in 69 patients with malignant lymphomas of the colon, 39 of which were located in the cecal or ileocecal region. Loehr et al (1969) reported 2 cases of appendiceal lymphomas among 100 cases of primary gastrointestinal lymphomas. Both occurred in women and were found incidentally during operation for unrelated diseases.

Helwig and Hansen (1951) compared the histological features of benign lymphoid polyps (70 patients) and malignant lymphomatous lesions of the rectum (17 out of a total of 395 patients with lymphomas). The characteristics of benign lymphoid polyps included primary follicles with reactive centers. Five of the 17 secondary lesions of the rectum showed nodular elevation of the mucosa; in the others, the lesion was flat or ulcerated. Occasionally a flat infiltration might encircle the bowel and lead to stenosis (Gechman et al 1956). Coller and Flotte (1957) reported 2 cases of lymphoma of the colon and 3 of the rectum. During the same time, they recorded 11 patients with benign lymphoma of the rectum. Dawson et al (1961) added the criteria that benign tumors should be entirely within the mucosa and submucosa and have at least two discrete germinal follicles present.

Scott (1958) commented that in the large bowel solitary lymphoma of the rectum is not rare, but occasionally a diffuse polypoid "reticulosarcoma" affects the entire colon. Diagnosis might be very difficult becasuse the symptoms suggesting ulcerative colitis and the radiological appearances defy interpretation. Warren (1959) pointed out that when lesions of the rectum and sigmoid appeared to be malignant by clinical examination but repeated biopsies were read as negative by the pathologist, the lesions probably were malignant. In particular, this was characteristic of lymphoma rather than adenocarcinoma. Two of his 8 patients who had malignant lymphomas of the rectum had long-standing ulcerative colitis. Dawson et al (1961) reported 37 cases of primary intestinal lymphomas: 14 of these were of rectum, 10 of colon, and 3 of both. Three of the 27 colonic cases were Hodgkin's disease. They said malignant lymphomas complicating ulcerative colitis were seen in 7 cases; all had poor prognosis.

Pack and Molander (1966) found no primary Hodgkin's disease of the colon in a series of 316 patients. Secondary involvement was found in 9 instances, and 3 patients had lesions within the reach of the sigmoidoscope. Complications included obstruction, perforation, and hemorrhage. One patient had palliative hemicolectomy for Hodgkin's disease of the splenic flexure, and he survived more than 4 years. In cases with malignant tumor involving the lower sigmoid or rectum that cannot have a resection, a simple decompressive loop colostomy should be done to facilitate administration of radiotherapy to the area (Lee 1968).

Naqvi et al (1969) found 14 cases involving the large intestine among 162 lymphomas of the gastrointestinal tract. There were 6 in the rectum; 2 each of the cecum, left colon, and sigmoid; and 1 each of the right and transverse colon. Only 8 of these 14 patients had primary lesions and their corrected 5-year survival rate was better than 50 percent. Six patients had colectomy without mortality, whereas lesions of the rectosigmoid area were treated with radiation and chemotherapy. Loehr et al (1969) included 10 lesions of large intestine among 100 cases of primary lymphomas of the gastrointestinal tract. Of 6 patients with cecal tumors, 4 had extirpative resection; of 4 patients with rectal lesions, 1 underwent abdominoperineal resection. Nonresectable lesions were treated with radiotherapy. An overall 5-year survival rate of 33 percent was attained.

Among 1555 adult patients with malignant lymphomas, Bush and Ash (1969) found 83 patients with involvement of the gastrointestinal tract. There were 8 patients with involvement of the ileocecal region, 5 of the colon, and 4 of the rectum; about half of the patients had primary lesions. Among 121 non-Hodgkin's lymphoma patients less than 16 years of age, Jenkin et al (1969) found 39 with primary sites in the gastrointestinal tract. Twenty-three of those 39 patients had colonic lesions. These included 10 cases of cecum, 8 of appendix, and 5 of ascending colon. They emphasized that surgical excision and adequate postoperative radiotherapy gave the best survival results. al-Bahrani and Bakir (1971) reported 45 patients with primary intestinal lymphomas presented with abdominal pain, 2 of whom had lesions involving the colon alone.

Perry et al (1972) reported 22 patients with malignant lymphomas of the rectum seen at St. Mark's Hospital, London. During the same time, 2900 patients were treated for carcinoma of the rectum. Only 3 patients had extrapelvic lymphadenopathy, and 19 had lesions confined to the gut and regional lymph nodes. There were 3 cases of Hodgkin's disease, 4 of reticulum cell sarcoma, and 15 of lymphosarcoma. The most common symptom was bleeding associated with diarrhea. Eight of the 10 patients who were treated with chemotherapy or radiotherapy alone died shortly.

Three patients had radiotherapy after sigmoid colostomy and 2 were alive and well. Nine patients had surgery, 8 by abdominoperineal resection and 1 by intrapelvic resection. Five of these patients were alive. They concluded that surgery, with or without radiotherapy, appeared to be the treatment of choice in operable cases.

SUMMARY OF EFSCH EXPERIENCE

In the present EFSCH series, about one-third of the patients with Hodgkin's disease and about half of those with other lymphomas had gastrointestinal x-ray studies at the time of the initial diagnosis. None of the 163 patients with Hodgkin's disease presented with lesions in the gastrointestinal tract; but 31 out of 364 patients with non-Hodgkin's lymphomas did, and 20 of these were probably primary lesions. These included 12 of the stomach, 4 of the ileum, and 4 of the cecum or right colon.

Table 7-1 lists the 7 patients who had subtotal gastrectomy for primary malignant lymphomas of the stomach and 2 patients who had stomach surgery 2–4 years after previous radiotherapy for malignant lymphomas of Waldeyer's ring. Among the 7 patients who had subtotal gastrectomies for primary disease of the stomach, 1 died postoperatively of gastrointestinal hemorrhage. Another 5 patients had postoperative radiotherapy and eventually died of their diseases at 6, 6, 11, 21, and 111 months after operation. The only patient (No. 21848) who had radical subtotal gastrectomy, with additional splenectomy and partial pancreatectomy, did not receive postoperative therapy. He died 15 years later without evidence of disease at the ripe old age of 87.

Three other patients (No. 04031, No. 20341, No. 24370) had only biopsy of the stomach lesion on exploration (p. 233). All 3 were treated with radiotherapy and 2 died 9 and 10 years later without evidence of malignant lymphomas. Two other patients (No. 20453, No. 20463) were treated with radiotherapy after gastrostomy and gastrojejunostomy (p. 234). Radiotherapy (4000 rads) alone controlled a histiocyctic lesion of the cardiac region of one patient; he died 5 years later without clinical evidence of recurrent lymphoma. From our limited experience, we have to say radiotherapy alone appears to be more effective than surgical resection in treating malignant lymphoma of the stomach (5-year survival rates: 60 percent versus 29 percent, or 3 of 5 versus 2 of 7).

Surgical resections of non-Hodgkin's lymphoma of the intestine were carried out in 8 patients (Table 7-2). These included 4 of the ileum and 4 of the cecum or right colon. Four patients had postoperative radiotherapy; only one (No. 24711) lived more than 10 years. Four did not receive postoperative radiotherapy, and 2 died 16 and 17 years later without recurrent malignant lymphomas. It appears that surgical resection alone, if encompassing all the lesions of the intestine and adjacent mesenteric nodes, can "cure" primary malignant lymphoma of the bowel in certain selected cases.

In the EFSCH series, 6 patients with Hodgkin's disease and 58 with other lymphomas had abnormal x-ray findings during the course of their disease. These figures are on the conservative side because special x-ray studies were done only when patients complained of gastrointestinal problems. Only 1 patient (No. 18934) with Hodgkin's disease had ileal resection for perforation, whereas 10 patients with non-Hodgkin's lymphomas had 11 operations for gastrointestinal complications secondary to malignant lymphomas (Table 7-3). Gastrointestinal obstruction is the most common problem (4 small intestine, 3 colon, 2 stomach), although 2 perforations (stomach, ileum) were noted. All patients had previous radiotherapy, and 7 of them had irradiation including the abdominal viscera. Thus, approximately 1 in 6 of those with documented abnormality of the gastrointestinal tract required palliative surgery in our series. Unfortunately, all patients had advanced diseases. It is difficult to evaluate the effectiveness of palliation in such cases since the postoperative survivals were relatively short.

SUMMARY

Gastrointestinal lymphomas can be divided into primary or secondary lesions. Dawson et al (1961) established five criteria for the diagnosis of primary lymphoma of the stomach and intestines (p. 244), and Naqvi et al (1969) proposed a staging system for malignant lymphoma of the gastrointestinal tract (p. 233).

About 2 percent of all gastrointestinal malignant lesions were of lymphomatous origin. The relative frequencies were 0.1 percent for those of the esophagus and rectum, 0.5 percent for the colon, 3 percent for the stomach, and over 20 percent for the small intestines.

Among patients with Hodgkin's disease, the gastrointestinal tract was the site of initial involvement in 2 percent; and the comparable figure for those with non-Hodgkin's lymphoma was 10 to 25 percent. Approximately half these lesions can be called primary lymphomas. About half the primary gastrointestinal lymphomas were gastric and half intestinal. More than half the intestinal lymphomas occurred in the ileocecal region. The preoperative diagnosis of gastrointestinal lymphoma is often difficult. The treatment of choice is nonradical surgical resection followed by postoperative radiotherapy.

In autopsy series, about 20–50 percent of the patients with malignant lymphoma had lesions of the gastrointestinal tract. For patients with Hodgkin's disease, about 12 percent had involvement of the stomach and 8 percent, of the small and large intestines. The comparable figures for those with non-Hodgkin's lymphomas were 30 percent and 25 percent respectively.

Table 7-1
Exploration and Gastrectomy for Non-Hodgkin's Lymphoma (EFSCH series)

Patient no.	Age	Sex	Date	Indication	Operation	Pathology			Postoperative		Survival (months) * = alive	Lymphoma at follow-up
						Diagnosis	Margin	Nodes (positive/total)	Radiotherapy (rads)	Chemotherapy		
11855	62	F	1-49	Antral mass	Subtotal gastrectomy	LPD	—	0/16	1500	+	111	+
19055	52	M	10-53	Pyloric mass	Subtotal gastrectomy	UC	+	—	2400	+	21	+
21848	72	M	2-56	Midstomach mass	Subtotal gastrectomy, splenectomy, partial pancreatectomy	UC	—	0/9	—	—	180	—(heart attack)
25768	70	M	6-60	Midstomach mass	Subtotal gastrectomy	Und	—	0/10	2300	—	6	+(? CVA)
28913	63	F	3-61	Bleeding ulcer and retroperitoneal mass	Subtotal gastrectomy and splenectomy, liver biopsy	Und	+	—	—	—	1	+(hemorrhage)
25467	45	F	3-62	Pyloric mass (3.5 yr after radiotherapy to tonsil)	Subtotal gastrectomy	LWD	—	1/10	—	—	11*	—

ID	Age	Sex	Date	Clinical presentation	Operation	Status						
38683	80	F	3-69	GI bleeding (2 yr after radiotherapy nasopharynx, 4 months after radiotherapy neck)	Subtotal gastrectomy	LWD	?	?	—	+	19	+
38879	59	M	3-70	Cardiac mass	Subtotal gastrectomy, splenectomy	HWD	+	0/11	6800	—	6	+(tracheo-esophgeal fistula)
40250	73	F	4-71	Pyloric mass	Subtotal gastrectomy	HPD	—	—	5400	—	11	+

Table 7-2
Exploration and Other Resections for Non-Hodgkin's Lymphoma (EFSCH series)

Patient no.	Age	Sex	Date	Indication	Operation	Pathology Diagnosis	Margin	Nodes (positive/total)	Postoperative Radiotherapy (rads)	Chemotherapy	Survival (months) * = alive	Lymphoma at follow-up
21126	24	M	12-54	Ileal stenosis mesentery node	Ileal resection	UC	—	2/4	—	—	205*	—
11910	78	F	6-56	Ileoileal intus-suception	Ileal resection	HPD	—	?	—	—	1	+
24711	35	F	12-57	Ileal, mesenteric mass	Ileal resection	MC	+	—	1000	+	128	+(stroke)
36583	9	M	6-67	Ileal, mesenteric mass	Ileal resection	LPD	?	?	3200	+	4	+
21075	4	F	8-55	R-colon mass	R-hemicolectomy	LPD	—	0/2	—	—	195*	—
23113	66	F	12-57	R-colon intus-suception	R-hemicolectomy	HWD	—	2/15	700	—	2	+
32236	58	F	1-64	Cecal mass	R-hemicolectomy	Und	—	12/16	3000	—	10	+
37788	54	M	10-68	Cecal mass	R-hemicolectomy	HPD	?	+	—	—	2	+

254

Table 7-3
Operation for Gastrointestinal Malignant Complications of Non-Hodgkin's Lymphoma (EFSCH series)

Patient no.	Age	Sex	Date	Diagnosis	Radiotherapy	Chemotherapy	Primary lesions Site	Interval to op	Complication	Operation	Survival	Lymphoma at follow-up
19430	37	M	12-54	LPD	+	—	Mesentery	6 M	Colon obstruction	Colostomy	1 mo	+
23162	67	M	12-56	LPD	+	+	Neck, axilla, groin, liver, marrow	15 M	Appendicitis	Appendectomy, cecostomy	2 mo	+
24775	62	M	3-58	Und	+	—	Axilla, scapula	2 M	Ileocecal intussuception	Resection of cecum	3 mo	+
24370	48	M	4-58	HWD	+	—	Stomach	6 M	Pyloric obstruction	Gastro-enterostomy	8 mo	+
29308	43	F	8-61	Und	+	—	Neck, bone, lung	7 M	Gastric perforation	Closure, gastrostomy	1 mo	+
27893	45	F	2-62	Und (N)	+	+	All nodes, bone	45 M	Bowel obstruction	Resection of small bowel, jejunostomy	2 mo	+
32144	45	M	1-64	HWD	+	—	Retroperitoneal	4 M	Pyloric obstruction	Gastro-enterostomy	14 days	+
			1-64	HWD	+	—	Retroperitoneal	5 M	Bowel obstruction	Tube enterostomy	3 days	+
35634	54	M	8-66	HWD	+	+	Axilla, neck, groin, mesentery, cecum, rectum	1 M	Colon obstruction	Ileocolostomy, sigmoid colostomy	4 mo	+
36583	9	M	9-67	LPD	+	+	Ileum	3 M	Ileal obstruction	Ileo-colostomy	1 mo	+
40250	73	F	12-71	HPD	+	—	Stomach	8 M	Perforated ileum and abscess	I and D, ileal resection	3 mo	+

Since such secondary lesions may cause obstruction, hemorrhage, or perforation, palliative resection is sometimes required. This can be performed in almost all of the small intestinal lesions, but was feasible only in about 50 percent of those of the stomach. Malabsorption syndrome may be antecedent to or mask the presence of lymphomatous involvement of the gastrointestinal tract.

Among autopsy series, the esophagus was involved in 2.5 percent of the patients with Hodgkin's disease and in 7.5 percent of those with non-Hodgkin's lymphoma. Invasion from adjacent mediastinal lymph nodes in Hodgkin's disease may result in fistula formations. Primary esophageal lymphoma is very rare.

Primary Hodgkin's disease of the stomach accounted for about 3 percent of all gastric neoplasms, and of all primary gastric lymphomas 18 percent. In early localized gastric lymphomas, surgical resection followed by radiotherapy appeared to be the treatment of choice, but radical or total gastrectomy did not improve the survival rate. Some felt resection of the gastric lymphoma should be carried out even though residual tumor must be left behind, since radiation therapy has proved its efficacy in treating residual disease, unresected lesions, and late recurrence. The 5-year survival rate of primary Hodgkin's disease of the stomach is about 30 percent, whereas that of the non-Hodgkin's lymphoma is better than 50 percent.

Malignant tumors of the small intestine are very rare (less than 0.1 percent in autopsy series). Primary lymphoma accounted for nearly half the small bowel neoplasms; and Hodgkin's lesions were present in 10 percent of the lymphoma cases. Symptoms of intestinal lymphoma included those of obstruction, perforation, hemorrhage, and intussception. Similiar to gastric lymphomas, multiple lesions are not rare and the possibility of pseudo-lymphoma should be ruled out. There is general agreement that wide surgical excision of the involved intestine and adjacent mesenteric lymph nodes, followed by radiotherapy, is the treatment of choice.

Lymphoma of the colon accounted for about 10 percent of the gastrointestinal malignant lymphomas. Lesions of the cecum are common, but those of the appendix are rare. Malignant lymphoma of the rectum may develop in cases with ulcerative colitis; it should also be differentiated from benign lymphoid rectal polyps, which are about 2 to 4 times more common. Whenever possible, extirpative resection (including abdominoperineal resection for rectal lesions) and adequate postoperative radiotherapy gave the best survival result (5-year 50 percent).

In the EFSCH series, 31 among the 364 patients with non-Hodgkin's lymphoma, had lesions of the gastrointestinal tract. There were 20 cases of primary lesions: 12 stomach, 4 ileum, and 4 cecum. For stomach lesions, 5 out of 12 survived 5 years after surgical resection or radiotherapy. For intestinal lesions, 3 of the 8 patients lived more than 10 years without recurrence. Palliative operation was required in about 1 in 6 of those patients who had abnormality documented by radiographic studies.

REFERENCES

Alexander JW, Altemeier WA: Association of primary neoplasms of the small intestine with other neoplastic growths. Ann Surg 167:958–964, 1968

Allen AW, Donaldson G, Sniffen RC, et al: Primary malignant lymphoma of the gastro-intestinal tract. Ann Surg 140: 428–438, 1954

Atlee J, Rowan PJ, Ziegler EE: Hodgkin's disease of the stomach with free perforation and apparent surgical cure. Ann Surg 134:1052–1057, 1951

Avent CH: Primary isolated lymphogranulomatosis (Hodgkin's disease) of stomach. Arch Surg 39:423–428, 1939

Azzopardi JG, Menzies T: Primary malignant lymphoma of the alimentary tract. Br J Surg 47:358–366, 1960

al-Bahrani ZR, Bakir F: Primary intestinal lymphoma: A challenging problem in abdominal pain. Ann R Coll Surg Engl 49:103–113, 1971

Bailey RJ Jr, Burgert EO Jr, Dahlin DC: Malignant lymphoma in children. Pediatrics 28:985–992, 1961

Ben-Asher H: The Radiology Corner: Hodgkin's disease of the stomach. Am J Gastroenterol 56:446–471, 1971

Berg JW: Primary lymphomas of the human gastrointestinal tract. Natl Cancer Inst Monogr 32:211–220, 1969

Berry GR, Mathews WH: Gastric lymphosarcoma and pseudolymphoma: Reappraisal of 12 cases of gastric lymphosarcoma. Can Med Assoc J 96: 1312–1316, 1967

Bichel J: Hodgkin's disease of the oesophagus. Acta Radiol [Ther] (Stockh) 35:371–374, 1951

Brunt PW, Sircus W, Maclean N: Neoplasia and the coeliac syndrome in adults. Lancet 1:180–184, 1969

Burman SO, van Wyk FA: Lymphomas of the small intestine and cecum. Ann Surg 143:349–359, 1956

Bush RS, Ash CL: Primary lymphoma of the gastrointestinal tract. Radiology 92:1349–1354, 1969

Caruso RD, Berk RN: Lymphoma of the esophagus. Radiology 95:381–382, 1970

Cathcart RS, Sutton JP, Gregorie HB Jr: Sarcomas of the stomach. Ann Surg 173: 398–402, 1971

Chioléro J: Un cas de lymphogranulomatose primitive de l'oesophage. Ann d'anat pathol 12:305–310, 1935

Cohen N: Lymphosarcoma of the stomach. Gastrointest Endosc 8:16–19, 1961

Cohen N, Canter JW: Hodgkin's disease of the small intestine: Report of six cases. Am J Dig Dis 4:361–377, 1959

Coller FA, Flotte CT: Lymphomas of the gastro-intestinal tract. Proceedings of Third National Cancer Conference. Philadelphia, Lippincott, 1957, pp 753–758

Cornes JS: Hodgkin's disease of the gastrointestinal tract. Proc R Soc Med 60:732–733, 1967

Craver LF: Treatment of Hodgkin's disease, in Pack GI, Ariel IM (eds): Treatment of Cancer and Allied Diseases (ed 2). New York, Hoeber, 1964, pp 168–191

Craver LF, Herrmann JB: Abdominal lymphogranulomatosis. Am J Roentgenol Radium Ther Nucl Med 55:165–172, 1946

Crile G Jr, Hazard JB, Allen KL: Primary lymphosarcoma of the stomach. Ann Surg 135:39–43, 1952

Cruveilheir J: Anatomie pathologique du corps human. Liv Sec 30:Part 2, I, 1827, Paris, 1829

Cupps RE, Hodgson JR, Dockerty MB, et al: Primary lymphoma in small intestine: Problems of roentgenologic diagnosis. Radiology 92:1355–1362, 1969

Dawson IM, Cornes JS, Morson BC: Primary malignant lymphoid tumours of the intestinal tract. Br J Surg 49:80–89, 1961

Deeb PH, Stilson WL: Roentgenologic manifestations of lymphosarcoma of the small bowel. Radiology 63:235–239, 1954

Dockerty MB, Dahlin DC: Classification and mode of spread of malignant neoplasms, in Pack GT, Ariel IM (eds): Treatment of Cancer and Allied Disease, vol 5 (ed 2). New York, Hoeber, 1962, pp 3–17

Dunn GD, Moeller D, Laing RR: Primary reticulum cell sarcoma of the stomach. Gastrointest Endosc 17:153–158, 1971

Dutz W, Asvadi S, Sadri S, et al: Intestinal lymphoma and sprue: A systematic approach. Gut 12:804–810, 1971

Ehrlich AN, Stalder G, Geller W, et al: Gastrointestinal manifestations of malignant lymphoma. Gastroenterology 54:1115–1121, 1968

Eidelman S, Parkins A, Rubin CE: Abdominal lymphoma presenting as malabsorption: A clinico-pathologic study of nine cases in Israel and a review of the literature. Medicine 45:111–137, 1966

Fairley NH, Mackie FP: Clinical and biochemical syndrome in lymphadenoma and allied diseases involving the mesenteric lymph glands. Br Med J 1:375–380, 1937

Faris TD, Saltzstein SL: Gastric lymphoid hyperplasia: A lesion confused with lymphosarcoma. Cancer 17:207–212, 1964

Faulkner JW, Dockerty MB: Lymphosarcoma of the small intestine. Surg Gynecol Obstet 95:76–84, 1952

Frazer JW Jr: Malignant lymphomas of the gastrointestinal tract. Surg Gynecol Obstet 108:182–190, 1959

Fu K. Stewart JR: Radiotherapeutic management of small intestinal lymphoma with malabsorption. Cancer 31:286–290, 1973

Fu YS, Perzin KH: Lymphosarcoma of the small intestine: A clinicopathologic study. Cancer 29:645–659, 1972

Fuller LM: Results of large volume irradiation in the management of Hodgkin's disease and malignant lymphomas originating in the abdomen. Radiology 87:1058–1064, 1966

Gall EA: The surgical treatment of malignant lymphoma. Ann Surg 118:1064–1070, 1943

Gall EA, Mallory TB: Malignant lymphoma: A clinicopathologic survey of 618 cases. Am J Pathol 18:381–415, 1942

Gechman E, Bluth I, Gross JM: Hodgkin's disease of the rectum. Arch Intern Med 97:483–491, 1956

Goldman LB: Hodgkin's disease: An analysis of 212 cases. JAMA 114:1611–1616, 1940

Hambly CK, Blundell JE: Hodgkin's disease of the oesophagus. Aust Radiol 12:43–48, 1968

Helwig EB, Hansen J: Lymphoid polyps (benign lymphoma) and malignant lymphoma of the rectum and anus. Surg Gynecol Obstet 92:233–243, 1951

Henderson M, Paterson WG: Perforation of jejunum by reticulum cell sarcoma in pregnancy. Am J Surg 115:385–389, 1968

Herter FP, Auchincloss H Jr: Total gastrectomy: Experience with ninety-one cases. Cancer 10:320–331, 1957

Hoerr SO: Malignant lesions of the stomach: An analysis of fifty-four five year survivors. Am J Surg 109:14–20, 1965

Hoskins EO: Unusual radiological manifestations of Hodgkin's disease. Proc R Soc Med 60:729–732, 1967

Irvine WT, Johnstone JM: Lymphosarcoma of the small intestine: With special reference to perforating tumours. Br J Surg 42:611–618, 1955

Jackson AS: Primary Hodgkin's disease of the stomach. Am J Surg 94:546–550, 1957

Jackson H Jr, Parker F Jr: Hodgkin's Disease and Allied Disorders. New York, Oxford University Press, 1947

Jacobs DS: Primary gastric malignant lymphoma and pseudolymphoma. Am J Clin Pathol 40:379–394, 1963

Jenkin RD, Sonley MJ, Stephens CA, et al: Primary gastrointestinal tract lymphoma in childhood. Radiology 92:763–767, 1969

Jones TE, Carmody MG: Lymphosarcoma of the stomach; report of case with a 19-year surgical cure. Ann Surg 101:1136–1138, 1935

Joseph JI, Lattes R: Gastric lymphosarcoma: Clinicopathologic analysis of 71 cases and its relation to disseminated lymphosarcoma. Am J Clin Pathol 45:653–669, 1966

Kahn LB, Selzer G, Kaschula RO: Primary gastrointestinal lymphoma: A clinicopathologic study of fifty-seven cases. Am J Dig Dis 17:219–232, 1972

Kane AA: Hodgkin's disease of the stomach. Am J Gastroenterol 40:504–513, 1963

Kaplan HS: Hodgkin's Disease. Cambridge, Mass, Harvard University Press, 1972

Kent TH: Malabsorption syndrome with malignant lymphoma. Arch Pathol 78:97–103, 1964

al-Khateeb AK: Primary malignant lymphoma of the small intestine. Int Surg 54:295–300, 1970

Lee HY, Cogbill CL: Primary lymphosarcoma of the stomach. Am Surg 37:256–262, 1971

Lee YN: Simple technic for fixing loop colostomy. Am J Surg 116:138–139, 1968

Loehr WJ, Mujahed Z, Zahn FD, et al: Primary lymphoma of the gastrointestinal tract: A review of 100 cases. Ann Surg 170:232–238, 1969

McNeer G, Berg JW: The clinical behavior and management of primary malignant lymphoma of the stomach. Surgery 46: 829–840, 1959

McNeer G, Pack GT: Malignant tumors of the stomach, in Pack GT, Ariel IM (eds): Treatment of Cancer and Allied Disease, vol. 5 (ed 2), New York, Hoeber, 1962, pp 296–305

Marcuse PM, Stout AP: Primary lymphosarcoma of the small intestine: Analysis of thirteen cases and review of the literature. Cancer 3:459–474, 1950

Marshall SF: Gastric tumors other than carcinoma: Report of unusual cases. Surg Clin North Am 35:693–702, 1955

Marshall SF, Adamson NE Jr: Sarcoma of the stomach: Tumors of lymphatic and reticuloendothelial origin (62 cases). Surg Clin North Am 39:711–718, 1959

Marshall SF, Brown L: Primary malignant lymphoid tumors of the stomach. Surg Clin North Am 30:885–892, 1950

Mestel AL: Lymphosarcoma of the small intestine in infancy and childhood. Ann Surg 149:87–94, 1959

Molander DW, Pack GT: Lymphosarcoma: Choice of treatment and end-results in 567 patients. Role of surgical treatment for cure and palliation. Rev Surg 20:3–31, 1963

Morioka WK, Starkloff GB: Tumors of the duodenum and jejunum. Mo Med 65: 211–214, 1968

Naqvi MS, Burrows L, Kark AE: Lymphoma of the gastrointestinal tract: Prognostic guides based on 162 cases. Ann Surg 170:221–231, 1969

Newall J, Friedman M: Reticulum-cell sarcoma. Part II. Radiation dosage for each type. Radiology 94:643–647, 1970

Newall J, Friedman M, Narvaez F de: Extra-lymph-node reticulum-cell sarcoma. Radiology 91:708–712, 1968

Novis BH, Bank S, Marks IN, et al: Abdominal lymphoma presenting with malabsorption. Q J Med 40:521–540, 1971

Pack GT, Molander DW: The surgical treatment of Hodgkin's disease. Cancer Res 26:1254–1263, 1966

Palmer ED: Sarcomas of the stomach. Am J Dig Dis 17:186–195, 1950

Papp JP, Penner JA: Esophagomediastinal fistula in Hodgkin's disease. Postgrad Med 48:180–183, 1970

Perry PM, Cross RM, Morson BC: Primary malignant lymphoma of the rectum (22 cases). Proc R Soc Med 65:72, 1972

Peters MV, Hasselback R, Brown TC: The natural history of the lymphomas related to the clinical classification, in Zarafonetis CJ (ed): Proceedings of the International Conference on Leukemia-Lymphoma. Philadelphia, Lea & Febiger, 1968, pp 357–371

Portmann UV, Dunne EF, Hazard JB: Manifestations of Hodgkin's disease of the gastrointestinal tract. Am J Roentgenol Radium Ther Nucl Med 72:772–787, 1954

Raiford TS: Treatment of Tumors of the Appendix, in Pack GT, Ariel IM (eds): Treatment of Cancer and Allied Disease, vol. 5 (ed 2). New York, Hoeber, 1962, pp 296–305

Ralston LS, Wasdahl WA: Gastrointestinal Hodgkin's disease. Am J Gastroenterol 29:537–544, 1958

Ramot B: Intestinal lymphoma with malabsorption in Mediterranean populations. Isr J Med Sci 7:1488–1490, 1971

ReMine WH: Gastric sarcomas. Am J Surg 120:320–323, 1970

Richmond J, Sherman RS, Diamond HD, et al: Renal lesions associated with malignant lymphomas. Am J Med 32:184–207, 1962

Rösch W, Hartwich G, Elster K, et al: Gastric lymphoma. Endoscopy 3:28–33, 1971

Rosenberg SA, Diamond HD, Jaslowitz B, et al: Lymphosarcoma: A review of 1269 cases. Medicine 40:31–84, 1961

Rubin CE, Massey BW: The preoperative diagnosis of gastric and duodenal malignant lymphoma by exfoliative cytology. Cancer 7:271–288, 1954

al-Saleem T, al-Bahrani Z: Malignant lymphoma of the small intestine in Iraq (Middle East lymphoma). Cancer 31:291–294, 1973

Salmela H: Lymphosarcoma of the stomach: A clinical study of 39 cases. Acta Chir Scand 134:567–576, 1968

Saltzstein SL: Extranodal malignant lymphomas and psuedolymphomas, in Sommers SC (ed): Pathology Annual, vol. 4. New York, Appleton-Century-Crofts, 1969, pp 159–184

Schamaun M: Surgical treatment in Hodgkin's disease, in Rüttimann A (ed): Progress in Lymphology, vol 1. Stuttgart, Thieme, 1967, pp 125–126

Schenkin JR, Burns EL: Gastrointestinal tract, in Anderson WA (ed): Pathology (ed 4). St. Louis, Mosby, 1961, pp 778–818

Schlagenhaufer F: Ueber Granulomatosis des Magendarmtrakts. Zentralbl Allg Pathol 24:965–966, 1913

Scott RB: The surgical aspects of the lymphomata. Ann R Coll Surg Engl 22:178–196, 1958

Shepard GH, Burko H, McSwain B: Sarcoma of the stomach: A review of 39 cases. South Med J 62:1064–1071, 1969

Sherman ED: Gastro-intestinal manifestations of lymphogranulomatosis (Hodgkin's disease). Arch Intern Med 61:60–82, 1938

Singer HA: Primary, isolated lymphogranulomatosis of the stomach. Arch Surg 22:1001–1017, 1931

Skrimshire JF: Lymphoma of the stomach and intestine. Q J Med 24:203–214, 1955

Smith JL Jr, Helwig EB: Malignant lymphoma of the stomach: Its diagnosis, distinction and biologic behavior. Am J Pathol 34:553, 1958 (Abstr)

Spratt JS Jr: Prevalence of neoplastic and pseudoneoplastic lesions of the small intestine. Geriatrics 21:231–238, 1966

Steindl H: Uber einen Fall von Lymphogranulomatose des Magens. Arch f Klin Chir 130:110–116, 1924

Stout AP: The results of treatment of lymphosarcoma. NY State J Med 47:158–164, 1947

Strauch M, Martin T, Remmele W: Case reports: Hodgkin's disease of the oesophagus. Endoscopy 3:207–209, 1971

Talvalkar GV: Primary malignant lymphoma of small and large intestines. Indian J Cancer 5:238–245, 1968

Teitelman SL, Brill NR: Localized Hodgkin's disease of the small intestine. Am J Surg 99:247–248, 1960

Ullman A, Abeshouse BS: Lymphosarcoma of the small and large intestines. Ann Surg 95:878–915, 1932

Vieta JO, Craver LF: Intrathoracic manifestations of lymphomatoid diseases. Radiology 37:138–158, 1941

Warren K: Malignant lymphoma of the duodenum, small intestine and colon. Surg Clin North Am 39:725–735, 1959

Warren KW, Littlefield JB: Malignant lymphomas of the gastrointestinal tract. Surg Clin North Am 35:735–746, 1955

Warren S, Lulenski CR: Primary solitary lymphoid tumors of the gastro-intestinal tract. Ann Surg 115:1–12, 1942

Weaver DK, Batsakis JG: Primary lymphomas of the small intestine. Am J Gastroenterol 42:620–625, 1964

Weaver DK, Batsakis JG: Pseudolymphomas of the small intestine. Am J Gastroenterol 44:374–381, 1965

Welborn JK, Ponka JL, Rebuck JW: Lymphoma of the stomach: A diagnostic and therapeutic problem. Arch Surg 90:480–487, 1965

Williams ER: Radiological study of intrathoracic lymphogranuloma and lymphosarcoma. Br J Radiol 8:265–279, 1935

Wychulis AR, Beahrs OH, Woolner LB: Malignant lymphoma of the colon: A study of 69 cases. Arch Surg 93:215–225, 1966

Wynne JW, Armstrong D: Clostridial septicemia. Cancer 29:215–221, 1972

Yamashiro KM, Gray GM: Primary intestinal lymphoma: Response to radiotherapy. Clin Res 20:183, 1972 (Abstr)

8

Nongastrointestinal Abdominal Lymphomas

SPLEEN

Spleen is the first recognized site of involvement in about 1 percent of the patients with non-Hodgkin's lymphoma, and some of these cases are primary lymphomas of the spleen. In 1923, Smith and Rusk reviewed 104 reported cases of primary splenic malignant neoplasms and stated that lymphomas were the most common form of splenic tumor. In 1939, Gerundo and Miller reported a case of reticulum cell sarcoma of the spleen with metastases confined to the lymph nodes. They mentioned that there were only about 120 well-authenticated primary tumors of the spleen published. Hausman and Gaarde (1943) added 1 case of lymphosarcoma of the spleen and found 9 others in the literature.

Gordon and Paley (1951) reported 2 patients with primary lymphosarcoma of the spleen treated by splenectomy. They found a total of 189 primary splenic tumors in the literature and estimated that 42 of these were lymphomas. In general, Willis (1953) said that cases of primary lymphomas of the spleen were rare; and Lumb (1954) listed only 1 patient in each of his groups of follicular lymphoma and reticulum cell sarcoma. Rappaport et al (1956) reported 3 apparently localized splenic tumors among 253 cases of follicular lymphoma.

On the other hand, splenic involvement during the course of lymphoma is very common. In 1229 patients with non-Hodgkin's lymphoma, Rosenberg et al (1961) noted that 0.8 percent had a palpable spleen as the initial manifestation, 36 percent had splenomegaly during the course of the disease, and 54 percent of those who were autopsied had lesions in the spleen. Even among enlarged spleens only 71 percent contained tumors at the autopsy.

261

There was no instance in which mechanical or hypersplenic manifestiations necessitated the operative removal of an enlarged spleen. Molander and Pack (1963) reviewed therapy of 567 patients with non-Hodgkin's lymphomas. Their series included 42 patients treated surgically for localized disease, including one splenectomy.

Hickling (1964) reported 5 patients with massive splenomegaly. Histology of the spleen showed giant follicle lymphomas in 2 and lymphatic leukemia in the other 3. After splenectomy, there was reversion of the circulating blood to normal pattern and all patients were in excellent health for 1, 4, 6, 10, and 13 years.

Das Gupta et al (1965) reported one case of primary splenic neoplasm and found 9 additional cases reported after Gordon and Paley (1951). Among the 10 added cases, 9 were malignant lymphomas (5 reticulum cell sarcoma and 4 lymphosarcoma). They specified the criteria for diagnosis of primary lymphoma of the spleen should be fourfold: "The prime symptomatic presentation is splenomegaly and associated mechanical discomfort. Clinical, biochemical, hematologic, and roentgenologic investigations must exclude any evidence of disease elsewhere. Results of intraabdominal examination during laparotomy must include negative formal biopsy of the liver and no evidence of lymphoma in mesenteric and para-aortic nodes. An arbitrary period of at least 6 months must elapse between the diagnosis of primary lymphoma of the spleen and detection of disease elsewhere." In one patient, evidence of lymphosarcoma of the parotid region developed 11 years after splenectomy and she was still living 23 years after the operation. Two patients in their series of 10 died of local extension of primary splenic lymphomas, one with fatal hematemesis and the other with a splenogastropleural fistula. Thus, they felt the possibility of local complications warranted palliative splenectomy whenever technically feasible, even though a particular tumor could not be classified as one of the primary splenic lymphomas.

Ahmann et al (1966) reported 49 cases of malignant lymphomas of the spleen; in all cases the diagnosis was made at the time of the splenectomy. The 5-year survival rate for the entire group was 31 percent. Eight of this group apparently had lymphomas only in the spleen, and another 9 had splenic hilar node disease also. The survival rates of these patients with stage I and II diseases (60 percent at 3 years, 45 percent at 5 years) were considerably better than those with stage III disease (25 percent at 3 years). In addition, they found that patients with a follicular pattern of lymphoma tended to have a better prognosis than those with diffuse infiltrations. The highest 5-year survival rate (60 percent) was seen in the group with lymphocytic lymphoma.

Hermann et al (1968) said that 52 out of 582 splenectomies done were for the diagnosis of splenomegaly (an incidence rate of 9 percent). The most common cause in these 52 patients was malignant lymphoma (15 cases, including 1 of Hodgkin's disease). Hyatt et al (1970) reported 7 patients undergoing splenectomy for lymphosarcoma who had primarily splenic involvement. All had splenomegaly and hypersplenism, and all had hematologic and clinical responses after splenectomy. Six of the 7 patients were alive and asymptomatic from 6 months to 10.5 years after operation without other therapy. This suggested that splenectomy might have a favorable effect, not only on hypersplenism but also on the basic disease process. It is not clear whether the long survival after splenectomy of patients with lymphosarcoma is because they have a different form of disease with a better prognosis, or because the splenomegaly and accompanying symptoms of hypersplenism might have resulted in earlier diagnosis and treatment.

Skarin et al (1971) reported the results of diagnostic splenectomy in 11 patients with lymphosarcoma primarily involving the spleen. Splenomegaly was the only finding in 3 patients; in the others, massively enlarged spleens with varying degrees of pancytopenia were present. Blood pictures compatible with lymphatic leukemia subsequently developed in 6 of the 11 patients. Follow-up time after surgery ranged from 1 to 16 years with a median of 3.5 years. Their experience supported the observation that patients with lymphosarcoma primarily involving the spleen tolerated splenectomy well and benefited from this procedure, despite the development of a leukemic blood picture in some cases.

LIVER

Hoster et al (1948) said the liver may be implicated in 50–60 percent of the patients with Hodgkin's disease at the time of death. Levitan et al (1959) reported 2 patients with esophageal varices secondary to portal hypertension caused by extensive intrahepatic Hodgkin's disease. Levitan et al (1961) found the liver had documented histological lesions in 66 percent of the necropsy cases. Diffuse involvement of the liver by Hodgkin's disease was the most common type of intrahepatic distribution (86.5 percent), whereas discrete nodular lesions were found in 10.8 percent, and the combined diffuse and nodular type was encountered in only 2.7 percent. In their series, the survival rates of patients who had clinical evidence of hepatic disease did not differ significantly from the surfvival rate of Hodgkin's disease in general. The presence or absence of hepatomegaly, the degree of hepatomegaly and splenomegaly, and sex did not significantly influence survival either. MacLeod and Stalker (1962) reported that aspiration biopsy of the liver gave valuable information in 11 cases of Hodgkin's disease in which the diagnosis could not be established by examination of a superficial lymph node.

In a review of 1229 patients with non-Hodgkin's lymphomas, Rosenberg et al (1961) found that the liver was palpably enlarged in 46 percent of the patients. However, in the autopsy series only 57 percent of the palpably enlarged livers had tumors upon histological examination.

Primary hepatic Hodgkin's disease apparently was first described by Goia in 1935 (cited by Loehry in 1964). Symmers (1944) reported a 40-year-old woman with symptoms of abdominal pain, ascites, and jaundice. At autopsy, two-thirds of the substance of the liver was replaced by Hodgkin's disease. The mesenteric and retroperitoneal lymph nodes were moderately increased in number and in size. He believed this case presented a unique feature in that the "primary" lesion of Hodgkin's disease was in the liver.

Loehry (1964) reported another case of a 15-year-old girl who had splenohepatomegaly at laparotomy. The liver biopsy was not diagnostic, but tissue at autopsy showed Hodgkin's disease of the liver and para-aortic nodes. Pack and Molander (1966) did not encounter such in their 316 patients. They also said none of the 60 hepatic lobectomies they performed was for Hodgkin's disease. However, among the 42 curative resections performed on 567 patients with non-Hodgkin's lymphomas, Molander and Pack (1965) included 1 patient who had segmental hepatic lobectomy and who survived more than 5 years.

Sahebjami (1971) reported an interesting case of generalized Hodgkin's disease of 6-years duration in combination with another extensive primary adenocarcinoma of the liver.

Hirsch (1937) described non-Hodgkin's lymphoma which presumably arose in the liver. Lumb (1954) listed 1 patient with lymphosarcoma in whom the primary site was the liver. Edmondson (1958) included a patient who had a single tumor replacing most of the liver; histologically it probably represented reticulum cell sarcoma. Torres and Bollozos (1971) reported another case of reticulum cell sarcoma which was truly primarily of the liver because, at autopsy, there was no evidence of spread to any other organ.

URINARY TRACT AND MALE GENITAL ORGANS

Baker and Mann (1939) pointed out that ureters might be obstructed by a lymphoid mass, and that, though very rarely, the bladder also might be involved in Hodgkin's disease. It is surprising that only 1 of their 65 patients died of uremia secondary to pressure on the ureter. The genitourinary tract is involved in 10 percent of patients with malignant lymphomas. (Gall and Mallory 1942). Watson et al (1949) found that 9.5 percent of 456 patients with lymphosarcomas had clinical involvement of the genitourinary system, whereas the figure was 61.9 percent for cases who had autopsies. Considerably lower incidences were found in patients with Hodgkin's disease: 1.3 percent clinically and 6.6 percent at postmortem.

In the 1229 non-Hodgkin's patients reported by Rosenberg et al (1961), 11 patients presented initially with genitourinary lesions (6 were testicular, others were bladder and prostate). About 3 percent of the patients had clinical evidence of genitourinary system involvement during the course of the disease, and 57 percent had genitourinary tumors in the autopsy series. They had one unusual case in which a rapidly fatal hypertension developed as a result of compromised renal circulation secondary to tumor invasion of one renal artery. This presentation was first reported by Blatt and Page (1939), and Kiely et al (1969) also saw a patient with this complication. Molander and Pack (1963) said 2 of their 567 non-Hodgkin's patients presented with uremia secondary to bilateral ureteral blockage without prodromal symptoms of retroperitoneal lymphoma of abdominal pain or backache.

Kidney

Richmond et al (1962) reviewed their autopsy series of 272 patients with Hodgkin's disease and 418 patients with other lymphomas. The incidence of lymphomatous infiltration of the kidneys in the whole series was 33.5 percent. The frequency with which the renal parenchyma was involved in the different lymphomas was as follows: 13 percent, Hodgkin's disease; 46 percent, reticulum cell sarcomas; 39 percent, lymphosarcomas without marrow involvement; and 63 percent with marrow involvement. Givler (1971) also did a retrospective study of the autopsy material on 703 patients with leukemia and lymphomas. He found the overall incidence of renal involvement to be 50 percent, including 13 percent for Hodgkin's disease and 41 percent for other lymphomas.

It was pointed out that the renal involvement was recognized in only 10 percent of the cases before death. For Hodgkin's disease, other than the lung, which was involved in 46 percent of the cases, the kidneys were infiltrated more frequently than any other organ or tissue (Richmond et al 1962). Amyloidosis, secondary to the underlying malignant process, was found only in patients with Hodgkin's disease, and occurred in only 2.8 percent of the cases. Winawer and Feldman (1959) reviewed 40 cases of amyloid nephrosis secondary to Hodgkin's disease. Amyloidosis is more likely to occur in patients with long-standing Hodgkin's disease and frequently involves the kidneys, liver, spleen, and adrenals (Kiely et al 1969).

Serial abdominal scout films and serial intravenous pyelograms in particular have been helpful in detecting renal involvement (Richmond et al 1962). But Hoskins (1967) said intravenous pyelography is not too helpful in detecting small deposits because they rarely produce any calyceal distortion. In bilateral renal involvement causing generalized enlargement of the organs, the appearance is rather characteristic of, or similar to, that of polycystic disease or renal hamartoma. Separated renal function studies have been useful in one case in which combination chemotherapy improved the concentrating ability of the disease kidney (Steel et al 1970). Pick et al (1971) studied the arteriographic findings of 2 patients with lymphomas involving the kidneys. They said the pattern of vascularity in these lesions, and in the others reviewed in the literature, was that of a relative paucity of pathologic vessels supplying the mass lesion. The arteriographic findings were unlike those seen in the classic hypernephroma.

Pack and Molander (1966) said Hodgkin's disease rarely originates in the kidney and that "nephrectomy is seldom applicable." Still, surgical procedure is often required in the diagnosis and occasional treatment of malignant lymphomas of the kidneys. Knoepp (1956) reported one case in which an apparently isolated lymphosarcoma of the kidney was removed, and no recurrence was noted at a second-look operation 2 years later. Follow-up examination 5 years after the original operation also showed no evidence of lymphoma. Kiely et al (1969) reported a case of reticulum cell sarcoma replacing the renal substance. The tumor was fixed to the aorta, and radiotherapy was given after a nephrectomy. Four years later an adenocarcinoma of the left transverse colon was removed, but no evidence of recurrence or residual of the original lymphoma was found.

Other renal complications of lymphoma not directly related to tumor invasion have been discussed by Kiely et al (1969). These include hypercalcemic nephropathy, complications of therapy (uric acid nephropathy and radiation nephritis), and immunologic reactions (nephrotic syndrome, amyloidosis, and retroperitoneal fibrosis). Occasionally, renal vein thrombosis and amyloidosis might be hard to differentiate.

Plager and Stutzman (1971) described 4 patients in whom an acute nephrotic syndrome was associated with a clinical relapse of Hodgkin's disease. They also reviewed 10 cases reported in the literature in which Hodgkin's idiopathic nephrotic syndromes were present. Since proteinemia was promptly relieved by effective treatment of Hodgkin's disease with either chemotherapy or radiotherapy delivered to areas distant to the renal bed, they postulated that there might be substances originating in the tumor which damaged the renal glomerular basement membrane, perhaps acting as an antigen–antibody complex. Subsequently, Lowry et al (1971), Jackson and Oo (1971), and Bichel and Jensen (1971) reported 7 more cases of nephrotic syndrome in Hodgkin's disease. Loughridge and Lewis (1971) reported 3 patients with extrarenal neoplasia who developed the nephrotic syndrome (2 had lung and 1 had breast cancer). Renal biopsies showed diffuse glomerular abnormalities, and they also postulated that the renal lesions might have resulted from an immune response to the tumors.

However, Hansen et al (1972) reported 3 patients, with Hodgkin's disease associated with the nephrotic syndrome, whose renal biopsies were without lesion when examined by light and electron microscopy. Two of the patients had a close time relationship between development of the syndrome and the activity of the disease, suggesting the two conditions might share a common pathogenetic mechanism. Bennett et al (1972) reported a new renal malfunction in advanced Hodgkin's disease. Two patients had hypouricemia secondary to excessive tubular secretion. In both cases, the abnormal renal handling of uric acid was corrected with therapy for Hodg-kin's disease, strongly suggesting that this disease was the causal factor.

Ureter, Bladder, and Prostate

In 1967, Smythe and Hwang reported a polypoid tumor of the ureter, probably a reticulum cell sarcoma. Braun et al (1972) reported an isolated plaque lesion of the upper ureter, containing Reed-Sternberg cells, which was treated with nephroureterectomy.

Apparently Chaffey (1885) reported the first case of primary malignant lymphoma of the urinary bladder. Bhansali and Cameron (1960) reported 8 cases and reviewed 23 patients reported in the literature. They pointed out the earliest and most outstanding symptom in malignant lymphoma of the bladder was usually periodic hematuria. An interesting feature was the common association of hematuria with frequency of micturition and/or dysuria, whereas in epithelial bladder tumors, such association occurred only in 12 percent of the cases.

In the autopsy series of 690 patients with lymphoma, Richmond et al (1962) found that the bladder was involved in 4.5 percent of those with Hodgkin's disease and in 10–19 percent of those with other lymphomas. Givler (1971) reported almost identical figures: 5.1 percent for Hodgkin's disease, 11.4 percent for non-Hodgkin's lymphoma, and 18–26 percent for leukemias. These represented an overall incidence of 19 percent with micro-scopic infiltrations, whereas only 2.8 percent had gross lesions of the bladder.

Wang et al (1969) reviewed 39 cases of primary malignant lymphoma of the bladder and added 2 cases of their own. One patient survived 5 years without recurrent disease after aggressive radiotherapy (4000 rads), and another was well 9 years after radical cystectomy without radiotherapy. Reymond et al (1971) reported 1 patient with no history of hematuria who had a tumor defect by x-ray and an intact mucosa on cystoscopy.

Tremann et al (1971) wrote about a patient with lymphatic leukemic infiltration of the bladder who had persistent chronic cystitis for 5 years after the initial biopsy. They commented that "whereas primary lymphosar-coma of the bladder demands aggressive surgical extirpation and/or radiation therapy, lymphoproliferative disorders that secondarily involve the bladder should be treated palliatively as symptoms indicate."

In the autopsy series of Richmond et al (1962), the prostate was involved in 0.5 percent of the patients with Hodgkin's disease, in 11.5 percent of those with reticulum cell sarcomas, and in 12–23 percent of those with lymphosarcomas. The seminal vesicle and vas deferens were involved in 0.5 percent of those with Hodgkin's disease and 4 percent of the other lymphomas. Molander and Pack (1963) said primary lymphosarcoma of the prostate had been reported, but prostatic lymphosarcoma was seen only as secondary involvement in 4 of their 378 male patients with non-Hodgkin's lymphomas. The seminal vesicle was involved in 2 instances.

Testes and Adrenals

In the autopsy study of 690 patients with lymphoma, Richmond et al (1962) found that testes were involved in 1 percent of those with Hodgkin's disease, in 15 percent with reticulum cell sarcoma and in 7–21 percent of those with lymphosarcomas (higher rate for those with marrow involvement).

Historically, the earliest report of lymphosarcoma of both testes was that of Hutchinson (1889). Varney (1955) pointed out that lymphosarcoma of the testis was a rare disease, and it usually occurred secondary to a primary lesion elsewhere. It might, however, present itself as a primary tumor of the testis.

Cohen et al (1955) reviewed the literature and found only 10 cases of reticulum cell sarcoma involving the testes among more than 2860 cases of testicular tumors reported in the English literature. They reported 4 cases, emphasizing the frequent finding of bilateral lesions, and pointed out that their biological behaviors were similar to seminomas. One case of the disease was arrested by radical orchiectomy and radiotherapy. Among a series of 343 patients with non-Hodgkin's lymphoma, Werf-Messing (1968) reported 11 patients with primary testicular lymphoma, 18 percent of whom survived more than 5 years after radiotherapy.

Kiely et al (1970) reviewed a series of 31 patients who underwent orchiectomy for lymphoma of the testis. Seventeen of the 31 patients were considered to have primary lesions of the testes (clinically no other evidence of lymphoma at orchiectomy), and 13 of the 17 were of the reticulum cell type. They pointed out that the prognosis of lymphoma clinically localized to the testis is relatively favorable after orchiectomy and radiation therapy to the regional lymph nodes (5-year survival, 29 percent). The previously held belief that life expectany is poor for men with testicular lymphoma was due to failure in most reports to separate survival of those with localized tumor from those with disseminated involvement at the time of orchiectomy. Histopathologically, all of the known 5-year survivors had reticulum cell lymphoma. In contrast to germ cell tumors, lymphoma of the testis occurs in an older age group, has no special propensity to develop in cryptorchid testes, and tends to involve the skin and nasopharynx when dissemination occurs. They reviewed the literature and found that although lymphoma comprised less than 5 percent of all testicular cancers, it was the most common type of testicular cancer after age 60, and approximately 50 percent of patients with bilateral tumors had lymphoma. Luce and Frei (1972) mentioned that secondary involvement of the testes occurred particularly often in children. Burkitt's lymphoma commonly involved the testes, ovaries, and kidneys.

Johnson et al (1972) studied the natural history of 13 patients with reticulum cell sarcoma presented as testicular tumors. All patients underwent orchiectomy initially. They pointed out that the diagnosis was often missed because in 8 cases the initial histologic diagnosis was erroneous. They felt the testicular lesions represented precocious development of an already disseminated disease because the lesions were bilateral at the time of diagnosis in 2 patients, subsequently involved opposite sides in 3 patients, and appeared in other tissues or distant sites in 7 (3, skin; 2, lymph nodes; and 2, head and neck area). The recommended treatment for reticulum cell sarcoma of the testes was "radical orchiectomy with thorough evaluation of the patient to exclude the presence of other forms of disease. Prophylactic radiotherapy may be given to the para-aortic lymph nodes when generalized disease has been excluded. Chemotherapy should be reserved for treatment of disseminated disease."

Hamlin et al (1972) reported 9 cases of lymphoma of the testicle (including 2 cases of Hodgkin's disease) and reviewed 57 cases reported in the literature (not including cases reported by Werf-Messing 1968, Kiely et al 1970, and Johnson et al 1972). They emphasized that although two-thirds of the patients had disease clinically confined to a single testicle, 11.3 percent had synchronous involvement of the opposite testicle, and an equal number presented evidence of superdiaphragmatic or extranodal disease. The first site of recurrence is often in a visceral organ or in a noncontiguous lymph node region. Thus, they felt that lymphoma of the testicle should be considered as part of a systemic disease, and radiotherapy to clinically uninvolved regions should not be recommended.

At autopsy, the adrenals are frequently found infiltrated by Hodgkin's disease, mainly by contiguous spread from the adjacent retroperitoneal nodes. Craver (1969) said the diagnosis of adrenal insufficiency may occasionally be established on account of severe asthenia, hypotension, skin pigmentation, and laboratory tests.

Sparagana (1970) reported the first case of reticulum cell sarcoma apparently confined to the adrenals. The patient presented with weakness, weight loss, fever, gastrointestinal symptoms, and postural hypotension. All the tests supported the diagnosis of Addison's disease. At necropsy, the adrenals were found to be completely replaced by reticulum cell sarcoma. The tumor had invaded the upper pole of both kidneys, but no tumor was found in the lymph nodes or in any other location.

EFSCH Experiences

In the EFSCH series, of those who had x-ray studies, about 5 percent of the patients with Hodgkin's disease showed abnormal kidneys and about 21 percent had overall abnormal intravenous pyelograms. During the course of the disease another 6 percent had abnormal x-rays recorded. The comparable figures for those with non-Hodgkin's lymphomas were 4, 56 and 11 percent. One (No. 23200) of the 163 patients with Hodgkin's disease originally had an exploration through a flank incision for a mistaken diagnosis of kidney tumor.

Subsequent abdominal exploration showed disease in the para-aortic and mesenteric lymph nodes (p. 142). Among the 364 patients with non-Hodgkin's lymphoma, 1 patient (No. 20894) had en-bloc resection of a retroperitoneal mass with attached left kidney, spleen, and tail of the pancreas (p. 247). The surgical specimen showed the excision was apparently adequate and three-fourths of the kidney was replaced by lymphosarcoma. The patient developed lesions in the lung and bone 5 months later and died 26 months after the operation. Testicular masses as the clinical presentation were seen in 5 patients with non-Hodgkin's disease, and one (No. 23207) had a bilateral orchiectomy before the nature of the disease was known (p. 153).

One patient (No. 37422) had an exploration for hydronephrosis and lower extremity edema 40 months after having had radiotherapy to the peria-ortic nodes and pelvis for Hodgkin's disease. Tissue biopsy showed only retroperitoneal fibrosis (p. 346). We listed the case under "Surgery for Radiotherapy Complication" for lack of a better category. Since Ormond first described this condition in 1948, many etiological factors were suggested to explain the common pathological picture of the retroperitoneal inflammatory response. Of special interest are the difficulties encountered in establishing the correct diagnosis since retroperitoneal lymphoma might present a clinical picture similar to that of idiopathic retroperitoneal fibrosis.

Trever (1958) described a patient who underwent exploration three times for a retroperitoneal fibrosing process. At the third laparotomy, the mesenteric lymph node showed reticulum cell sarcoma. Kendall and Lakey (1961) reported a patient who had exploratory surgery for bilateral ureteral obstruction. A biopsy of a peripheral lymph node had been read as nonspecific inflammation 1 year previously. The slide was reviewed with the retroperitoneal biopsy and both were compatible with Hodgkin's disease. Longley et al (1965) reported 2 cases in which there were retroperitoneal ureteral obstructions initially. In each case, the biopsy was reported as a nonspecific inflammation with fibrosis, but later a peripheral node biopsy demonstrated lymphosarcoma. Kiely et al (1969) also reported a patient who had an exploratory laparotomy for bilateral hydroureters and hydronephrosis. The biopsy specimen showed fatty and fibrous tissue with lymphoid infiltration. Subsequently, an inguinal node biopsy showed follicular lymphoma. The diagnosis of the initial retroperitoneal biopsy was changed into lymphoma when it was reviewed.

FEMALE GENITAL ORGANS

Hellwig (1947) reported a patient with "lymphocytoma" of the uterus treated by radical surgery alone who was living and well 6 years later. In the large series of Rosenberg et al (1961), the genital tract was involved in 5 out of 470 non-Hodgkin's female patients seen clinically and in 38.8

percent autopsied. In the necropsy study of Richmond et al (1962), the female genital system was involved in nearly one-third of those with Hodgkin's disease, and in half of those with other lymphomas. Ovaries, tubes, and the uterus were positive in about equal frequencies (approximately 10 percent of the patients with Hodgkin's disease and 20 percent in other lymphomas), and the vagina was least often involved (1 percent).

In the EFSCH series, 144 of the 364 patients with non-Hodgkin's lymphomas were females. Two patients (No. 14157, No. 16694) had abdominal hysterectomies and salphingo-oophorectomy for retrouterine and tubo-ovarian masses (Table 8-1). The resections were carried out before the true nature of the disease was known, and the surgical margins showed lymphomatous infiltrations. These pointed out the necessity for abdominal and gynecological surgeons to be aware of the possibility that lymphomatous lesions can present initially as abnormalities of the pelvic organs.

Lathrop (1967) said that the frequency with which the gynecologist saw malignant lymphoma clinically as a primary or secondary disorder of the female genital tract was rare. Five such patients were seen in his department over 7 years; about 1000 were admitted each year. He studied the genital involvement, at autopsy, of 33 female patients with Hodgkin's disease and 72 with other lymphomas. Involvement of the female organs was found in 28 percent of the total group, and in 33 percent of those who did not have prior pelvic operations. Of the patients with intact reproductive systems, 42 percent of the lymphosarcoma patients and 14 percent of the women with Hodgkin's disease had demonstrable pelvic metastases. Overall, the ovaries were involved in 79 percent; uterus, 31 percent; cervix, 17 percent; vagina, 7 percent; vulva, 4 percent; and multiple genital sites, 45 percent.

Several reports have been published which emphasize the gynecological aspects of Hodgkin's disease and other malignant lymphomas (Hennessy and Rottino 1956; Johnson and Soule 1957; Hahn 1958; Weingold et al 1961). Heller and Palin reported ovarian involvement in Hodgkin's disease in 1946. Bare and McCloskey (1961), and Long and Patchefsky (1971) found primary Hodgkin's disease of the ovaries in specimens from total hysterectomies and bilateral salphingo-oophorectomies for cystic ovarian masses. Hodgkin's disease primarily limited to the uterine cervix has been reported by Retikas (1960), Nasiell (1964), and Anderson (1967). Nasiell's case was interesting because the initial diagnosis was suggested by cervical smears. The patient was treated with radium, followed by a total abdominal hysterectomy and salphingo-oophorectomy. The patient reported by Anderson was operated upon for uterine myoma, and a diagnosis of Hodgkin's disease was made on the hysterectomy specimen. Knobel (1971) added a fourth patient who was treated with a total abdominal hysterectomy and bilateral oophorectomy with simultaneous exploration of the upper abdomen, splenectomy, liver and para-aortic lymph node biopsy. All the surgical specimens showed the disease was confined only to the cervix.

Table 8-1
Exploration and Other Resections for Non-Hodgkin's Lymphoma (EFSCH series)

| Patient No. | Age | Sex | Date | Indication | Operation | Pathology | | | Postoperative | | Survival (months) | Lymphoma at follow-up |
						Diagnosis	Margin	Nodes (positive/total)	Radiotherapy (rads)	Chemotherapy		
14157	47	F	8-50	Rectal and uterine mass	Hysterectomy and oophorectomy	LWD	+	—	2000	—	5	+
16694	57	F	8-51	L-tuboovarian mass	Hysterectomy and oophorectomy	LPD	+	—	2500	—	12	+
20894	17	F	2-54	Anemia, flank pain, fever, splenomegaly	En-bloc resection of retroperitoneal mass, kidney, spleen, tail of pancreas	UC	—	—	1500	+	26	+
38435	65	F	9-69	Anemia, spleno-hapatomegaly	Splenectomy liver biopsy	LPD	—	0/3	1500	+	2	+ (septicemia)

Non-Hodgkin's lymphoma of the uterus was reported by Walton (1953), Johnson and Soule (1957), Welch and Hellwig (1963), and Vieaux and McGuire (1964). Buckingham and McClure (1955) reported reticulum cell sarcoma of the vulva, and McElin and Wagner (1971) reported a case of possible primary malignant lymphoma of the vagina.

Lathrop (1967) reviewed 14 patients thought to have unicentric pelvic lymphomas reported since 1937 in the American literature and added 2 cases of his own. One patient had a Wertheim hysterectomy and bilateral pelvic node dissection for reticulum cell sarcoma of the cervix. It is interesting to note that cytological examination was done in 7 cases and was positive for tumor cells in 4. Among the 11 patients who had surgical treatment, he said it was probably curative in 2, possibly curative in 3, and of no value in 6. He suggested that unicentric pelvic lymphoma should be treated initially with surgical excision followed by full pelvic irradiation.

PREGNANCY AND MALIGNANT LYMPHOMA

There are many publications discussing the problem of pregnancy in Hodgkin's disease. In 1950 Bichel reported that 73 of their 81 women with Hodgkin's disease were between the age of 16 and 45 years and 11 of them became pregnant. He also reviewed the details of 46 women with typical Hodgkin's disease complicated by pregnancy reported in the literature. Only one case was recorded in which the mother died during the seventh month of pregnancy after receiving "spray radiation" to the whole body. His final comment was that "from an obstetric point of view, the pregnancy, parturition, and puerperium run a normal course in the great majority of cases. The exacerbation of Hodgkin's disease is at any rate not essentially more frequent during the pregnancy than could be expected spontaneously . . . Generally, there will be no indication for interruption of pregnancy in patients with Hodgkin's disease."

Reviewing the literature on familial incidence of Hodgkin's disease, Mazar and Straus (1951) cited four mother–daughter pairs involving newborn infants reported before 1948. Since the characteristic histopathology of Hodgkin's disease was not clear until the publication of the monograph of Jackson and Parker (1947), the authenticity of many of the earlier cases was in doubt.

Gilbert (1951) pointed out that pregnancy occurring after radiotherapy and during the symptom-free period had no influence whatsoever on Hodgkin's disease. Even in "alarming evolutive" forms the child could often be saved, and the benefit that one hoped to attain for the mother by interrupting pregnancy usually turned out to be a vain hope. Hultberg (1954) reemphasized there was no reason to interrupt pregnancy, except in the exceptional cases where the disease was localized in the inguinal or pelvic regions requiring radiotherapy or in patients who had received nitrogen mustard or radiomimetic drugs. Lactation may be permitted if the patient is in good condition and does not require radiotherapy.

Gellhorn (1955) was rather pessimistic when he said that "since the mean life expectancy of a patient with Hodgkin's disease is about 3 years, it is apparent that, even if pregnancy does not accelerate the course of Hodgkin's disease, the child born has a very high likelihood of losing his mother early in his life. Unless there are some very compelling reasons to the contrary, the known sociologic problems of a motherless child suggest that interruption of an early pregnancy should be seriously considered."

Southam et al (1956) studied 59 patients who had 83 pregnancies concurrent with Hodgkin's disease. The mean survival time of 26 patients in whom the onset of Hodgkin's disease occurred during pregnancy was significantly shorter (46 months) than in 33 patients (91 months) in whom onset of the disease occurred before conception. Prognosis for long survival was best if Hodgkin's disease was inactive for at least 9 months prior to conception. They pointed out that spontaneous abortions occurred in Hodgkin's disease only in those patients having active disease before and during pregnancy and more frequently in patients with intraabdominal or disseminated disease, or both.

Peters and Middlemiss (1958) reported a large series of 291 patients with Hodgkin's disease including 13 cases complicated by pregnancy either at the onset of the disease or following the initial control of the disease (3 patients had both). The 8 patients who were pregnant when the disease was first noted responded to treatment somewhat better than expected: one patient lived 25 years and died of an extraneous disease. They found that pregnancy, subsequent to the control of the disease, did not alter the expected survival according to the stage on admission. Peters et al (1966) even commented that "The slightly superior survival rates of Hodgkin's disease in females could be attributed to the large proportion of females in stage IIA who had pregnancies subsequent to the initial control of the disease. But further study is required in this area before any conclusions may be drawn."

Smith et al (1958) reported pregnancy occurred in 18 of their 56 Hodgkin's patients (an overall incidence of 33 percent). In addition, they reviewed 40 publications and compiled the experiences of 603 females with Hodgkin's disease, 18 percent of whom had pregnancies. The onset of Hodgkin's disease during pregnancy was not found to be incompatible with long survival. Pregnancy had no deleterious effects on Hodgkin's disease or vice versa, and therapeutic abortion was not indicated. They analyzed the data of 56 patients who received irradiation during pregnancy and showed that treatment of lesions away from the uterus produced no apparent harmful effect on the fetus. They also summarized the experiences of 21 patients who received cytotoxic agents during pregnancy and found that conventional doses could be tolerated at least during the last two trimesters. However, the use of chemotherapy in the first trimester should be avoided. The cytotoxic agents used included nitrogen mustard, trimethylene melamine, mercaptopurine, ^{32}P, myleren, and urethen.

Barry et al (1962) reexamined their data from 1910 to 1959 and revised some of the conclusions reported by Southam et al (1956). A total of 347 patients with Hodgkin's disease were between the ages of 18 and 40; of these, 84 had pregnancy recorded. (The pregnancy status of 35 patients was unknown.) They found that the survival curves of these 84 patients were more favorable than the 228 nonpregnant control patients (median survival 9 months versus 52 months, Fig. 8-1). Even the onset of Hodgkin's disease during pregnancy or following a recent pregnancy did not affect survival adversely (median survival was 64 months versus 59 months for the total 347 patients). The incidence of exacerbation during a 9-month pregnancy plus a 3-month postpartum was not greater than that which would be expected during a comparable 12-month period in a group of nonpregnant women. They did point out, though, that active disease during the first and second years after diagnosis carried a grave prognosis. Thus, they recommended that women wanting to become pregnant be urged to wait until they had quiescence of Hodgkin's disease for at least 2 years. Hennessy and Rottino (1963) confirmed these findings and pointed out that in no instance did Hodgkin's disease per se lead to difficult labor.

Lützenberger and Brandenburg (1966) reviewed the world literature since the first publication in 1925 and said there were 548 women with Hodgkin's disease with a total of 693 pregnancies reported. Poliwoda et al (1967) analyzed 378 patients collected from 75 papers in the literature who had the disease during pregnancy. They found that patients with Hodgkin's disease prior to pregnancy had a more prolonged survival, and that the survival of patients who had first symptoms of the disease during or shortly after pregnancy was the same as the nonpregnant control sample.

Crépin et al (1969) reported 9 Hodgkin's cases associated with 15 pregnancies. They found the evolutive character of the disease was not noticeably changed by its association with pregnancy, nor were the pregnancy and delivery disturbed by the disease. Lactation did not aggravate the disease and involved no risk for the child, but it led to increased fatigue which might have been harmful to the mother. Phelan (1969) also felt that breast feeding by mothers with malignant conditions was not advisable.

With the development of newer chemotherapeutic agents several reports concerning their use during pregnancy have appeared. Armstrong et al (1964), Lacher (1964), Rosenzweig et al (1964) and Goguel et al (1969), reported no obvious deleterious effects on off-spring whose mothers received vinblastine during pregnancy even during the first trimester. The mothers treated by Armstrong and Rosenzweig et al also had vinblastine prior to and throughout pregnancy. Lacher and Geller (1966) reported a patient who received

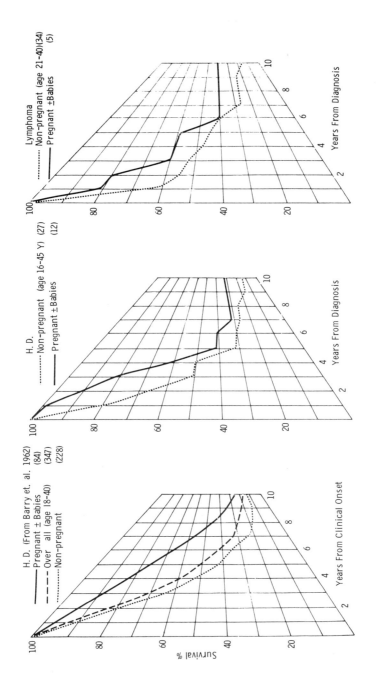

Fig. 8-1. Survival curves of patients who had associated pregnancy with or without child birth versus those who had no pregnancy. (a) adapted from Barry et al (1962), with permission from the author and the publisher; (b) 39 patients with Hodgkin's disease (EFSCH series); (c) 39 patients with other lymphomas (EFSCH series).

both vinblastine and cyclophosphamide from the second trimester on; a normal baby was delivered by caesarian section at term. Procarbazine administered to a patient with Hodgkin's disease during the first trimester of her pregnancy resulted in no adverse effect on the infant (Wells et al 1968). Coopland et al (1969) found that high doses of antileukemic agents (prednisone, methotraxate, and vincristine) were used safely in the second and third trimesters of pregnancy. However, Greenberg and Tanaka (1964) and Toledo et al (1971) reported two cases of multiple fetal anomalies, especially of the fingers and toes, when the mothers received cyclophosphamide during the first trimester of pregnancy. Thus the advice of Lacher and Geller (1966) seems sound: "Because of the meager experience with chemotherapeutic agents during pregnancy . . . it is desirable to avoid treatment in all trimesters in all cases whenever possible."

Kaplan (1972) discussed his current therapeutic approach to patients who had Hodgkin's disease diagnosed during pregnancy. When the disease was localized, histologically favorable and the pregnancy was at or beyond the seventh month, he said it was probably best simply to observe the patient, deferring both the diagnostic evaluation and the treatment until after delivery. In cases with accelerated conditions, induction of labor or caesarian section was indicated. When the diagnosis of Hodgkin's disease is made during the first half of the pregnancy, his policy is to recommend therapeutic abortion followed by diagnostic evaluation of the extent of the disease and the initiation of appropriate treatment. As mentioned elsewhere (p. 98), the treatment of choice for patients with stage I to III Hodgkin's disease, as defined by Kaplan, was megavoltage radiotherapy to all of the lymph node areas.

Craver (1964) emphasized that the "treatment of Hodgkin's disease during pregnancy, or vice versa, is a matter for individualization and calls for close cooperation between therapist and obstetrician. If pregnancy must be allowed to go on, the family may be assured that there is little reason statistically to fear the development of Hodgkin's disease in the offspring." Absolute assurance of this last point would not be possible, since Razis et al (1959) reviewed 1102 cases of Hodgkin's disease and calculated that the probability for the immediate relatives of a Hodgkin's disease patient to develop the same diseasee was about three times as great as that of the general population.

Reported cases of the mother's malignant condition involving the fetus or gestational product are extremely rare. Boronow (1964) surveyed this problem, finding 24 documented cases reported in the literature where the placenta or fetus was involved with a tumor. Melanoma and Hodgkin's disease made up the majority of such cases. Stephenson et al (1971) reported the seventh known case of a malignant melanoma "metastasizing" from the mother to the placenta, and the fourth instance in which melanoma cells invaded placenta villi. They carried out an exchange transfusion, in which the son's blood was given to the mother, with the hope of passively transferring immunologic factors to reject the mother's tumor. The mother died but the son was well 2 years later. Stephenson (1972) also found in the literature one case of lymphosarcoma involving the fetus.

The problem of pregnancy occurring in a patient with non-Hodgkin's lymphoma is not too great, since most patients with other lymphomas are older and their prognoses in general are not as good as those with Hodgkin's disease. The median age in the EFSCH series of 364 non-Hodgkin's patients was 62 years, versus 40 years for those with Hodgkin's disease. Palen (1950) reported the first case of retroperitonal lymphosarcoma complicating pregnancy. Henderson and Paterson (1968) said that only 9 cases of reticulum cell sarcoma occurring prior to or during pregnancy were found in the literature. They added a patient who had perforation of the jejunum during pregnancy. Di Re et al (1969) reported 18 patients who had malignant lymphomas associated with pregnancy (8 had non-Hodgkin's lymphomas). Four patients without retroperitoneal adenopathies were treated prophylactically with endolymphatic radiotherapy and became pregnant afterwards. All babies were normal. Two patients treated during the first 4 months with antiproliferative agents (chlorambucil, vinblastine) delivered normal infants, while a third patient treated during the third month of pregnancy had a miscarriage. They pointed out the importance of using diagnostic lymphangiogram to define the stage of disease and to plan appropriate therapy. When disease of the lymph node and/or viscera was found below the diaphragm during the first trimester, they felt therapeutic abortion was indicated.

There was one pregnant patient among the series of 52 cases of reticulum cell sarcomas of the bone reported by Miller and Nicholson (1971). All the patients received bacterial toxin alone or as part of the therapy. They found that patients who had such adjuvant therapy had a 50 percent better survival rate than those who were treated by surgery or radiotherapy alone. In this particular patient, who had generalized bone symptoms during the eighth month of her twin pregnancy, there was fever before and after blood transfusions. In addition to radiotherapy, she also received a hormone supplement for menopausal symptoms. The patient was in good health 29 years after diagnosis, and the authors commented, "the possible effect of the pregnancy and confinement must also be considered."

The experience at EFSCH with pregnancy and lymphoma was similar to that of Barry et al (1961)(Fig. 8-1). Among 163 patients with Hodgkin's disease, 64 were females, and 39 were between the ages of 16 and 45. Of these 39, 3 had the onset of Hodgkin's disease during pregnancy, 4 had pregnancies over 1 year after the diagnosis, and 5 had both. The survival curves of these 12 patients were not any worse than those of the 27 patients without pregnancies. Among the 364 patients with non-Hodgkin's lymphomas, 144 were females. Thirty-nine belonged to the age group of 21 to 40, 4 had the onset of disease during pregnancy, and 1 had subsequent pregnancies. As with patients having Hodgkin's disease, pregnancy occurring either at the onset of symptoms or after diagnosis does not seem to adversely affect survival.

One Hodgkin's patient (p. 387) noted upper neck adenopathy during the last trimester. One month after the diagnosis was made, she underwent a planned caesarian section. Her obstetrician was not familiar with the literature on staging laparotomy for lymphomas; consequently her upper abdomen was not explored. Since recent advances in radiotherapy have achieved a substantial cure rate and improved the already good prognosis of young female patients, more patients might have pregnancies during follow-up. And since exploratory laparotomies and oophoropexis have shown to be valuable as part of the pretreatment staging procedures, it is conceivable that obstetricians and general surgeons could cooperate and perform necessary tissue biopsies during planned caesarian sections and thus avoid a second major operation for selected patients.

SUMMARY

The spleen and liver are eventually involved in more than 50 percent of the patients with malignant lymphoma. About 1 percent of the patients with non-Hodgkin's lymphomas had localized splenic tumors, and Das Gupta et al (1965) had specified 4 criteria for diagnosis of primary lymphoma of the spleen. Up to 1965, over 210 cases of primary splenic tumors were reported; one-fourth of the lesions were lymphomas (non-Hodgkin's). Primary lymphoma of the spleen, presenting as splenomegaly and hypersplenism, required splenectomy both for diagnosis and treatment. Primary hepatic lymphoma is very, very rare; possibly 3 cases of Hodgkin's disease and 4 of non-Hodgkin's lymphoma have been reported in the literature.

Initially, patients with malignant lymphoma might have clinical evidence of urinary system involvement in about 10 percent of the cases; and eventually, in about 60 percent. In the autopsy series, the kidney was involved in 13 percent of those with Hodgkin's disease and in nearly 50 percent of those with non-Hodgkin's lymphomas. The bladder was the second most commonly involved organ (in 5 percent and 15 percent respectively). Microscopic infiltration of the bladder was 7 times more common than gross lesions.

Primary lymphoma of the kidney is very rare. However, retroperitoneal lymphoma might present as kidney tumors or idiopathic retroperitoneal fibrosis. Over 40 cases of primary malignant lymphoma of the urinary bladder have been reported in the literature. Malignant lymphoma of the testes has been reported in more than 120 patients. It is probably the initial presentation of a systemic disease, and accounted for less than 5 percent of all testicular cancers. Bilateral involvement is frequent and it is the most common type of testicular malignancy after age 60. In early lesions, orchiectomy and radiotherapy can achieve a 5-year survival rate of 30 percent.

Female genital organs may be the initial sites of involvement in about 1 percent of the patients with malignant lymphomas. Autopsy studies showed that the female genital tract might have Hodgkin's disease in nearly one-third of the patients, and non-Hodgkin's lymphoma in half of the patients. The most common sites are the ovaries and the uterus. Several cases of primary lymphomas of these organs have been reported, and the treatment of choice in unicentric lesions is surgical excision followed by pelvic irradiation.

About one-fourth of the Hodgkin's patients of child-bearing age do become pregnant. Pregnancy occurring either at the onset of symptoms or after the diagnosis had no deleterious effect on the natural history of Hodgkin's disease. The treatment of malignant lymphoma during pregnancy, or vice versa, should be individualized. Therapeutic abortion may be suggested when the pregnancy is early and/or when the progression of the disease is accelerated. The survival curves of patients who had pregnancies are not any worse than those who did not become pregnant.

REFERENCES

Ahmann DL, Kiely JM, Harrison EG Jr, et al: Malignant lymphoma of the spleen: A review of 49 cases in which the diagnosis was made at splenectomy. Cancer 19: 461–469, 1966

Anderson GG: Hodgkin's disease of the uterine cervix: Report of a case. Obstet Gynecol 29:170–172, 1967

Armstrong JG, Dyke RW, Fouts PJ, et al: Delivery of a normal infant during the course of oral vinblastine sulfate therapy for Hodgkin's disease. Ann Intern Med 61:106–107, 1964

Baker C, Mann WN: Hodgkin's disease: Study of 65 cases. Guys Hosp Rep 89: 83–107, 1939

Bare W, McCloskey JF: Primary Hodgkin's disease of the ovary: Report of a case. Obstet Gynecol 17:477–485, 1961

Barry RM, Diamond HD, Craver LF: Influence of pregnancy on the course of Hodgkin's disease. Am J Obstet Gynecol 84:445–454, 1962

Bennett JS, Bond J, Singer I, et al: Hypouricemia in Hodgkin's disease. Ann Intern Med 76:751–756, 1972

Bhansali SK, Cameron KM: Primary malignant lymphoma of the bladder. Br J Urol 32:440–454, 1960

Bichel J: Hodgkin's disease and pregnancy. Acta Radiol [Ther] (Stockh) 33:427–434, 1950

Bichel J, Jensen KB: Nephrotic syndrome and Hodgkin's disease. Lancet 2:1425–1426, 1971

Blatt E, Page IH: Hypertension and constriction of renal arteries in man: Report of case. Ann Intern Med 12:1690–1699, 1939

Boronow RC: Extrapelvic malignancy and pregnancy. Obstet Gynecol Surv 19:1–29, 1964

Braun E, Manley C, Liao K, et al: Intrinsic Hodgkin's disease of the ureter. J Urol 107:952–954, 1972

Buckingham JC, McClure JH: Recticulum cell sarcoma of vulva: Report of case. Obstet Gynecol 6:138–143, 1955

Chaffey WC: Lymphosarcoma of the bladder (cord specimen). Trans Pathol Soc Lond 36:285, 1885

Cohen BB, Kaplan G, Liber AF, et al: Reticulum-cell sarcoma with primary manifestations in the testis. Cancer 8: 136–142, 1955

Coopland AT, Friesen WJ, Galbraith PA: Acute leukemia in pregnancy. Am J Obstet Gynecol 105:1288–1289, 1969

Craver LF: Hodgkin's disease, in Tice F (ed): Practice of Medicine, vol 6. Hagerstown, Md, Harper & Row, 1969, pp 1017–1063

Craver LF: Treatment of Hodgkin's disease, in Pack GT, Ariel IM (eds): Treatment of Cancer and Allied Diseases (ed 2). New York, Hoeber, 1964, pp 168–191

Crépin G, Gardez C, Demaille A: L'association maladie de Hodgkin et grossesse (a propos de 9 observations de maladie de Hodgkin associee a l'evolution de 15 grossesses). Rev Fr Gynecol Obstet 64:235–249, 1969

Das Gupta T, Coombes B, Brasfield RD: Primary malignant neoplasms of the spleen. Surg Gynecol Obstet 120:947–960, 1965

Di Re F, Fossati Bellani F, Monfardini S: Diagnosi e terapia dei linfomi maligni durante la graviaza. Tumori 55:1–8, 1969

Edmondson HA: Tumors of the liver and intrahepatic bile ducts. Atlas of Tumor Pathology, Section VII, Fassicle 25. Armed Forces Institute of Pathology, 1958

Gall EA, Mallory TB: Malignant lymphoma: Clinico-pathologic survey of 618 cases. Am J Pathol 18:381–429, 1942

Gellhorn A: Management of the patient with Hodgkin's disease. J Chron Dis 1:698–705, 1955

Gerundo M, Miller MB: Reticulum-cell sarcoma of spleen. Am J Cancer 35:528–533, 1939

Gilbert R: The problem of pregnancy in Hodgkin's disease. Acta Radiol [Ther] (Stockh) 35:71–75, 1951

Givler RL: Involvement of the bladder in leukemia and lymphoma. J Urol 105:667–670, 1971

Goguel A, Helpt-Eppinger M, Teillet F, et al: Maladie de Hodgkin et grossesese. Nouv Rev Fr Hematol 9:581–600, 1969

Gordon JD, Paley DH: Primary malignant tumors of the spleen. Surgery 29:907–913, 1951

Greenberg LH, Tanaka KR: Congenital anomalies probably induced by cyclophosphamide. JAMA 188:423–426, 1964

Hahn GA: Gynecologic considerations in malignant lymphomas. Am J Obstet Gynecol 75:673–683, 1958

Hamlin JA, Kagan AR, Friedman NB: Lymphomas of the testicle. Cancer 29:1352–1356, 1972

Hansen HE, Skov PE, Askjaer SA, et al: Hodgkin's disease associated with the nephrotic syndrome without kidney lesion. Acta Med Scand 191:307–313, 1972

Hausman PF, Gaarde FW: Malignant neoplasms of the spleen. Surgery 14:246–255, 1943

Heller EL, Palin W: Ovarian involvement in Hodgkin's disease. Arch Pathol 41:282–289, 1946

Hellwig CA: Malignant lymphoma: Value of radical surgery in selected cases. Surg Gynecol Obstet 84:950–958, 1947

Henderson M, Paterson WG: Perforation of jejunum by reticulum cell sarcoma in pregnancy. Am J Surg 115:385–389, 1968

Hennessy JP, Rottino A: Hodgkin's disease as it affects physiology and anatomy of female generative tract. Am J Obstet Gynecol 72:153–159, 1956

Hennessy JP, Rottino A: Hodgkin's disease in pregnancy. Am J Obstet Gynecol 87:851–853, 1963

Hermann RE, DeHaven KE, Hawk WA: Splenectomy for the diagnosis of splenomegaly. Arch Surg 168:896–900, 1968

Hickling RA: Giant follicle lymphoma of the spleen. A condition closely related to lymphatic leukaemia but apparently curable by splenectomy. Br Med J 2:787–790, 1964

Hirsch EF: Primary lymphosarcoma of the liver with metastases to marrow and secondary anemia. Arch Pathol 23:674–678, 1937

Hoskins EO: Unusual radiological manifestations of Hodgkin's disease. Proc R Soc Med 60:729–732, 1967

Hoster HA, Dratman MB, Craver LF, et al: Hodgkin's disease—1832–1947. Cancer Res 8:1–48, 49–78, 1948

Hultberg S: Pregnancy in Hodgkin's disease. Acta Radiol [Ther] (Stockh) 41:277–289, 1954

Hutchinson J: Lymphosarcoma of both testes with considerable interval of time. Br Med J 1:413, 1889

Hyatt DF, Skarin AT, Moloney WC, et al: Splenectomy for lymphosarcoma. Surg Gynecol Obstet 131:928–932, 1970

Jackson H Jr, Parker F Jr: Hodgkin's Disease and Allied Disorders. New York, Oxford University Press, 1947

Jackson RH, Oo M: Nephrotic syndrome with Hodgkin's disease. Lancet 2:821–822, 1971

Johnson CE, Soule EH: Malignant lymphoma as a gynecologic problem: Report of 5 cases including one primary lymphosarcoma of the cervix uteri. Obstet Gynecol 9:149–157, 1957

Johnson DE, Butler JJ, Luce JK: Histiocytic reticulum cell sarcoma presenting as a testicular tumor. J Urol 107:425–428, 1972

Kaplan HS: Hodgkin's Disease. Cambridge, Mass. Harvard University Press, 1972 pp. 268–269

Kendall AR, Lakey WH: Sclerosing Hodgkin's disease vs idiopathic retroperitoneal fibrosis. J Urol 86:217–221, 1961

Kiely JM, Wagoner RD, Holley KE: Renal complications of lymphoma. Ann Intern Med 71:1159–1175, 1969

Kiely JM, Massey BD Jr, Harrison EG, et al: Lymphoma of the testis. Cancer 26:847–852, 1970

Knobel J, Gage NC: Hodgkin's disease of the uterine cervix. S Afr J Obstet Gynaecol 9:70–72, 1971

Knoepp LF: Lymphosarcoma of the kidney. Surgery 39:510–514, 1956

Lacher M: Use of vinblastine sulfate to treat Hodgkin's disease during pregnancy. Ann Intern Med 61:113–115, 1964

Lacher MJ, Geller W: Cyclophosphamide and vinblastine sulfate in Hodgkin's disease during pregnancy. JAMA 195:486–488, 1966

Lathrop JC: Malignant pelvic lymphomas. Obstet Gynecol 30:137–145, 1967

Levitan R, Diamond HD, Craver LF: Esophageal varices in Hodgkin's disease involving the liver. Am J Med 27:137–143, 1959

Levitan R, Diamond HD, Craver LF: The liver in Hodgkin's disease. Gut 2:60–71, 1961

Loehry CA: Hodgkin's disease limited to the liver. Br Med J 2:1594, 1964

Long JP, Patchefsky AS: Primary Hodgkin's disease of the ovary: A case report. Obstet Gynecol 38:680–682, 1971

Longley JR, Bush J, Brunsting OD: Occult neoplasm causing syndrome of retroperitoneal fibrosis. Calif Med 103:279–282, 1965

Loughridge LW, Lewis MG: Nephrotic syndrome in malignant disease of nonrenal origin. Lancet 1:256–258, 1971

Lowry WS, Munzenrider JE, Lynch GA: Nephrotic syndrome in Hodgkin's disease. Lancet 1:1127, 1971

Luce JK, Frei E III: Lymphomas, in Mengel CE, Frei E III, Nachman R (eds): Hematology: Principles and Practice. Chicago, Year Book, 1972, pp 445–489

Lumb G: Tumours of Lymphoid Tissue. Edinburgh & London, Livingston, 1954

Lützenberger P, Bradenburg J: Lymphogranulomatose und Schwangerschaft. Zentralbl Gynaekol 88:1355–1361, 1966

MacLeod M, Stalker AL: Diagnosis of Hodgkin's disease by liver biopsy. Br Med J 1:1449–1451, 1962

McElin TW, Wagner AL Jr: Primary malignant vaginal lymphoma: Case report. Am J Obstet Gynecol 110:883–885, 1971

Mazar SA, Straus B: Marital Hodgkin's disease. Arch Intern Med 88:819–830, 1951

Miller TR, Nicholson JT: End results in reticulum cell sarcoma of bone treated by bacterial toxin therapy alone or combined with surgery and/or radiotherapy (47 cases) or with concurrent infection (5 cases). Cancer 27:524–548, 1971

Molander DW, Pack GT: Lymphosarcoma: Choice of treatment and end-results in 567 patients. Role of surgical treatment for cure and palliation. Rev Surg 20:3–31, 1963

Molander DW, Pack GT: Management and survival of 883 patients with malignant lymphoma. Am J Roentgenol Radium Ther Nucl Med 93:154–159, 1965

Nasiell M: Hodgkin's disease limited to the uterine cervix. Acta Cytol 8:16–18, 1964

Ormond JK: Bilateral ureteral obstruction due to envelopment and compression by an inflammatory retroperitoneal process. J Urol 59:1072–1079, 1948

Pack GT, Molander DW: The surgical treatment of Hodgkin's disease. Cancer Res 26:1254–1263, 1966

Palen GM: Retroperitoneal lymphosarcoma complicating pregnancy. J Int Coll Surgeons 13:376–382, 1950

Peters MV, Alison RE, Bush RS: Natural history of Hodgkin's disease as related to staging. Cancer 19:308–316, 1966

Peters MV, Middlemiss KC: A study of Hodgkin's disease treated by irradiation. Am J Roentgenol Radium Ther Nucl Med 79:114–121, 1958

Phelan JT: Cancer and pregnancy. CA 19: 85–93, 1969

Pick RA, Castellino RA, Seltzer RA: Arteriographic findings in renal lymphoma. Am J Roentgenol Radium Ther Nucl Med 111:530–534, 1971

Plager J, Stutzman L: Acute nephrotic syndrome as a manifestation of active Hodgkin's disease. Am J Med 50:56–66, 1971

Poliwoda H, Stolte H, Voth H, et al: Hodgkin's disease and pregnancy. Arch Klin Med 213:255–277, 1967

Rappaport H, Winter WJ, Hicks EB: Follicular lymphoma: A re-evaluation of its position in the scheme of malignant lymphoma, based on a survey of 253 cases. Cancer 9:792–821, 1956

Razis DV, Diamond HD, Craver LF: Familial Hodgkin's disease: Its significance and implications. Ann Intern Med 51:933–971, 1959

Retikas DG: Hodgkin's sarcoma of the cervix: Report of a case. Am J Obstet Gynecol 80:1104–1107, 1960

Reymond R, Hazra T, Lott S, et al: Primary malignant lymphoma of the bladder: A case report. J Can Assoc Radiol 22: 170–172, 1971

Richmond J, Sherman RS, Diamond HD, et al: Renal lesions associated with malignant lymphomas. Am J Med 32:184–207, 1962

Rosenberg SA, Diamond HD, Jaslowitz B, et al: Lymphosarcoma: A review of 1269 cases. Medicine 40:31–84, 1961

Rosenzweig AI, Crews QE Jr, Hopwood HG: Vinblastine sulfate in Hodgkin's disease in pregnancy. Ann Intern Med 61: 108–112, 1964

Sahebjami H: Hodgkin's disease and hepatoma. South Med J 64:117–118, 1971

Skarin AT, Davey FR, Moloney WC: Lymphosarcoma of the spleen: Results of diagnostic splenectomy in 11 patients. Arch Intern Med 127:259–265, 1971

Smith CE, Rusk GY: Endothelioma of the spleen: A study of two cases, with review of the literature of primary malignancy of the spleen. Arch Surg 7:371–414, 1923

Smith RB, Sheehy TW, Rothberg H: Hodgkin's disease and pregnancy: Case reports and a discussion of the treatment of Hodgkin's disease and leukemia during pregnancy. Arch Intern Med 102:777–789, 1958

Smythe CA, Hwang MZ: Ureteral tumor in childhood: A case report. J Urol 97: 837–839, 1967

Southam CM, Diamond HD, Craver LF: Pregnancy during Hodgkin's disease. Cancer 9:1141–1146, 1956

Sparagana M: Addison's disease due to reticulum-cell sarcoma apparently confined to the adrenals. J Am Geriatr Soc 18:550–554, 1970

Steele TH, Presant CA, Serpick AA: A reversible concentrating defect in predominantly unilateral renal Hodgkin's disease. Am J Med 48:375–381, 1970

Stephenson HE: Malignant melanoma metastatic to the products of maternal gestation. Presented at the annual meeting of the Missouri Academy of Science, Oncology Section, Columbia, April 28, 1972

Stephenson HE Jr, Terry CW, Lukens JN, et al: Immunologic factors in human melanoma "metastatic" to products of gestation (with exchange transfusion of infant to mother). Surgery 69:515–522, 1971

Symmers D: Clinical significance of deeper anatomic changes in lymphoid diseases. Arch Intern Med 74:163–171, 1944

Toledo TM, Harper RC, Moser RH: Fetal effects during cyclophosphamide and irradiation therapy. Ann Intern Med 74:87–91, 1971

Torres A, Bollozos GD: Primary reticulum cell sarcoma of liver. Cancer 27:1489–1492, 1971

Tremann JA, Norris HT, McRoberts JW: Lymphoproliferative disease of the bladder. J Urol 106:687–691, 1971

Trever RW: Reticulum-cell sarcoma producing retroperitoneal and periureteric fibrosis: Report of a case. N Engl J Med 258–268, 1958

Varney DC: Lymphosarcoma of testis. J Urol 73:1081–1088, 1955

Vieaux JW, McGuire DE: Reticulum cell sarcoma of the cervix. Am J Obstet Gynecol
89:134–135, 1964
Walton LL: Lymphosarcoma of uterus: Report of two cases. Conn Med J 17:819–
821, 1953
Wang CC, Scully RE, Leadbetter WF: Primary malignant lymphoma of the urinary
bladder. Cancer 24:772–776, 1969
Watson EM, Sauer HR, Sadugor MG: Manifestations of lymphoblastomas in the
genito-urinary tract. J Urol 61:626–645,
1949
Weingold AB, Stone ML, Parente JT:
Gynecologic aspects of malignant lymphoma. Obstet Gynecol 18:461–467, 1961
Welch JW, Hellwig CA: Reticulum cell sar-

coma of the uterine cervix: Report of a
case. Obstet Gynecol 22:293–294, 1963
Wells JH, Marshall JR, Carbone PP: Procarbazine therapy for Hodgkin's disease
in early pregnancy. JAMA 205:935–937,
1968
Werf-Messing, B van der: Reticulum cell sarcoma and lymphosarcoma: A retrospective study of potential survival in locoregional disease. Eur J Cancer 4:549–557,
1968
Willis RA: Pathology of tumours (ed 2).
London, Butterworth, 1953
Winawer SJ, Feldman SM: Amyloid nephrosis
in Hodgkin's disease: Presentation of a
case and review of the literature. Arch
Intern Med 104:793–796, 1959

9
Head, Neck, and Chest Lymphomas

HEAD AND NECK

Incidence and Diagnosis

The actual frequency of primary or secondary malignant lymphomas of the head and neck area, excluding cervical adenopathy, is difficult to assess. In the report of Sugarbaker and Craver (1940), 22.5 percent of 196 patients had apparent extranodal non-Hodgkin's lymphoma of the head and neck structures. Over half of these (14 percent) involved the tonsils. In a large series of 1269 cases of non-Hodgkin's disease, Rosenberg et al (1961) found that 8.7 percent of the lesions were present in the head and neck first. In many instances the disease apparently originated in these sites. They also showed that the most common extranodal primary focus in such cases is in the Waldeyer's ring. Molander and Pack (1963) also reported that primary lymphosarcomas of the head and neck region occurred in 6 percent of the patients, and secondary involvement of these structures occurred in 20 percent.

In a series of 1467 patients reported to have localized extranodal non-Hodgkin's lymphomas, Freeman et al (1972) reported that lesions in the head and neck region accounted for 28 percent. (Details of specific sites of involvement are given on p. 170.) In 249 patients with lymphomas involving the head and neck region reported by Catlin (1966), the histopathological distribution was as follows: reticulum cell sarcoma, 48 percent; lymphosarcoma, 30 percent; and Hodgkin's disease, 22 percent. Other than cervical adenopathy (107 patients, 43 percent), the most common site was the Waldeyer's ring (70 patients, 28 percent), which included the tonsil

(39 patients), nasopharynx (17 patients), base of the tongue (9 patients), and palate (5 patients). Eighteen patients had involvement of the thyroid gland and 16, the parotid gland. Other sites were the maxillary antrum (11 patients); submaxillary gland, nasal cavity, and orbit (5 patients each); skin of the head (4 patients); extrinsic larynx (3 patients); ethmoid sinus (2 patients); mandible (2 patients); and pharynx (1 patient). He reported a total of 101 definitive operations performed on 91 patients. The four most common operations were neck dissection (49), parotidectomy (15), node excision (14), and thyroidectomy (7). In addition, 6 partial resections of the maxilla were done for lymphomas of the nasal cavity, paranasal sinuses, and orbit. Seven posterior mouth lymphomas of the tonsil, tongue, palate, and pharynx were resected.

In a series of 95 patients with reticulum cell sarcomas reported by Newall et al (1968), 69 patients presented with extranodal disease. Eight patients had lesions of the head and neck region: antrum (3); tonsil (2); and 1 each in the pharynx, tongue, and nasal cavity. They specifically excluded patients with primary tumors of the nasopharynx since some pathologists called lymphomas of this area "lymphoepithelioma." They found that malignant lymphoma in the head and neck area behaved more like a primary carcinoma in that metastasis progressed along lymphatic drainage areas. Such tumors are highly curable but require large doses of radiotherapy, ranging from 5000 to 6500 rads in 25 to 35 days (Newall and Friedman 1970).

The symptoms which accompany head and neck lymphomas are primarily the result of the presence of tumor masses. About 50 percent of the patients with facial and lingual lymphomas were seen with advanced bulky lesions; and most patients complained of throat irritation, soreness or foreign body association. A few patients experienced dysphagia and dyspnea. Patients with nasopharyngeal lymphomas complained of hearing loss, with or without otitis media, and nasal obstruction (Wang 1970). Occasionally, the tumor may invade the nasal cavity, paranasal sinuses, orbit, and cranial nerves (Lascelles and Burston 1962).

Nobler (1969) emphasized that malignant lesions of the head region could present as mental nerve palsy secondary to direct pressure of the tumor mass on either the inferior dental or mental nerves. The syndrome is manifested primarily by numbness and/or anesthesia of the skin and mucous membranes of the lower lip and chin extending to the midline; secondarily by painless ulceration present in the same region. Of the 8 cases reported by Nobler, 1 was Hodgkin's disease and 1 was lymphosarcoma. Both patients had isolated mental nerve palsy without other abnormal physical findings. Robbins (1971) presented 7 cases of malignant lymphomas with involvement of the buccinator node. (This node is present in less than 20 percent of all individuals.) In 3 patients this particular facial adenopathy was the sole manifestation of the disease. May and Lucente (1972) pointed out that Hodgkin's disease affecting facial nerves could be misdiagnosed as Bell's palsy.

Elias and Mittelman (1971) reported a series of 150 patients with non-Hodgkin's lymphomas who had major surgical procedures; 25 had unusual head and neck manifestations. Only 10 patients had palpable cervical nodes, and none had distant adenopathy or masses at the time of diagnosis. Many lesions grossly simulated carcinomas. They had indurated and everted edges around necrotic centers and regional invasion. This misdiagnosis occurred especially often for masses in the tonsil, thyroid, parotid, and submaxillary salivary glands. Even the pathologist may have difficulty in making a correct tissue diagnosis. Thus, they emphasized that the histological diagnosis of anaplastic carcinoma, if made in an ulcerating lesion in the oropharynx, should be questioned and all efforts exerted to rule out the possibility of lymphoma. Similarly, reticulum cell sarcoma must be considered in the differential diagnosis when a biopsy specimen of the cervical lymph node is read as anaplastic carcinoma with unknown primary.

Larsen et al (1972) said only 4 of 379 (0.8 percent) malignant tumors of the head and neck region seen in a 10-year period (1958–1967) were malignant lymphomas; 3 cases were reticulum cell sarcomas involving the nasopharynx, tongue, and salivary gland; the fourth case was lymphosarcoma of the tongue. During the same period, 3 of the 43 cases (7 percent) of reticulum cell sarcomas diagnosed at their hospital were first observed in the head and neck region. They presented 2 patients who had radical neck dissection and excision of lesions in the tonsil and maxillary sinus because the preliminary diagnosis was undifferentiated carcinoma. Echoing the advice of Elias and Mittelman, they commented, "When the diagnosis is made from a small piece of tissue removed by punch biopsy forceps, the distinction of these two diseases may be nearly impossible for the pathologist."

Waldeyer's Ring

Waldeyer's ring includes the circular series of lymphoid tissues formed by the lingual, pharyngeal, and facial tonsils. Among 316 patients with Hodgkin's disease, Pack and Molander (1966) found that 1.9 percent had lesions presenting in the nasopharyngeal area. Among the 117 Hodgkin's disease patients who had staging exploratory laparotomies (Kadin et al 1971), one had a lesion involving the lymphoid tissue of the nasopharynx. Rosenberg et al (1961) found the nasooropharynx to be the site of initial manifestation in 7.4 percent of 1269 patients with non-Hodgkin's lymphomas. In the EFSCH series, only 1 patient of 163 with Hodgkin's disease had involvement of the tonsil initially (0.6 percent). By contrast, 4 percent of the 364 patients with non-Hodgkin's lymphomas had lesions in the tonsil and 1 percent in the nasopharynx at diagnosis.

However, other reports recorded a much higher incidence rate. Of the 343 patients with reticulum cell sarcomas and lymphosarcomas reported by Werf-Messing (1968), 50 percent of 142 patients with stage I and II disease had lesions primarily in the structures of Waldeyer's ring. The sites of disease in the 74 patients were as follows: tonsils, 44; tongue, 11; nasopharynx, 9; maxillary antrum, 6; nasal cavity, 4. Banfi et al (1970, 1972) conducted systematic biopsies of the whole Waldeyer's ring in all patients with non-Hodgkin's lymphoma, irrespective of the clinical presentation, and found involvement in 55 percent of those with reticulum cell sarcoma and 21 percent of those with lymphosarcoma. They summarized the world literature from 1935 to 1969, showing that non-Hodgkin's lymphoma constituted 1.2 percent to 43.9 percent of the malignant tumors of the nasopharynx, 2 percent to 41.6 percent of lesions of the tonsil, and 1.2 percent to 4.6 percent of the malignancies of the base of the tongue. They presented a series of 292 patients with non-Hodgkin's lymphomas of Waldeyer's ring. The distributions according to site were: tonsil, 36.9 percent; nasopharynx, 36.3 percent; base of tongue and soft palate, 5.8 percent; oropharyx, 2.1 percent; and other sites, 18.9 percent.

Clinically, in 20 percent of the patients,where the lesions were localized to the Waldeyer's ring, 44 percent had spread to contiguous nodes, 24 percent to distant nodes, and 12 percent to extranodal tissues. Many of the patients with lymphoma of the Waldeyer's ring had occult disease below the diaphragm, and lymphangiograms showed abnormal retroperitoneal lymph nodes in 38.3 percent of the cases (Banfi et al 1972). A surprising finding reported by Banfi et al (1970) was the high rate (20 percent) of lymphomatous infiltration of the stomach in patients with lymphomas of the head and neck region. This suggests the possibility that a certain number of patients could have non-Hodgkin's lymphomas arise concomitantly in Waldeyer's ring and in the gastrointestinal tract. Since the lymphomatous lesions of the stomach tend to bleed, they felt that surgical resection should be carried out if possible before further treatment and that chemotherapy should be added to radiotherapy to control the probable diffuse disease (Banfi et al 1972).

Banfi et al (1970) found no case of secondary involvement of the nasopharynx if the lymphomas originated as primary lesions in the lymph nodes, even when the disease became widespread. Werf-Messing (1968) also said there was no regional extension to Waldeyer's ring in patients having high cervical primaries; and in only 1 of 65 patients who presented with tonsillar or lingual primaries was extension to nasopharynx noted.

Radical surgery for treatment of malignant lymphoma of Waldeyer's ring has been done occasionally in the past. In 1947, Hellwig reported 3 patients with non-Hodgkin's malignant lymphomas involving the tonsils; they were treated by radical surgery and the patients lived free of disease for 7, 12, and 20 years, respectively. Stout (1947) reported 1 case of tonsil involvement and 2 of buccal mucosa lesions treated with surgery and post-operative radiotherapy; both patients were well for 10 to 14 years. Catlin (1966) listed 5 patients with lymphomas of the head and neck who survived more than 5 years after surgery with or without radiotherapy. Of these 5 there were 3 with tonsillar lesions and 1 each with tumors of the hard palate and nasopharynx. In addition, he said partial resections of lymphomas of the nasal cavity and paranasal sinus were done because of painful masses and obstruction. In a few patients, surgery was performed on lesions which failed to respond to x-ray therapy. Klopp (1968) commented that removal of malignant tumors in the regions of the nasal cavity, sinuses, tonsil, and nasopharynx is not justified because of the need for extensive surgery and its associated disability and deformity. However, surgery does have an adjunct role as a means of promoting drainage and as an aid in controlling infection.

With localized radiotherapy, Werf-Messing (1968) reported that the 5-year survival rates for non-Hodgkin's lymphoma of the Waldeyer's ring were 67 percent for stage I_1 lesions, 36 percent for stage I_2, and 31 percent for stage II lesions. Wang (1969) reported on the radiotherapeutic management and results of 75 cases of malignant lymphomas of Waldeyer's ring. Pathological classification showed 50 percent with reticulum cell sarcomas; 36 percent, lymphosarcomas; and 14 percent, unclassified. The principal anatomical locations were 53 percent, facial; 23 percent, nasopharyngeal; and 16 percent, lingual tonsils. In contrast to squamous cell carcinoma of the head and neck, lymphomas occurred relatively more often in females, although the male-to-female ratio in his study was 1.8 : 1. Treated by aggressive supervoltage radiotherapy, the 5-year survival rates for stages I and II lesions were 79 percent and 48 percent, respectively. The most important single factor that affected survival was the presence or absence of lymph node metastasis.

al-Saleem et al (1970) presented 52 malignant lymphomas of Waldeyer's ring: tonsils, 30; nasopharynx, 10; tongue, 9; pharyngeal wall, 2; and soft palate, 1. Three patients had Hodgkin's disease (tonsil, 2; nasopharynx, 1). They correlated survival results with histological types, showing that reticulum cell sarcoma had an overall 5-year survival rate of 38 percent and was highly curable in patients with no involvement of the cervical nodes (7 out of 9). Well differentiated lymphocytic lymphomas showed more tendency to disseminate, but recurrences were relatively easy to control by radiotherapy or chemotherapy and 57 percent survived 5 years. All 3 patients with nodular lymphomas were living for more than 5 years, and only 1 had evidence of disseminated disease. With high-energy radiotherapy and prophylactic treatment to both sides of the neck, Banfi et al (1972) reported an overall 5-year survival rate of 42 percent. The incidence of recurrence and new manifestation of the disease was highest during the first year after treatment.

Thyroid and Parotid Gland

Thyroid tumors, as the initial manifestation of generalized lymphosarcomas, have been known since Kundrat presented two such examples in 1893. Hodgkin's involvement of the thyroid is rare, but primary lymphoma of the thyroid gland of other types, occurring most frequently in elderly women, is not uncommon. Such lesions need to be differentiated from small cell carcinomas and advanced struma lymphomatosa. Apparently some evidence of struma lymphomatosa might be seen in up to 40 percent of the patients with primary malignant lymphomas of the thyroid (Luce and Frei 1972); and conversely, malignant lymphomas could develop in a small proportion of patients with struma lymphomatosa (Lindsay and Dailey 1955).

Tumor of the thyroid gland was the initial manifestation of lymphosarcoma in 2 of the 1269 patients of Rosenberg et al (1961). Another patient had proven involvement of the thyroid gland during the course of the disease, and 9.1 percent of the cases autopsied had such involvement. In no case was thyroid dysfunction detected clinically. Among 567 patients with lymphosarcomas, Molander and Pack (1963) said the thyroid gland was involved in 1 case initially and in 4 cases subsequently. Respiratory embarrassment was the main problem, and the lesion often extended into the larynx.

Walt et al (1957) reported 21 cases of primary malignant lymphomas of the thyroid. Seventeen of these were managed by resection and postoperative x-ray. Eight patients survived more than 4 years. The authors recommended that as much of the involved tissue as possible be resected and extensive contralateral subtotal thyroidectomy performed. Infiltration of perithyroid tissues and the symptom of voice change appeared to be correlated with a poor prognosis. Among the patients who had postmortem examinations, they found a high proportion with metastases in the gastrointestinal tract.

There were 108 cases of lymphomas of the thyroid reported in the world literature before 1961 (Smith and Klopp 1961). Woolner (1966) reviewed another 46 cases and emphasized that the presence or absence of locally invasive tendencies appeared to have major prognostic importance. Ten patients had inoperable lesions and only 4 were living 1 to 4 years after radiotherapy. Twenty patients had extrathyroid invasion of positive lymph nodes. All had surgical resection followed by irradiation; only 4 survived. In contrast, 15 of 16 patients who had lymphomas confined within the capsule were cured by complete surgical excision and radiotherapy.

Among 249 patients with head and neck lymphomas, Catlin (1966) said 101 operations were performed on 91 patients (36 percent). Operations were done for curative, palliative, or diagnostic purposes. Next to radical neck dissection (49 operations), the most common procedures were parotidectomies (15 operations) and thyroidectomies (7 operations). Eight parotidectomy and 2 thyroidectomy patients survived 5 years. Catlin commented that surgery was the treatment of choice for most tumors of these two glands, and most of the operations were performed without a preoperative pathological diagnosis. Klopp (1968) also felt surgery was a good method of treatment, and postoperative irradiation was not indicated when the removal had apparently been complete.

Scott (1971) reported 29 patients with malignant lymphomas of the thyroid gland seen at a radiotherapy department from 1930 to 1970. All patients were over 50 years of age. The treatment was thyroidectomy and radiotherapy (3500–4500 rads) in all operable cases, and radiotherapy alone following biopsy in inoperable cases. About 33 percent were alive and well over 5 years after treatment, and only 1 out of 4 had complete surgical removal. Scott also pointed out that in 3 of the 6 patients who had postmortem examination, there was definite evidence of gastrointestinal involvement.

Azzopardi and Evans (1971) reported 5 patients who had malignant lymphomas (reticulum cell sarcoma or Hodgkin's disease) of the parotid gland associated with the benign lymphoepithelial lesion of Mikulicz's disease. The two conditions were either discovered simultaneously or the malignant lymphoma was detected subsequently. These cases suggested that autoimmune disorders in men could be followed by the development of malignant lymphomas.

In the EFSCH series, no thyroidectomy or parotidectomy was performed on any of the 527 patients with malignant lymphomas. For comparison, from 1940 to 1962, 43 patients had either partial or total parotidectomy for metastatic disease among 2802 patients with epidermoid cancer of the skin of the head and neck area (Ridenhour and Spratt 1966).

Larynx

Sarcoma constitutes less than 1 percent of laryngeal neoplasms, and fibrosarcoma accounts for one-half of the mesenchymal tumors. Lymphomas of the larynx are even rarer than fibrosarcomas. MacKenty (1934) gave the first description of laryngeal lymphosarcoma in English; the patient survived 10 years after laryngectomy.

DeSanto and Weiland (1970) reported 9 patients treated at the Mayo Clinic from 1952 to 1968, 6 having lymphosarcomas and 3 with reticulum cell sarcomas. During the same period, 5319 patients were seen for malignant lymphoma. Thus, the overall incidence of malignant lymphoma involving the larynx was less than 0.2 percent. They reviewed the world literature and found only 19 other patients with laryngeal lymphomas, all were non-Hodgkin's. Thirteen patients had laryngeal involvement as part of their advanced disease. One had laryngectomy and postoperative irradiation and was followed for only 3 months. Five patients had local laryngeal disease without subsequent dissemination and had long survivals of 4.5, 10, 10, 12, and 13.5 years, respectively.

Dickson (1971) also searched the world literature. Eight of his 14 cases were not reviewed by DeSanto and Weiland, and he added two new cases (one, lymphosarcoma; one, reticulum cell sarcoma). Podoshin et al (1971) reported a 19-year-old woman with lymphosarcoma whose lesion presented as a benign cyst. They emphasized that the symptoms of both sarcoma and carcinoma of the larynx are similar.

Seven of the 9 patients reported by DeSanto and Weiland (1970) had tumors in the supraglottic larynx. Grossly, the tumors were of a gray-white, fish-flesh color and texture. Three had distinctly local laryngeal growths; 2 had disease limited to the area above the clavicle; 3 had disease presented in the larynx, followed by distant sites; and 1 had laryngeal disease as part of the disseminated disease. When a biopsy taken through the laryngoscope could not establish the diagnosis, laryngofissure and excisional biopsies of the lesion were required. They concluded that irradiation to curative dose levels was the treatment of choice and all patients should have careful follow-up for distant disease. With persistence in treatment, 2 of the patients were cured and 5 were 5-year survivals. Wang (1972) reported 4 cases of malignant lymphomas of the larynx. He commented that the lesions tended to be smooth, submucosal, and massive; a tracheostomy was often required during the course of their management. Using megavoltage radiotherapy and doses ranging between 4500 and 5000 rads, Wang's patients were free of disease for 4, 8, 8.5, and 12 years, respectively.

Among the combined total of 43 cases with malignant lymphomas of the larynx reported in the literature, only 2 patients had Hodgkin's disease (Mills et al 1947; Norris and Peale 1961). In the EFSCH series of 527 patients with malignant lymphomas, one patient (p. 387) required a tracheostomy for respiratory distress secondary to an abscess over the thyroid cartilage. At autopsy, 8 months later, the only site with Hodgkin's disease was in the larynx.

Eye and Orbit

In 1–2 percent of patients with malignant lymphomas, the lesions may occur initially in the conjunctiva, orbit, or retro-orbital areas. Of the 1269 patients with non-Hodgkin's lymphoma, Rosenberg et al (1961) found conjunctival lesions were the initial manifestations in 6 patients, and developed subsequently in 19 additional patients. Among another 567 patients, Molander and Pack (1963) reported 3 with initial involvement of the orbit (2 lacrimal gland and 1 conjuntiva), and in one, the retro-orbital space, which presented as severe proptosis. Secondary involvement occurred in 22 patients (6 each of lacrimal gland and retro-orbital space, and 10 of the conjunctiva).

McGavic (1955) found 21 cases of malignant lymphomas of the eye, 17 of which were primarily in the region of the eye; in the other 4, ocular involvement was part of a generalized disease. Hogan and Zimmerman (1962) collected 171 cases of lymphomatous lesions involving the orbit, lacrimal apparatus, conjunctiva, lids, brows, iris, and ciliary body. The eye lesions occurred insidiously so that the patients presented themselves not because of symptoms, but because of an unexplained mass under the conjunctiva or skin or because of an exophthalmos indicating orbital involvement. Malignant lymphoma of the lacrimal sac might give the picture of an acute inflammatory process, and the orbital lesions were sometimes diagnosed as chronic granulomas, especially in the early stages. Reese (1963) saw two instances in which Hodgkin's disease was responsible for Horner's syndrome; 3 other patients had papilledema due to intracranial disease. However, intraocular Hodgkin's disease must be very rare, because Higgins (1968) mentioned he had not found such a case in the record file of the New York Eye and Ear Infirmary.

Catlin (1966) recorded 1 patient with reticulum cell sarcoma of the orbit who was successfully treated by surgery and was well for over 5 years. In the 150 non-Hodgkin's lymphoma patients who had surgical procedures, Elias and Mittleman (1971) included 1 patient with exophthalmos and 1 with an infraorbital nodule presented as carcinoma.

Currie and Henson (1971) reviewed 774 patients with "reticulosis" (Hodgkin's disease, non-Hodgkin's lymphoma, myeloma, polcythemia vera, and various leukemias), and found 246 neurological episodes occurring in 200 patients. Among the 200, there were 51 patients with Hodgkin's disease and 34 with lymphosarcomas. They mentioned 7 cases of orbital lymphosarcomas; 2 were primary. Among those with Hodgkin's disease, one had intraocular infiltration and one had orbital disease. The last case showed no evidence of recurrence during the 18 years after surgery.

Neault et al (1972) reported that uveitis was the initial clinical sign in 7 of the 17 patients who underwent craniotomy at the Mayo Clinic between 1956 and 1968 for reticulum cell sarcoma of the brain. The uveitis was primarily a posterior segment process and eventually became bilateral. None of the 7 patients had evidence of systemic malignant lymphomas. They pointed out that, "The clinician must consider reticulum cell sarcoma of the eye and brain in the differential diagnosis of uveitis in any patient who is more than 40 years old, and especially in one who has neurologic symptoms or signs."

Among 1467 patients reported to have extranodal and nondisseminated non-Hodgkin's lymphomas, Freeman et al (1972) reported that connective tissue was the site of primary disease in 122 patients. Among these 122, 32 had disease in the orbit. The 5-year relative survival rate of these 122 patients was 57 percent, and the 10-year rate was 50 percent. The details of therapy were not given, but in the whole series, surgery was the common initial treatment, although radiotherapy was used just as often.

Oral Cavity and Surrounding Structures

Hellwig (1947) reported one case of "reticulocytoma" of the jaw treated by radical surgery without radiation. The patient was living and without disease for 10 years. In the 50 cases of lymphosarcoma of the head and neck reported by Catlin (1948), 2 involved the palate; there was 1 case each involving the tongue, gingiva, and pharynx. In a subsequent series of 249 patients with various malignant lymphomas reported by Catlin (1966), there were 9 cases of tongue involvement, 5 each of palate and submaxillary gland, 2 of mandible and 1 of the pharynx. Lymphosarcoma of the base of tongue can be controlled with radiotherapy, especially when the disease is diagnosed before it has spread beyond the limits of the neck; 5 of 12 patients were well 5 years after therapy (Ackerman and Del Regato 1970).

Tillman (1956) reported 12 cases of malignant lymphomas with oral manifestations, 7 of which were primary. These lesions affected the maxilla, tongue, tonsil, soft palate, and sublingual salivary gland. Only 1 patient had Hodgkin's disease, and he had gingival involvement. Tillman pointed out that the various presenting symptoms included swelling of the mucobuccal fold, the hard and soft palate; enlargment of the maxilla, mandible or the major and minor salivary glands; pain or parasthesia of the maxillary or mandibular areas; loose teeth or unhealed tooth sockets; chronic hypertrophic gingivitis: and segmental herpes zoster of one side of the face. A biopsy must be performed to establish the diagnosis of malignant lymphomas.

In the literature of the oral surgeons, Steg et al (1959) reviewed 21 reported cases of malignant lymphoma of the mandibular and maxillary region and added 47 cases of their own (34 involved maxilla; 12, mandible; and 1, both). Histologically, 10 were lymphosarcomas; 14, reticulum cell sarcomas; 2, Hodgkin's disease; and 21, transitional types. They pointed out that the majority of these patients had a prolonged delay in their diagnoses because they were treated for benign processes with procedures such as tooth extraction, antral operations, incision and drainage, and so forth. Cook (1961) also reviewed 34 cases of oral lymphomas reported in the literature and added 6 more. He found the maxilla and mandible were affected about equally. The common presenting sign of these lesions was swelling, with or without accompanying pain. Often anesthesia or hyperesthesia of the skin following a regional distribution is seen. This is of the utmost diagnostic importance and should not be ignored.

Barclay (1971) said that in the 10 years since Cook's report, there were 5 other reports of reticulum cell sarcomas of the jaw in the dental literautre. He added a case which presented as a periapical abscess. Sippel and Samartano (1971) cited 3 cases of lymphosarcomas of the gingiva, 1 of the submaxillary gland, and presented 1 case of leukemia manifested as lymphosarcoma of the mandible. They commented that the maxilla seems to be affected by lymphosarcoma more frequently than the mandible.

Wang (1971) reported a series of 37 patients with extranodal malignant lymphomas arising from the oral cavity and paranasal sinuses. The frequency of involvement of various structures were as follows: antrum and/or malar bone, 54 percent; buccogingival sulcus, 38 percent; nasal cavity, 30 percent; gingiva and cheek, 27 percent each; ethmoid sinus, 24 percent, and maxillary plate, 22 percent. The 5-year survival rates were 65 percent for stage I lesions (28 patients) and 33 percent for stage II (9 patients). The treatment recommended was radiotherapy in a dose of 5000 rads over a period of 5 weeks. Due to the relative infrequency of regional metastases, the advisability of elective nodal irradiation was doubtful. However, Wang recommended that the regional lymphatic drainage areas be irradiated from the mastoid process to the supraclavicular area if lymph node involvement was present.

Other Tissues

Cahn (1948) and Lautz (1958) reported Hodgkin's disease involving the nose. Invasion of the nasal fossa and the associated sinus cannot be separated from each other because the involvement of one extends into the other along the soft tissue or through the thin bony plates which separate them. Such invasion is nearly always associated with cervical lymphadenopathy (Higgins 1968).

Stewart and Stuart (1971), after reviewing the literature, found only 7 recorded cases of Hodgkin's disease involving the nose and added 2 cases of their own. In one case, the lesion was a nasal polyp with metastases to the parotid gland; in the other, the nasopharynx was involved during the course of the disease.

Paparella and el-Fiky (1972) studied 16 temporal bones of 8 patients with lymphomas and said that the ear was commonly involved. In 5 patients with lymphosarcoma and 1 with reticulum cell sarcoma, there were tumor cell infiltration and bleeding in the external auditory canal; eustachian tube and middle ear; the cochlear, vestibular, and facial nerves; and the modiolus, submacular, and subcristal areas. Clinical problems were mainly ascribed to the eustachian tube and middle ear, although inner ear dysfunction could not be ruled out. Facial palsy occurred in one patient, although in 6 others facial nerves had tumor infiltration but no neurological dysfunction.

Eleven cases involving soft tissues were included in the 50 cases of lymphosarcoma of the head and neck region reported by Catlin (1948). Among 81 patients with stage I and II lesions of reticulum cell sarcoma, Musshoff et al (1971) reported 35 patients who had primarily extranodal involvement (an incidence rate of 43 percent). Five of the 35 had lesions of the skin and soft tissue of the face. They pointed out that patients with primary organ involvement had almost the same prognosis as that of the lymph node if they received the same treatment.

Molander and Pack (1963) found that the skin of the scalp was the most common site involved in lymphosarcoma of the skin. Among 567 patients, 8 had scalp lesions initially and 32, secondarily. In the 249 patients with malignant lymphomas of the head and neck areas, 4 patients initially presented with scalp involvement (Catlin 1966). In patients who have lesions in the scalp controlled, follow-up examinations should be maintained, with particular attention paid to adenopathy in the neck, especially those nodes in the suboccipital area and posterior accessory spinal chain (Bloedorn 1971).

CHEST AND INTRATHORACIC LESIONS

Incidence and Diagnosis

Apparently, O'Donnell was the first to write about lymphosarcoma of the lung in 1926. Moolten (1934) reported one patient who had hemoptysis secondary to a polypoid growth of the main bronchus. Falconer and Leonard (1936) studied 29 patients with Hodgkin's disease and showed that the lungs were involved in 37.6 percent, and 71 percent of those with lung lesions had pleural effusion. Charr and Wascolomis (1941) reported a case of Hodgkin's disease with extensive lesions limited almost entirely to the right lung.

Baker and Mann (1939) described a case of spontaneous pneumothorax in their series of 65 cases of Hodgkin's disease. Jackson and Parker (1947) did not observe this complication in their 245 patients, but they encountered 2 pericardial effusions occurring terminally.

Radiological evidence of pulmonary involvement was seen in 7 percent of 715 cases of malignant lymphomas (Robbins 1953). At necropsy, lymphomatous pulmonary deposits were found in 25 percent of the cases. A higher figure was reported in another autopsy series: Richmond et al (1962) found that the lung was involved in 46 percent of 272 patients with Hodgkin's disease, and pleura in 10.5 percent. Among the 418 patients with non-Hodgkin's disease, the comparable figures were 45 percent and 18.5 percent for reticulum cell sarcomas, and 24 percent and 8 percent for lymphosarcomas without bone marrow involvement.

Rosenberg et al (1961) found that intrathoracic lesions were the presenting sites in 4 percent of 1269 patients with non-Hodgkin's lymphomas. The figures for specific sites included 3.2 percent for mediastinal or hilar nodes, 0.4 percent each for pleura and lung parenchyma. However, intrathoracic structures were involved in 50.8 percent during the course of the disease and 21.4 percent had pulmonary parenchyma disease. In a series of 567 patients with lymphosarcoma, Molander and Pack (1963) found 22 patients presented with mediastinal nodes, 4 had pleural effusion, and 2 presented with lung lesions (an overall incidence of 5 percent). Subsequently, 30 percent of the patients had mediastinal disease, 20 percent had pleural effusion, and 15 percent had infiltration of lung parenchyma.

Clinically, lung parenchyma is involved more often in cases with Hodgkin's disease than in other lymphomas. Fisher et al (1962) said lung disease was present in about 30 percent of their 154 Hodgkin's cases, but was the presenting feature in none. About two-thirds of the patients had intrapulmonary involvement within 2 years after the initial diagnosis. Nickau and Reeves (1958) pointed out that intrapulmonary involvement in Hodgkin's disease was not necessarily ominous. The average survival after the onset of parenchymal disease was 30.3 months. The prognosis in patients who were relatively asymptomatic when first seen was better. Stolberg et al

(1964) stressed that next to disease in the lymph nodes, the lung ranks with the liver and spleen as one of the more commonly affected organs. They also indicated that one of the outstanding types of localized intrathoracic manifestations is involvement of the subpleural lymphatics in the form of plaques or lymph nodes. Involvement of the diaphragm was found in 14 percent of the Hodgkin's cases at postmortem examination. Loss of the normal diaphragmatic outline in the absence of pleural effusion and abnormalities in diaphragmatic mobility are valuable diagnostic findings.

Since 1945, when Papanicolaou studied a sputum specimen from an obscure case in which there was x-ray and clinical suspicion of cancer of the lung (Watson 1968), cytological examination of sputum and bronchial washings has become an important diagnostic procedure for pulmonary lesions. Even in patients with metastatic lesions, Rosenberg et al (1959) found cancer cells present in the sputum in 38 percent of 50 patients, and Parker and Reid (1960) found them in 73 percent of 30 such patients. Koss (1961) and Suprun and Koss (1964) described several cases of Hodgkin's disease with pulmonary lesions which had identifiable malignant cells. They also encountered a second malignancy of bronchiolar carcinoma which developed in a patient with Hodgkin's disease. In the EFSCH series, among the 364 patients with non-Hodgkin's lymphomas, 1 had coexisting lung cancer and 2 had additional lung cancer diagnosed at autopsy.

Koss (1970) mentioned that pulmonary changes resulting from radiotherapy or chemotherapy, especially the multinucleated giant cells, might be mistaken for cancer cells by an inexperienced observer. Melamed (1963) described cytological characteristics typical of those found in malignant lymphomas. Burke and Melamed (1968) described 2 cases of reticulum cell sarcoma of the lung and said that malignant lymphoma and leukemia had an almost equally unique cytologic pattern. Fullmer and Morris (1972) reported 1 patient with unsuspected mediastinal Hodgkin's disease, and Levij (1972) reported 1 patient with cavitary lesions of the lung; both cases were first diagnosed by malignant cells in the sputum and later confirmed by tissue biopsy. Variakojis et al (1972) described the diagnosis of Hodgkin's disease by brush biopsy when the cytologic examination was negative.

The most frequent pathway of lymphomatous involvement of the lung is through the peribronchovascular lymphatics (Stolberg et al 1964). Roentgenologically, the most common finding of lymphomatous involvement of the lung is bilateral perihilar streaks radiating out from the mediastinum in a fanlike distribution (Fisher et al 1962). Other findings of secondary pulmonary deposits of Hodgkin's disease may take the form of (1) a solitary nodule resembling a deposit of secondary carcinoma, (2) miliary nodules scattered throughout both lungs, (3) a large mass occupying the whole or major part of a lobe, (4) pleural plaques, and (5) very rarely, nodular deposits in the walls of the large bronchi (Spencer 1967). Strickland (1967) pointed out that peripheral deposits did not occur before mediastinal glandular enlargement. Some of the pulmonary lesions underwent cavitation (Efskind and Wexels 1952; Steel 1964), although the incidence was said to be less than 1 percent (Korbitz 1970). Diaphragmatic paralysis is uncommon, and this distinguishes it from carcinoma in which it is relatively more frequent (Cremin 1971).

In 29 patients with Hodgkin's disease involving the lung, Whitcomb et al (1972) reported that the most common radiographic abnormalities were confluent infiltration (13 patients), discrete nodule(s) and fibronodular infiltration (6 patients each). Fourteen of the 29 had additional intrathoracic complications including pleural effusion (7), superior vena cava obstruction and phrenic nerve paralysis (2 each). Twenty-six of the 29 patients had nodular sclerosis subtype. In 18 patients, the lung abnormality was seen at the time of the initial diagnosis; their mean survival was 30 months. In the other 11, lung involvement developed between 1 and 13 years after Hodgkin's disease was recognized, and they had a mean survival of 17 months after detection of the pulmonary lesion. Confirming the results of others, in all patients who had not previously received anterior mediastinal radiation or systemic chemotherapy, hilar adenopathy was present when lung involvement was recognized. In addition, at least one-third of the patients also had other evidence of stage IV disease.

Peters et al (1967) felt chest tomography should be performed on all patients who presented with supraclavicular adenopathy but with negative chest x-rays. Davidson and Clarke (1968) showed that routine tomography was required to detect hilar or mediastinal adenopathy and lung lesions. In 82 examinations, 44 showed additional lesions which could not be seen on plain radiographs. The most common lesions were subcarinal nodes, unilateral involvement of the lung hilum, small nodular opacities, and infiltration of the lung. Feldman et al (1969) described simultaneous use of arterial and venous angiography in the evaluation of anterior mediastinal tumors. In 2 patients, bilateral extension of the lymphoma not seen on routine films was strongly suggested on the basis of angiographic studies. Valenca et al (1970) studied pulmonary functions in patients with secondary malignant lymphomas and found an interstitial pattern of dysfunction (decreased lung volume, low carbon monoxide diffusing capacity, hypoxemia, and hyperventilation).

Blank and Castellino (1972) studied the normal patterns of pleural reflections of the left superior mediastinum. They suggested that diagnosis of early mediastinal adenopathy could be made by studying this pleural reflection since it lay in close relationship to the left prevascular group of lymph nodes. Castellino and Blank (1972) presented 5 cases of Hodgkin's disease who had enlargement of the diaphragmatic lymph nodes adjacent to the pericardium and cardiophrenic angles. They pointed out that these nodes not only could be the site of recurrent disease, but on occasion might be involved during the initial presentation of malignant lymphomas. Two of the 5 patients had thoracotomy and biopsy for tissue diagnosis.

An increased incidence of malignancy in organ transplant recipients surviving over a prolonged period has appeared in the literature in recent years. Pierce et al (1972) reported 3 cases of reticulum cell sarcoma occurred in their 151 renal allotransplant recipients. None of the 3 patients had peripheral lymph adenopathy, and 1 had two separate 3-cm nodules in the right lung.. Statistically, 15 lymphomas have occurred during the course of 3631 man-years of patients with functioning renal transplants, giving an annual rate of occurrence of lymphoma in all renal transplant recipients of 0.4 percent. On the other hand, the annual mortality rate from non-Hodgkin's lymphoma for white males of comparable age groups (0–44 years, 1955 U.S. data) ranged from 0.001 to 0.003 percent. Thus, it was estimated that the probability of patients, who received renal transplants, dying from malignant lymphoma was 100 to 400 times as great as that observed in the general population.

Palliative Thoracic Procedures

There are situations where palliative resection of intrathoracic lymphoma is needed. Williams et al (1951) reported 5 exploratory thoracotomies performed in a series of 240 patients hospitalized for Hodgkin's disease. In 3 patients, tissue biopsies established the diagnosis for the first time. Two patients had tracheal compression, and the tumor was removed to relieve the symptom as well as to establish diagnosis. Craver (1964) said a right upper lobectomy might be indicated when repeated and worsening hemoptysis arose from an eroded bronchus.

Russell et al (1970) pointed out that direct extension to the lung, secondary to nodular sclerosing Hodgkin's disease, should be considered as a localized process. Depending upon the location, removal may be the treatment of choice. Other investigators would utilize radiotherapy. Mincer et al (1970) used moving strip irradiation for palliative treatment of extensive metastatic lesions in one or both lungs when the primary tumor was under control. Short-term regression was noted in 60 percent of the advanced lymphomas, though survival was not notably prolonged.

Another infrequent thoracic procedure is aspiration or even thoracotomy with biopsy, culture, and drainage for lung abscesses. Nocardial abscesses sometime occur in patients who have been on long-term steroid therapy (Pack and Molander 1966). Grossman et al (1970) presented 12 cases; of these, 3 patients had a single cavitating mass, 2 had infiltration, and 4 had both. At Memorial Hospital in New York, the opportunistic pulmonary fungal pathogens were, in decreasing order of frequency, aspergillosis, candidiasis, mucormycosis, cryptococcosis, and nocardiosis. Williams et al (1971) pointed out that 6 of 45 renal transplant patients, who were on steroid and immunosuppressive therapy, developed serious mycotic infections of the lung. Of the 3 patients who survived, each had a resection of his diseased lung. Pathological specimens showed abscesses of corynebacterium, histoplasmona, and aspergilloma. Thus, he felt early aggressive surgical extirpative therapy is most important for localized pulmonary lesions in immunosuppressed patients.

Pneumocystis pneumonia also can be a complication in patients who receive unusually long-term prednisone therapy. Goodell et al (1970) showed that pneumocystis carinii had become the most common cause of diffuse progressive pneumonia, especially in patients with immunologic deficiency and with treated reticuloendothelial neoplasa. Williams et al (1972) discussed a lymphoma patient with acute respiratory distress who had pneumocystis carinii infection diagnosed by lung biopsy. Forrest (1972) described the characteristic radiographic findings as diffuse perihilar distribution of pulmonary infiltrates, frequently sparing the peripheral lung fields in the early stages. Unusual findings included initial lobar distribution, pleural effusion, and relative sparing of previously irradiated areas of the lung. Pentamidine therapy is frequently successful if initiated in the early stages of the disease. This protozoan infection is unique in that spontaneous remission has been reported (Dominy and Lucas 1965), and reinfection following apparent recovery has been described (Hughes and Johnson 1971).

Mediastinal Lesion

Fisher et al (1962) said mediastinal adenopathy occurred in 85 of their 154 patients with Hodgkin's disease; about 10 percent had stage I disease at the time of diagnosis. They pointed out that enlargement of the paratracheal nodes preceded any change in the hilar node. In another 316 patients with Hodgkin's disease, Pack and Molander (1966) found 52 patients (16.4 percent) had intrathoracic, but extrapulmonary, mediastinal adenopathy initially. The mediastinal nodes were especially common during childhood.

Meese et al (1964) reported 3 cases of localized Hodgkin's involvement of the thymus in young individuals 15 to 23 years of age. All patients were asymptomatic, diagnosed by routine chest x-rays, and treated by surgical extirpation followed by radiotherapy. Fechner (1969) showed that so-called granulomatous thymoma was actually the nodular sclerosing subtype of Hodgkin's disease, in which diagnostic Reed-Sternberg cells were present but extremely sparse. Katz and Lattes (1969) studied 24 patients with granulomatour thymoma. Of the 17 treated, 10 were apparently free from disease 2 to 9 years later. Radiation therapy alone or with associated surgical procedures appeared to be better treatment than operation alone. Six patients developed extrathoracic lesions which were either typical of Hodgkin's disease or acceptable as a mixture of classic Hodgkin's disease and pleomorphic reticulum cell sarcoma. Thus, these studies suggested that granulomatous thymoma is basically a peculiar manifestation of Hodgkin's disease, primarily involving the thymus and eliciting in it a unique tissue response.

In 12 patients with stage I Hodgkin's disease involving the mediastinum,

Burke et al (1967) reported that complete excision was possible in 7. The thymus was part of the surgical specimen in 4, and all showed Hodgkin's disease. Eight of the 12 patients survived from 5 to 12 years. The authors pointed out that Hodgkin's disease of the mediastinum is best treated by a combination of surgery and radiotherapy. During the same time period, 10 patients were encountered who had x-ray evidence of a mediastinal mass together with histologically proved Hodgkin's disease involving supra-clavicular or scalene lymph nodes. Among patients with such stage II disease, 50 percent were alive from 2 to 11 years after the onset. In the discussion of this paper, Baisch reported that he had treated 9 similar patients with excision followed by irradiation. He felt that "the disease should be excised as widely as technical capabilities will safely permit, preferably including the lymph nodes from both pulmonary hili, from the lower cervical areas, and from the supraclavicular fossae. This type of excision of necessity requires a median sternotomy."

Van Heerden et al (1970) reviewed 97 patients with malignant lymphomas presented in the mediastinum. Fifty-seven had Hodgkin's disease and 61 percent survived 5 years; 40 had other lymphomas and only 15 percent survived 5 years. Sixteen patients had thoracotomies with curative resections followed byf radiation therapy; 13 of these survived 5 years and 7 survived 10 years. Five patients who had palliative resections also survived for more than 5 years. The 5-year survival rate of the remaining 76 was 36 percent. They pointed out that radical surgery has a distinct place in the therapy of selected patients with mediastinal lymphomas. Munnell (1971) listed 3 patients who had resections of mediastinal lymphomas. One died 2 months after the operation; the others, with Hodgkin's disease, were living and well 6 and 8 years after surgery and irradiation.

Levinsky et al (1971) presented the case of a 21-year-old girl with right and left hilar lymph nodes who had insignificant glands in both axillae and inguinal regions. Hodgkin's disease was diagnosed and treated by radical excision through bilateral thoracotomy performed 2 weeks apart, followed by intensive radiotherapy. Follow-up examination 27 months later revealed no recurrence. Boyd (1971) commented that "with improved knowledge about clinicopathological factors that influence the prognosis and decision-making process regarding management of patients with malignant lymphomas, surgery, like radiotherapy, is being extended and courageous advancement of an accepted technique is being tried."

Kaplan (1972) remarked that "thoracotomy may be required in an occasional patient for biopsy of mediastinal adenopathy when no enlarged peripheral nodes are available for biopsy or for biopsy of pleural or pulmonary nodules." But he felt, since postoperative radiotherapy is indicated for all Hodgkin's lesions and for virtually all other neoplasma as well, "major attempts at resection are seldom warranted and simple diagnostic removal of representative tissue samples for histopathologic diagnosis is usually the wisest procedure."

Malignant Lymphoma of the Lung

Sugarbaker and Craver (1940) studied 196 patients with lymphosarcoma and only one had its origin in the lung. Churchill (1947) was one of the first to employ resectional therapy for pulmonary lymphosarcoma. Beck and Reganis (1951) reported disease-free survival ranging up to 30 months postoperatively in 11 out of 15 patients with primary pulmonary lymphosarcomas treated by surgical extirpation (lobectomy or pneumonectomy). They stated that these lymphomas were usually slow-growing, did not metastasize until very late, and tended to spread locally to involve mediastinal structures.

Hochburg and Crastnopol (1956) reviewed 9 patients reported in the literature from 1944 to 1956 who had resections for pulmonary lesions of Hodgkin's disease and found only one who survived for 2 years. Cooley et al (1956) reviewed 9 cases of primary lymphomas of the lung (4 each of Hodgkin's and lymphosarcoma, 1 of reticulum cell sarcoma) and emphasized that these lesions frequently (30 percent) masquerade as pneumonia or lung abscesses. Of the 6 patients on whom resections were possible at the time of exploration, 3 were living without evidence of disease at 8.5 years, 2 years, and 3 months, respectively, with added postoperative radiotherapy.

Rose (1957) reported 2 cases of primary lymphosarcoma of the lung. He also updated the follow-up information on 15 patients reported by Beck and Reganis (1951) and added 6 additional cases from the literature. Of these 23 patients, 17 were treated surgically (8 by pneumonectomy and 9 by lobectomy); 7 survived between 5 and 12 years and 10 lived less than 5 years. There was only 1 patient who died of his lymphomatous disease, although several of the long-term survivors had repeated radiotherapy for lesions in the lung or elsewhere. The six patients who could not be operated upon, but were treated by irradiation alone, were dead within 12 months. Rose emphasized the similarity between the clinical course of these lesions and that of lymphosarcoma of the stomach, which often remained localized for long periods and might be cured by operation.

Sternberg et al (1959) reported 7 cases of primary lymphoma of the lung including the only case of follicular lymphoma reported in the literature. Hall and Blades (1959) reported 3 cases of primary lymphosarcoma of the lung. One patient treated by pneumonectomy was well 8 years after the operation, apparently without additional therapy. In the other 2 patients, the lesions were not suitable for surgical extirpation.

Kern et al (1961) described 4 patients who had Hodgkin's disease mainly of the lung with minimal hilar or mediastinal involvement. Three patients were treated with pneumonectomy or lobectomy followed by radiotherapy. They found 14 other patients met this stricter criteria reported in the literature since 1937 (including 3 cases reported by Cooley et al 1956). Seven of these had surgical resections and postoperative radiotherapy. Meese et al (1964) reported a case of primary Hodgkin's disease of the lung treated by left upper lobectomy. Ellison et al (1964) reported 4 cases of primary lymphosarcomas of the lung. They showed it could be of multifocal origin and suggested that the lesion arose from lymphatics of the lung parenchyma.

It is important to realize the rarity of resections done for pulmonary malignant lymphomas. Out of 1822 lung tumors treated surgically at the Mayo Clinic (Clagett et al 1964), about 1 percent was done for malignant lymphomas, (10 were lymphosarcomas, 5 Hodgkin's disease, and 2 reticulum cell sarcomas). Papaioannou and Watson (1965) reported that the incidence of primary pulmonary lymphoma was only about 0.5 percent of that of bronchogenic carcinoma. In about one-third of the patients, the disease was discovered on routine chest films, and the diagnosis was difficult to make by bronchoscopy or sputum cytologic examination because bronchial obstruction and ulceration were not common.

Papaioannou and Watson (1965) reported on 7 cases and established specific criteria for the diagnosis of primary lymphoma of the lung: "The disease had to be confined to one lung, with or without hilar involvement, but without mediastinal disease." They found no report of Hodgkin's disease met this criteria, but 93 cases of non-Hodgkin's lymphomas did. Of these cases, 82.6 percent were lymphosarcomas and 17.4 percent, reticulum cell sarcomas. They pointed out that this lymphosarcoma versus reticulum cell sarcoma ratio was substantially higher than that in the combined series of 1836 cases from all sites as reported by Rosenberg et al (1961) and Molander and Pack (1963) in which lymphosarcomas accounted for 59 percent of the cases and reticulum cell sarcomas for 41 percent. The treatment results of these 93 patients could be summarized as follows: "Surgery and radiation therapy, either alone or in combination, effect a 45.2 percent 5-year survival rate. Local recurrences are frequent, regardless of the therapeutic modality employed initially. Fatal recurrences usually occur early; those occurring late are usually controlled by radiation therapy." They felt that "even though radio-sensitive, these tumors should be treated initially by operation in view of the likelihood of repeated recurrences and the limited resistance of the lung to radiation. And following adequate resection, prophylactic radiation therapy does not seem to be indicated."

Monahan (1965) published a case history of Hodgkin's sarcoma primary in the lung in which a 10-year disease-free survival period was achieved by pneumonectomy, resection of adjacent pericardium, and postoperative irradiation with 2800 rads. Pack and Molander (1966) commented that "when technically feasible, resection of the involved lobe or lobes and mediastinal dissection with or without postoperative irradiation are usually done." Among 312 patients of Hodgkin's disease, one had segmental excision of a solitary nodular lung lesion with postoperative radiotherapy (3400 rads). The patient died 2.5 years later. Schamaun (1967) found that 3 out of 5 patients with lung lesions of Hodgkin's disease were unresectable at thoracotomy. One of the 2 who had a resection was free of symptoms 5 years after lobectomy.

Hilbun and Chavez (1967) reported a case of lymphocytic lymphoma, believed to be primary, of the right lung because careful examination and tests, including a lymphangiogram, revealed no other disease. Rubin (1968) reported a personal series of 11 cases of primary lymphomas of the lung (6 lymphosarcoma; 3 Hodgkin's disease; 2 reticulum cell sarcoma). Ten patients had thoracotomy and 3 of the 4 patients who had the lesions resected lived free of disease for 3, 9, and 11 years; the fourth died of disease 6 years after the operation. Four of the other 6 treated with radiotherapy were well 1, 3, 14 and 15 years later; two died less than 6 months with disease. Rubin believed that the most important prognostic factor is the presence or absence of disease in the hilar node. The nodes were found to be uninvolved in 7 of the 10 patients who had thoracotomy; 6 of these were free of disease 3.5 to 15 years after biopsy.

McNamara et al (1969) reported 3 cases of primary lymphoma of the lung. One patient died 5 years after wedge resection with widely disseminated reticulum cell sarcoma. The other 2 were well 10 and 14 years after surgery. They reviewed the literature, pointing out that primay Hodgkin's disease of the lung is rare and usually fatal, being the most malignant lymphoma occurring in the lung. Reticulum cell sarcoma, though unusual, is more common than Hodgkin's disease and is associated with a greater than 50 percent cumulative 5-year survival. Lymphosarcoma accounts for more than 80 percent of primary pulmonary lymphomas, over 100 cases having been reported. Five-year survival rate reported is greater than 70 percent.

Valenca et al (1970) described 1 patient who had a mass in the right lung. At thoracotomy, large hilar nodes and lesions involving the upper and middle lobes with pleural and pericardial extension were found. Upper and middle lobectomies were performed because the histopathology report was undifferentiated bronchogenic carcinoma. Postoperative radiotherapy was given for residual disease. Four years later the slides were reviewed and found to be more consistent with Hodgkin's disease. Seven years after this review, recurrent disease appeared in the breast, and the patient died 16 years after thoracotomy.

In 1963, Saltzstein introduced the term ''pseudolymphoma'' to designate a benign inflammatory process with true germinal centers which may be found in the lung or other areas, and is manifested by infiltrates of mature lymphocytes and other inflammatory cells. He maintained that ''pseudo-lymphomas'' are benign lesions and that their prognosis is invariably good. However, Papaioannou and Watson (1965) emphasized that it is impossible to differentiate between true lymphoma and ''pseudolymphoma'' and that long-term survival alone does not exclude neoplasia. McNamara et al (1969) also felt that attempts to distinguish benign from malignant lymhosarcoma were not helpful. Jenkins and Salm (1971) pointed out that the ''starry-sky'' pattern of true follicules, typical of reactive lymphoid hyperplasia, were not present in any of their cases regarded as pseudolymphomas. Thus, they rejected Saltzstein's concept, regarding all such cases as neoplastic. They presented 4 cases to illustrate the variable natural history of primary lymphosarcoma of the lung, Two patients died (one had the lung lesion for over 13 years without any specific treatment) and 2 survived (one had a lung lesion for 25 years and was well 5 years after pneumonectomy and one lived 18 years after a lung biopsy and radiotherapy). The patient who survived 18 years is of interest, because she had two small bowel resections for perforated lymphoma 1 and 2.5 years after radiotherapy to the chest.

In the present EFSCH series of 527 patients, none had pulmonary resection for malignant lymphoma; 3 out of 364 non-Hodgkin's disease patients had thoracotomies for diagnosis of intrathoracic lesions (p. 149). However, another patient (No. 36188), who was not included in the present series, did have a lobectomy for pseudolymphoma. From 1940 to 1969, 117 patients had thoracotomies for histologically confirmed malignancies of the lung at the EFSCH (Lee 1973). Ninety-four had bronchogenic cancer and 23 had metastatic pulmonary neoplasma. Thus, similar to the report of Clagett et al (1964), lymphoma of the lung occurred in less than 1 percent of the patients who required thoracic surgery for lung tumors.

Pleural Effusion

Among 312 patients with Hodgkin's disease, Pack and Molander (1966) reported 52 patients with mediastinal adenopathy, and of these, 12 (23 percent) had associated pleural effusion. Another 5 had pleural effusion without detectable mediastinal involvement. Thus, pleural effusion occurred as an initial manifestation of Hodgkin's disease in 5.4 percent of the patients, and secondarily in 18 percent. Fisher et al (1962) reported that 44 of 154 patients had pleural effusion (28.5 percent): none was present at onset, 8 occurred within 3 months of diagnosis, and the remainder were fairly evenly distributed between 18 months and 10 years after diagnosis. MacMurray et al (1950) described eosinophilia, defined as 5 percent or more of the leucocytes being eosinophiles, in pleural fluid of Hodgkin's disease. However, this finding is not diagnostic since 1–5 percent of all pleural fluids may be eosinophilic anyway (Sulavik and Katz 1963).

In patients with non-Hodgkin's lymphoma, Rosenberg et al (1961) reported an incidence of 29 percent pleural involvement. In the 567 lymphosarcoma patients reported by Molander and Pack (1963) 4 presented with pleural effusion and 22 had mediastinal adenopathy. Eventually, 20 percent of the patients had pleural effusion and 30 percent had mediastinal nodes. On the other hand, Bruneau and Rubin (1965) said that the incidence of mediastinal adenopathy was less than that of pleural fluid (26 percent versus 33 percent). In particular, 15 out of 21 patients (71 percent) with effusions were without overt mediastinal disease on film, and only 8 out of the 15 were symptomatic. They pointed out that if the fluid is a transudate (specific gravity below 1.015), mediastinal lymphatic obstruction would be a logical etiological factor and irradiation would be required. If the fluid is an exudate (specific gravity above 1.018), pleural seeding probably occurred and should be treated with direct intrapleural instillation of radioactive gold or cytotoxic agents. However, their experience showed this latter method was usually ineffective, and mediastinal irradiation was advisable for all types of pleural fluid.

In some patients the pleural effusion might appear after radiotherapy to the mediastinum. Whitcomb and Schwarz (1971) reported on 3 patients; 2 had Hodgkin's disease. In one, thoracotomy had to be carried out to accomplish decortication of the pleural fibrosis and creation of a pericardial window. The patient had marked clinical improvement. Surgical biopsy of this patient and autopsy examination of 2 others showed only pleural fibrosis without any other abnormality that could explain the presence of the effusion. Since fluid and particles in the pleural space normally drain toward the lung roots, they believed that obstruction of the lymphatic channels of the pleural space secondary to intensive radiation of the mediastinum was the cause of pleural effusion. Other problems, such as constrictive pericarditis or superior vena caval obstruction, were all complications of mediastinal irradiation and should be considered in the differential diagnosis of pleural effusion.

Bruneau and Rubin (1965) questioned the value of pleurectomy in the treatment of pleural fluid, while Munnell (1971) reported pleurectomy for effusion with excellent results in 2 patients (one with reticulum cell sarcoma, one with chronic lymphatic leukemia). In addition, Munnell listed that tube thoracostomy was used in 15 patients (9 effusions, 3 pneumothorax, 3 chylothorax). Twelve of the 15 had fair to excellent results, i.e., no recurrence of fluid for more than 6 months.

Nitrogen mustard was first used in 1949 for the intracavitory treatment of malignant pleural effusion. Since at least one-half to two-thirds of the patients showed response, this agent is the initial treatment of choice for the local management of malignant effusion in most situations. Recently, quinacrine (Atebrine), which was reported to be useful in 1961, has gained popularity because its response rate was higher (64–88 percent) and more predictable. It produces an intense inflammatory reaction, lasting from weeks to months, resulting in adhesions and fibrothorax. Quinacrine also has the advantage of not depressing the hematopoietic system, and thus it is useful in patients who have impaired bone marrow function due to disease or treatment. Other chemotherapeutic agents, radioactive isotopes, anciliary and novel surgical approaches are rarely used (Dollinger 1972)

In the EFSCH series, about 7 percent of the 163 patients with Hodgkin's disease had pleural effusion at the time of diagnosis, and 37 percent of all patients had mediastinal involvement. The comparable figures for 364 patients with non-Hodgkin's lymphomas were 9 percent and 20 percent, respectively. During the course of the disease, another 20 percent developed pleural effusion, but only about half of the patients required pleurocentesis and/or thoracostomy for palliation.

At EFSCH before 1967, patients with symptomatic pleural effusion requiring chest tube insertion were treated with 20 mg of nitrogen mustard instilled into the chest cavity after the pleural fluid was removed. The tube was clamped for 2 hr, reopened to water-sealed drainage, and removed when all fluid was drained and the lung expanded, usually 24 to 72 hours after insertion (Spratt 1967). Leininger et al (1969) reported a similar method but used only 10 mg nitrogen mustard instilled twice and left the tube clamped for 24 hr after each administration. Among 18 patients who had malignancy confirmed either by cytology or pleural biopsy (including lymphosarcoma), and who had recurrent, symptomatic fluid after repeated needle aspirations, there was only one failure. Presently at EFSCH, quinacrine (Atebrine) is being used almost exclusively for intractable pleural effusions secondary to various malignant tumors. Borja and Pugh (1973) reported a high response rate of 70 percent in a series of 27 patients (6 had malignant lymphomas). The method recommended is using a single dose (400–800 mg) given through a thoracostomy tube.

Weick et al (1973) reported 303 of 4500 patients with lymphoma seen had pleural effusion, as judged from roentgenograms of the thorax. They studied 159 patients in detail; 40 had Hodgkin's disease. The presence of underlying parenchymal lung involvement or a chylous type of effusion does not further alter the poor prognosis; but the presence of malignant cells in the fluid, which occurred in 10 percent of the cases, probably shortens survival. Obstruction of lymphatic drainage is probably the most common cause of non-chylous pleural effusion. In contrast to patients with metastatic carcinoma, pleural involvement by lymphomas is uncommonly the major factor in fluid formation. They feel that radiation therapy to the mediastinum or to the affected hemithorax is more likely to relieve lymphomatous effusion than is intrapleural therapy or systemic chemotherapy alone.

Chylothorax

Chylothorax is of special interest because it is found more often in patients with lymphomas and can be particularly troublesome due to the rapidity of its reaccumulation. Rarely it is the presenting sign of lymphoma. Williams and Burford (1964) noted a case which required multiple thoracenteses and intercostal tube drainages over a 5-year period. Exploratory thoracotomy was done with double ligation of the thoracic duct. Not until autopsy was reticulum cell sarcoma discovered.

Bower (1964) reported 20 cases of chylothorax; 6 of these were due to malignant lymphomas. In 4 of the 6, ascites were present, and the ascitic fluid was chylous in 2. Roy et al (1967) reported 58 patients with chylothorax (diagnosed by the criteria of fat content greater than 400 mg-percent). The cause of chylothorax in 23 of the patients was malignant lymphomas. None of the patients with neoplastic disease was successfully treated by drainage alone. Radiation therapy resulted in adequate control of the chylothorax for the remainder of the patients' lives in 68 percent of those with lymphomas. However, Macfarlane and Holman (1972) reported that chylothorax persisted after radiotherapy in 6 out of 7 cancer patients: 2 had Hodgkin's disease and 2 had lymphosarcomas (details of radiotherapy were not given).

Swensson et al (1966) reported 2 cases of chylothorax complicating lymphosarcoma with ascites which regressed completely following cobalt radiotherapy delivered only to the abdomen. Lowe et al (1972) reported 2 cases of stage IV lymphosarcoma which were not controlled by chemotherapeutic agents. Because of life-threatening complications of chylous ascites and chylothorax, the patients were treated with irradiation to the main masses in the abdomen and, in one patient, to the lower part of the mediastinum. The patients were then maintained on chemotherapeutic agents for longer than 1 year without evidence of tumor or further respiratory complications. Thus, they recommended that "the treatment of choice for patients with chylothorax secondary to lymphoma is repeated thoracenteses and prompt radiotherapy to the abdominal or mediastinal masses followed by systemic chemotherapy."

In the EFSCH series, one patient with Hodgkin's disease (No. 39646) and another with other lymphoma (No. 39025) developed chylothorax (p. 387, 392). In addition to appropriate radiotherapy, chemotherapy, and repeated thoracentesis and thoracostomy drainage, ancillary measures used included strict bed rest, low salt and fat intake, limitation of fluid and food, sedation, diuretics, and intravenous hyperalimentation (Dudrick and Rhoads 1971). Our experience is too limited to know which therapy offered the greatest benefit, but one patient died 2 months later, and at autopsy only radiation pneumonitis without residual Hodgkin's disease was found.

Sternum, Pericardium, and Heart

Fleischner et al (1948) first pointed out that retrosternal malignant lymphoma can present as "boardlike" or lobulated "padlike" soft tissue masses, with or without evidence of sternal erosion or other manifestations of intrathoracic lymphoma. Goldman (1971) reported 2 patients who presented with parasternal chest wall masses at the time of diagnosis and 4 other patients who developed pectoral masses later. In all the cases, the mass was associated with contiguous intrathoracic disease and responded well to localized radiotherapy.

Arnold et al (1966) reported Hodgkin's disease presented as a localized sternal tumor which was treated by total sternectomy. The defect was covered with Marlex mesh. This was done on a mistaken properative diagnosis of chondrosarcoma, and the lesion apparently originated in the right internal mammary chain of lymph glands. Meher-Homji et al (1972) reported a patient who presented with a sternal mass 2 months before axillary adenopathy, and without any retrosternal or mediastinal adenopathy.

Pilcher and Zubair (1970) reported one case of Hodgkin's disease which presented solely as pericarditis with pericardial effusion. They found 10 other cases reported in the world literature. When the pericardial effusion did not respond to chemotherapy, thoracotomy was attempted but the patient died during induction of anesthesia.

Pericardial fibrosis and effusions may occur after intensive radiotherapy for malignant diseases involving the mediastinum or lung parenchyma. Pierce et al (1969) did a retrospective review of all chest roentgenograms of patients who received mediastinal irradiation for Hodgkin's disease. When the cardiac transverse diameter showed an increase of 1.5 cm or more, the finding was considered significant. Of 87 patients, 22 (25 percent) showed radiographic evidence of pericardial effusions secondary to irradiation 4 to 18 months after treatment. Clinical evidence of tamponade was noted in 7 patients; of these, 3 died before surgery could take place and 4 had pericardiectomies. Three of the other 15 patients had elective pericardiectomies for persistent effusions. The pericardium was removed anteriorly to the atrioventricular groove on the right, superiorly to the base of the pulmonary artery, posterolaterally to the inferior pulmonary vein, inferiorly over the diaphragm, and posteriorly to the inferior vena cava (Kagan et al 1969). Three of the 7 patients who underwent surgery received further radiotherapy or chemotherapy; the other 4 were well without evidence of disease from 3 to 16 months postoperatively. The authors felt that, even in asymptomatic patients, pericardiectomy was desirable because constrictive pericarditis would probably result.

Malignant tumors of the heart are not common, but cardiac involvement with malignant lymphoma occurs relatively frequently. At autopsy, approximately 1 in 3 patients with reticulum cell sarcomas, 1 in 5 with lymphosarcomas, and 1 in 10 with Hodgkin's disease had tumors involving the heart (Javier et al 1967). Clinical findings of cardiac metastases were often not specific, and electrocardiographic changes were usually nondiagnostic even in patients with pericarditis. Roberts et al (1968) showed that the incidence of dyspnea, chest pain, effusion into body cavities, precordial murmurs, ventricular gallops, edema, and electrocardiographic distrubances were similar in patients with or without cardiac lymphomas. The clinical findings most often seen were the result of intrathoracic lymphoma, anemia, hypoalbuminemia, or an underlying cardiac condition. Only 10 percent of the cases of lymphomatous involvement of the heart showed signs or symptoms of cardiac dysfunction. Nearly half of the heart lesions were not grossly visible (cardiac involvement was diagnosed only on histologic sections in 21 of 48 patients).

Leidtke et al (1971) reported a patient with known lymphoblastic lymphoma who developed dyspnea secondary to a tumor mass obstructing the pulmonary outflow tract. After a total dose of 3800 rads radiotherapy to the pulmonary artery and 2400 rads to the pericardium, the tumor reduced in size and the patient was well 8 months after treatment. Fayos and Lampe (1971) described 3 cases of Hodgkin's disease which manifested as a mass near the apex of the heart. In one case, the mass was controlled for 16 years by radiotherapy. They believed that the cardiac apical mass is a pleural plaque located so as to stimulate a pericardial fat pad. Castellino and Blank (1972) described diaphragmatic lymph nodes adjacent to the pericardium and the cardiophrenic angle. Two of 5 Hodgkin's patients had thoracotomy and tissue biopsy for diagnosis.

In Hodgkin's disease, the pathological findings show the lesions infiltrating the pericardium and the epicardium more frequently than the endomyocardium. Ultmann and Moran (1973) found three cases reported in the literature who had myocardial infarction due to intramyocardial nodules. Although there is no good correlative clinicopathologic study concentrating on the association of pericardial Hodgkin's disease with mediastinal involvement, they felt that the pericardium became involved secondarily to mediastinal disease by contiguous spread.

SUMMARY

In patients with non-Hodgkin's lymphoma, about 6–9 percent of the lesions presented in the extranodal structures of the head and neck region initially; and about 20 percent could have secondary lesions involvement of these structures. Such lesions often are erroneously diagnosed as anaplastic or undifferentiated carcinoma.

The most common site of involvement is the Waldeyer's ring, especially the tonsils and nasopharynx. These structures were involved in about 2 percent of those with Hodgkin's disease. But they were found to contain non-Hodgkin's lymphomas in over 50 percent of those with reticulum cell sarcomas when systemic biopsy was taken from these areas irrespective of the clinical presentations. In patients with malignant lymphomas of the Waldeyer's ring, retroperitoneal disease was common (38 percent) and concomitant lesions of the gastrointestinal tract, especially the stomach, were found in about 20 percent of the cases. Treated by aggressive supervoltage radiotherapy, the overall 5-year survival rate of malignant lymphoma of the Waldeyer's ring should be better than 50 percent.

Malignant lymphomas might appear as primary or localized lesions of the thyroid and parotid glands. In operable cases, surgical excision followed by radiotherapy appears to give a better survival rate. When malignant lymphoma involved larynx, eye, orbit, oral, and other structures, radiotherapy alone offered the best treatment of choice.

Malignant lymphoma occasionally presented as intrathoracic visceral lesions (about 0.5 percent). And eventually over 50 percent of the patients had involvement of the lung, pleura, pericardium, and heart. Routine tomograms of the chest could detect early lesions which cannot be seen on plain x-rays. Palliative operations, such as resection of pulmonary abscess or for control of massive hemoptysis, might be life-saving in certain cases. Thoracotomy for biopsy and occasionally resection may be required in patients who had mediastinal adenopathy or parenchymal lesions of the lung without enlarged peripheral lymph nodes.

The incidence of primary pulmonary lymphoma was only about 0.5 percent of that of bronchogenic carcinoma, but lymphomatous lesions of the lung constituted about 1 percent of those patients who had thoracotomy for lung neoplasms. The most common histological type was lymphosarcoma; the rarest, Hodgkin's disease. Papaioannou and Watson (1965) established specific criteria for the diagnosis of primary lymphoma of the lung (p. 303). Although Saltzstein (1963) designated a benign form as "pseudolymphoma," others doubted this entity. Many patients who had primary malignant lymphoma of the lung are long-term survivors after lobectomy or pneumonectomy, with or without added postoperative radiotherapy.

In about 20–30 percent of the patients with malignant lymphoma, pleural effusion may appear, with or without mediastinal adenopathy. And in half of the cases, pleurocentesis and thoracostomy, and very rarely pleurectomy, are required for palliation. Chylothorax is a special interesting problem in patients with malignant lymphoma, and radiotherapy could give palliation. Postirradiation constrictive pericarditis needed pericardiectomy. Only about 10 percent of the patients with lymphomatous involvement of the heart had cardiac signs or symptoms.

REFERENCES

Ackerman LV, del Regato JA: Cancer: Diagnosis, Treatment and Prognosis (ed 4). St. Louis, Mosby, 1970, p. 289

Arnold HS, Meese EH, D'Amato NA, et al: Localized Hodgkin's disease presenting as a sternal tumor and treated by total sternectomy. Ann Thorac Surg 2:87–93, 1966

Azzopardi JG, Evans DJ: Malignant lymphoma of parotid associated with Mikulicz disease (benign lymphoepithelial lesion). J Clin Pathol 24:744–752, 1971

Baker C, Mann WN: Hodgkin's disease: Study of 65 cases. Guys Hosp Rep 89: 83–107, 1939

Banfi A, Bonadonna G, Carnevali G, et al: Lymphoreticular sarcoma with primary involvement of Waldeyer's ring: Clinical evaluation of 225 cases. Cancer 26:341–351, 1970

Banfi A, Bonadonna G, Ricci SB, et al: Malignant lymphomas of Waldeyer's ring: Natural history and survival after radiotherapy. Br Med J 3:140–143, 1972

Barclay JK: Reticulum cell sarcoma: Report of case. J Oral Surg 29:734–736, 1971

Beck WC, Reganis JC: Primary lymphoma of lung. J Thorac Surg 22:323–328, 1951

Blank N, Castellino RA: Patterns of pleural reflections of the left superior mediastinum. Radiology 102:585–589, 1972

Bloedorn FG: Treatment after excision of scalp lymphosarcoma. JAMA 218:602, 1971

Borja ER, Pugh RP: Single-dose quinacrine (Atabrine) and thoracostomy in the control of pleural effusions in patients with neoplastic diseases. Cancer 31:899–902, 1973

Bower GC: Chylothorax: Observations in 20 cases. Dis Chest 46:46–468, 1964

Boyd DP: Aggressive therapy for Hodgkin's disease. Chest 59:357–358, 1971

Bruneau R, Rubin P: The management of pleural effusions and chylothorax in lymphoma. Radiology 85:1085–1092, 1965

Burke MD, Melamed MR: Exfoliative cytology of metastatic cancer in lung. Acta Cytol 12:61–74, 1968

Burke WA, Burford TH, Dorfman RF: Hodgkin's disease of the mediastinum. Ann Thorac Surg 3:287–296, 1967

Cahn HL: Hodgkin's disease involving the nose. NY State J Med 48:2622–2624, 1948

Castellino RA, Blank N: Adenopathy of the cardiophrenic angle (diaphragmatic) lymph nodes. Am J Roentgenol Radium Ther Nucl Med 114:509–515, 1972

Catlin D: Lymphosarcoma of the head and neck. Am J Roentgenol Radium Ther Nucl Med 59:354–358, 1948

Catlin D: Surgery for head and neck lymphomas. Surgery 60:1160–1166, 1966

Charr R, Wascolomis A: Pulmonary lesions in Hodgkin's disease. JAMA 116:2013–2014, 1941

Churchill ED: Malignant lymphoma of lung and pulmonary coccidioidomycosis: Clinic on surgical lesions of lung with consolidation. Surg Clin North Am 27:1113–1120, 1947

Clagett OT, Allen TH, Payne WS, et al: The surgical treatment of pulmonary neoplasms: A 10-year experience. J Thorac Cardiovasc Surg 48:391–400, 1964

Cook HP: Oral lymphomas. Oral Surg 14:690–704, 1961

Cooley JC, Mc Donald JR, Clagett OT: Primary lymphoma of the lung. Ann Surg 143:18–28, 1956

Craver LF: Treatment of Hodgkin's disease, in Pack GT, Ariel IM (eds): Treatment of Cancer and Allied Diseases (ed 2) New York, Hoeber, 1964, pp 168–191

Cremin BJ: The radiological appearance and incidence of lymphoma. South Afr Med J 45:1360–1363, 1971

Currie S, Henson RA: Neurological syndromes in the reticuloses. Brain 94:307–320, 1971

Davidson JW, Clarke EA: Influence of modern radiological techniques on clinical staging of malignant lymphomas. Can Med Assoc J 99:1196–1204, 1968

DeSanto LW, Weiland LH: Malignant lymphoma of the larynx. Laryngoscope 80:966–978, 1970

Dickson R: Lymphoma of the larynx. Laryngoscope 81:578–585, 1971

Dollinger MR: Management of recurrent malignant effusions. CA 22:138–147, 1972

Dominy DE, Lucas RN: Pneumocystis carinii infection diagnosed by ante-mortem lung biopsy. Ann Thorac Surg 1:305–310, 1965

Dudrick SJ, Rhoads JE: New horizons for intravenous feeding. JAMA 215:939–949, 1971

Efskind L, Wexels P: Hodgkin's disease of lung with cavitation: Report of 3 cases. J Thorac Surg 23:377–387, 1952

Elias EG, Mittelman A: Lymphoma of head and neck masquerading as carcinoma. Am J Surg 122:424–426, 1971

Ellison RG, Bailey AW, Yeh TJ, et al: Primary lymphosarcoma of the lung. Am Surg 30:737–744, 1964

Falconer EH, Leonard ME: Hodgkin's disease of lung. Am J Med Sci 191:780–788, 1936

Fayos JV, Lampe I: Cardiac apical mass in Hodgkin's disease. Radiology 99:15–18, 1971

Fechner RE: Hodgkin's disease of the thymus. Cancer 23:16–23, 1969

Feldman F, Kanter IE, Fleming RJ, et al: Simultaneous arterial and venous angiography in the evaluation of anterior mediastinal tumors. Radiology 93:1281–1289, 1969

Fisher AM, Kendall B, van Leuven BD: Hodgkin's disease: A radiological survey. Clin Radiol 13:115–127, 1962

Fleischner FG, Bernstein C, Levine BE: Retrosternal infiltration in malignant lymphoma. Radiology 51:350–357, 1948

Forrest JV: Radiographic findings in Pneumocystis carinii pneumonia. Radiology 103:539–544, 1972

Fullmer CD, Morris RP: Primary cytodiagnosis of unsuspected mediastinal Hodgkin's disease: Report of a case. Acta Cytol 16:77–81, 1972

Freeman C, Berg JW, Cutler SJ: Occurrence and prognosis of extranodal lymphomas. Cancer 29:252–260, 1972

Goldman JM: Parasternal chest wall involvement in Hodgkin's disease. Chest 59: 133–137, 1971

Goodell B, Jacobs JB, Powell RD, et al: Pneumocystis carinii: The spectrum of diffuse interstitial pneumonia in patients with neoplastic diseases. Ann Intern Med 72:337–340, 1970

Grossman CB, Bragg DG, Armstrong D: Roentgen manifestations of pulmonary nocardiosis. Radiology 96:325–330, 1970

Hall ER Jr, Blades B: Primary lymphosarcoma of the lung. Chest 36:571–578, 1959

Hellwig CA: Malignant lymphoma: The value of radical surgery in selected cases. Surg Gynecol Obstet 84:950–958, 1947

Higgins GK: Pathologic anatomy, in Molander DW, Pack GT (eds): Hodgkin's Disease. Springfield, Ill, Thomas, 1968, pp 20–63

Hilbun BM, Chavez CM: Lymphoma of the lung. J Thorac Cardiovasc Surg 53:721–725, 1967

Hochburg LA, Crastnopol P: Primary sarcoma of the bronchus and lung. Arch Surg 73:74–98, 1956

Hogan MJ, Zimmerman LE: Ophthalmic Pathology, an Atlas and Textbook (ed 2). Philadelphia, Saunders, 1962

Hughes WT, Johnson WW: Recurrent pneumocystis carinii pneumonia following apparent recovery. J Pediatr 70:755–759, 1971

Jackson H Jr, Parker F Jr: Hodgkin's Disease and Allied Disorders. New York, Oxford University Press, 1947

Jackson H Jr, Parker F Jr: Hodgkin's disease: Involvement of certain other organs. N Engl J Med 233:369–376, 1945

Javier BV, Yount WJ, Crosby DJ, et al: Cardiac metastasis in lymphoma and leukemia. Chest 52:481–484, 1967

Jenkins BA, Salm R: Primary lymphosarcoma of the lung. Br J Dis Chest 65:225–237, 1971

Kadin ME, Glatstein E, Dorfman RF: Clinicopathologic studies of 117 untreated patients subjected to laparotomy for the staging of Hodgkin's disease. Cancer 27:1277–1294, 1971

Kagan AR, Morton DL, Hafermann MD, et al: Evaluation and management of radiation-induced pericardial effusion. Radiology 92:632–634, 1969

Kaplan HS: Hodgkin's Disease. Cambridge, Mass., Harvard University Press, 1972, p. 103

Katz A, Lattes R: Granulomatous thymoma or Hodgkin's disease of thymus? A clinical and histologic study and reevaluation. Cancer 23:1–15, 1969

Kern WH, Crepeau AG, Jones JC: Primary Hodgkin's disease of the lung: Report of 4 cases and review of the literature. Cancer 14:1151–1165, 1961

Klopp CT: Surgical treatment of primary lymphoma. Cancer Management: A special graduate course on cancer, sponsored by American Cancer Society. Philadelphia, Lippincott, 1968, pp 393–397

Korbitz BC: Massive cavitation of the lung in Hodgkin's disease. Chest 58:542–545, 1970

Koss LG: Diagnostic Cytology and Its Histopathologic Bases. Philadelphia, Lippincott, 1961

Koss LG: Progress in cytologic diagnosis of lung cancer. Proc Natl Cancer Conf 6: 817–819, 1970

Kundrat H: Ueber Lympho-Sarkomatosis. Wien klin Wochenschr 6:211–213, 1893

Larsen RR, Hill GJ II, Ratzer ER: Reticulum cell sarcoma in head and neck surgery. Am J Surg 123:338–342, 1972

Lascelles RG, Burston J: Hodgkin's disease: Disease presenting with symptoms of cranial nerve involvement. Arch Neurol 7:359–364, 1962

Lautz HA: Nasal and laryngeal involvement in abdominal Hodgkin's disease. Arch Otolaryngol 67:78–80, 1958

Lee YN: Thoracotomy for lung cancer: Review of experiences at one cancer hospital. Am Surg 39:410–418, 1973

Leininger BJ, Barker WL, Langston HT: A simplified method for management of malignant pleural effusion. J Thorac Cardiovasc Surg 58:758–763, 1969

Levij IS: A case of primary cavitary Hodgkin's disease of the lungs, diagnosed cytologically. Acta Cytol 16:546–549, 1972

Levinsky L, Lewinski U, Vries A de et al: Bilateral thoracotomy for Hodgkin's disease involving the hilar nodes. Chest 59:446–448, 1971

Liedtke AJ, Adams DF, Weber ET, et al: Remission of cardiac lymphoma with supervoltage radiation. Am J Med 50:816–822, 1971

Lindsay S, Dailey ME: Malignant lymphoma of the thyroid gland and its relation to Hashimoto disease: Clinical and pathologic study of 8 patients. J Clin Endocrinol 15:1332–1352, 1955

Lowe DK, Fletcher WS, Horowitz IJ, et al: Management of chylothorax secondary to lymphoma. Surg Gynecol Obstet 135:35–38, 1972

Luce JK, Frei E III: Lymphomas, in Mengel CE, Frei E III, Nachman R (eds): Hematology: Principles and Practice. Chicago, Year Book, 1972, pp 445–489

Macfarlane JR, Holman CW: Chylothorax. Am Rev Respir Dis 105:287–291, 1972

MacKenty JE: Malignant disease of larynx. Arch Otolaryngol 20:297–328, 1934

MacMurray FG, Katz S, Zimmerman HJ: Pleural-fluid eosinophilia. N Engl J Med 243:330–334, 1950

McGavic JS: Lymphomatous tumors of eye. Arch Ophthalmol 53:236–247, 1955

McNamara JJ, Kingsley WB, Paulson DL, et al: Primary lymphosarcoma of the lung. Ann Surg 169:133–140, 1969

May M, Lucente FE: "Bell's Palsy" caused by basal cell carcinoma. JAMA 220:1596–1597, 1972

Meese EH, Doohen DJ, Elliott RC, et al: Primary organ involvement in intrathoracic Hodgkin's disease. Chest 46:699–705, 1964

Meher-Homji DR, De Souza LJ, Mohanty B, et al: Unusual sternal mass in Hodgkin's disease. J Bone Joint [Br] Surg 54-A:402–404, 1972

Melamed MR: The cytological presentation of malignant lymphomas and related diseases in effusions. Cancer 16:413–431, 1963

Mills WH, Dominguez R, McCall JW: Simultaneous carcinoma and malignant lymphoma of larynx: Case report and review of literature. Laryngoscope 57:491–500, 1947

Mincer F, Botstein C, Schwarz G, et al: Moving strip irradiation in treatment of extensive neoplastic disease in the chest. Am J Roentgenol Radium Ther Nucl Med 108:278–283, 1970

Molander DW, Pack GT: Lymphosarcoma: Choice of treatment and end-results in 567 patients. Role of surgical treatment for cure and palliation. Rev Surg 20:3–31, 1963

Monahan DT: Hodgkin's disease of the lung. J Thorac Cardiovasc Surg 49:173–175, 1965

Moolten SE: Hodgkin's disease of the lung. Am J Cancer 21:253–294, 1934

Munnell ER: Current concepts of thoracic surgery in the management of lymphoma. Ann Thorac Surg 11:151–159, 1971

Musshoff K, Schmidt-Vollmer H, Merten D: Reticulum cell sarcoma: An oncologic model for a system of classifying the malignant lymphomas. Eur J Cancer 7:451–457, 1971

Neault RW, Van Scoy RE, Okazaki H, et al: Uveitis associated with isolated reticulum cell sarcoma of the brain. Am J Ophthalmol 73:431–436, 1972

Newall J, Friedman M: Reticulum cell sarcoma. Part II. Radiation dosage for each type. Radiology 94:643–647, 1970

Newall J, Friedman M, Narvaez F de: Extralymph-node reticulum-cell sarcoma. Radiology 91:708–712, 1968

Nickau RH, Reeves RJ: The pulmonary manifestations of Hodgkin's disease. J Fla Med Assoc 44:1224–1228, 1958

Nobler MP: Mental nerve palsy in malignant lymphoma. Cancer 24:122–127, 1969

Norris CM, Peale AR: Sarcoma of the larynx. Ann Otol Rhinol Laryngol 70:894–909, 1961

O'Donnell TJ: Two cases of lymphosarcoma of lung. Ir J Med Sci 1:324, 1926

Pack GT, Molander DW: The surgical treatment of Hodgkin's disease. Cancer Res 26:1254–1263, 1966

Papaioannou AN, Watson WL: Primary lymphoma of the lung: An appraisal of its natural history and a comparison with other localized lymphomas. J Thorac Cardiovasc Surg 49:373–387, 1965

Paparella MM, el-Fiky FM: Ear involvement in malignant lymphoma. Ann Otol Rhinol Laryngol 81:352–363, 1972

Parker RE, Reid JD: Five-year survey of results of cytological examination for lung cancer. NZ Med J 59:68–72, 1960

Peters MV, Brown TC, Davidson JW, et al: The value of locating occult disease in the treatment of Hodgkin's disease, in Rüttimann (ed): Progress in Lymphology, vol 1. Stuttgart, Thieme, 1967, pp 119–125

Pierce JC, Madge GE, Lee HM, et al: Lymphoma: A complication of renal allotransplantation in man. JAMA 219:1593–1597, 1972

Pierce RH, Hafermann MD, Kagan AR: Changes in the transverse cardiac diameter following mediastinal irradiation for Hodgkin's disease. Radiology 93:619–624, 1969

Pilcher J, Zubair M: Hodgkin's disease and pericardial effusion. Thorax 235:631–633, 1970

Podoshin L, Fradis M, Schalit M: Lymphosarcoma of the larynx. J Laryngol Otol 85:1063–1068, 1971

Reese AB: Tumors of The Eye (ed 2). New York, Hoeber, 1963

Richmond J, Sherman RS, Diamond HD, et al: Renal lesions associated with malignant lymphomas. Am J Med 32:184–207, 1962

Ridenhour CE, Spratt JS Jr: Epidermoid carcinoma of the skin involving the parotid gland. Am J Surg 112:504–507, 1966

Robbins JP, Fitz-Hugh S, Constable WC: Involvement of buccinator node in facial malignancy. Arch Otolaryngol 94:356–358, 1971

Robbins LL: The roentgenological appearance of parenchymal involvement of the lung by malignant lymphoma. Cancer 6:80–88, 1953

Roberts WC, Glancy DL, DeVita VT Jr: Heart in malignant lymphoma (Hodgkin's disease, lymphosarcoma, reticulum cell sarcoma and mycosis fungoides). Am J Cardiol 22:85–107, 1968

Rose AH: Primary lymphosarcoma of the lung. J Thorac Surg 33:254–263, 1957

Rosenberg BF, Spjut HJ, Gedney MM: Exfoliative cytology in metastatic cancer of the lung. N Engl J Med 261:226–231, 1959

Rosenberg SA, Diamond HD, Craver LF: Lymphosarcoma: Survival and the effects of therapy. Am J Roentgenol Radium Ther Nucl Med 85:521–532, 1961

Rosenberg SA, Diamond HD, Jaslowitz B, et al: Lymphosarcoma: A review of 1269 cases. Medicine 40:31–84, 1961

Roy PH, Carr DT, Payne WS: The problem of chylothorax. Mayo Clin Proc 42:457–467, 1967

Rubin M: Primary lymphoma of lung. J Thorac Cardiovasc Surg 56:293–303, 1968

Russell WO, Race GJ, Butler JJ, et al: Leukemia-Lymphoma. Chicago, Year Book, 1970, pp 375–385

al-Saleem T, Harwick R, Robbins R, et al: Malignant lymphomas of the pharynx. Cancer 26:1383–1387, 1970

Saltzstein SL: Pulmonary malignant lymphomas and pseudolymphomas: Classification, therapy, and prognosis. Cancer 16:928–955, 1963

Schamaun M: Surgical treatment in Hodgkin's disease, in Rüttimann A (ed): Progress in Lymphology, vol 1. Stuttgart, Thieme, 1967, pp 125–127

Scott JS: Malignant lymphoma of the thyroid gland. Br J Radiol 44:820, 1971 (Abstr)

Sippel HW, Samartano JG: Leukemia manifested as lymphosarcoma of the mandible: Report of a case. J Oral Surg 29:363–366, 1971

Smith DF, Klopp CT: The value of surgical removal of localized lymphomas. Surgery 49:469–476, 1961

Spencer H: Pathology of intrathoracic Hodgkin's disease. Proc R Soc Med 60:738–739, 1967

Spratt JS Jr: Surgical techniques for the management of mammary cancer, in Spratt JS, Donegan WL (ed): Cancer of the Breast. Philadelphia, Saunders, 1967, pp 88–116

Steel SJ: Hodgkin's disease of the lung with cavitation. Am Rev Respir Dis 89:736–744, 1964

Steg RF, Dahlin DC, Gores RJ: Malignant lymphoma of the mandible and maxillary region. Oral Surg 12:128–141, 1959

Sternberg WH, Sidransky H, Ochsner S: Primary malignant lymphomas of the lung. Cancer 12:806–819, 1959

Stewart IA, Stuart AE: Hodgkin's disease in the nose. J Laryngol Otol 85:1069–1073, 1971

Stolberg HO, Patt NL, MacEwen KF, et al: Hodgkin's disease of the lung: Roentgenologic-pathologic correlation. Am J Roentgenol Radium Ther Nucl Med 92:96–115, 1964

Stout AP: Results of treatment of lymphosarcoma. NY State J Med 47:158–164, 1947

Strickland B: Intra-thoracic Hodgkin's disease. Part II. Peripheral manifestations of Hodgkin's disease in the chest. Br J Radiol 40:930–938, 1967

Sugarbaker ED, Craver LF: Lymphosarcoma: Study of 196 cases with biopsy. JAMA 115:17–23, 112–117, 1940

Sulavik S, Katz S: Pleural Effusion: Some infrequently emphasized causes. Springfield, Ill, Thomas, 1963

Suprun H, Koss LG: The cytological study of sputum and bronchial washings in Hodgkin's disease with pulmonary involvement. Cancer 17:674–680, 1964

Swensson NL, Kurohara SS, George FW III: Complete regression, following abdominal irradiation alone, of chylothorax complicating lymphosarcoma with ascites. Radiology 87:635–640, 1966

Tillman HH: Malignant lymphomas involving the oral cavity and surrounding structures: Report of 12 cases. Oral Surg 19:60–72, 1965

Ultmann JE, Moran EM: Clinical course and complications in Hodgkin's disease Arch Intern Med 131:332–353, 1973

Valenca LM, Aisenberg AC, Kazemi H: Abnormalities of lung function in malignant lymphoma. Cancer 26:154–161, 1970

Van Heerden JA, Harrison EG Jr, Bernatz PE, et al: Mediastinal malignant lymphoma. Chest 57:518–529, 1970

Variakojis D, Fennessy JJ, Rappaport H: Diagnosis of Hodgkin's disease by bronchial brush biopsy. Chest 61:326–330, 1972

Walt AJ, Woolner LB, Black BM: Primary malignant lymphoma of the thyroid. Cancer 10:663–677, 1957

Wang CC: Malignant lymphoma of the larynx. Laryngoscope 82:97–100, 1972

Wang CC: Malignant lymphoma of Waldeyer's ring. Radiology 92:1335–1339, 1969

Wang CC: Management of malignant lymphoma of the Waldeyer's ring by irradiation. Eye Ear Nose Throat Mon 49:375–377, 1970

Wang CC: Primary malignant lymphoma of the oral cavity and paranasal sinuses. Radiology 100:151–153, 1971

Watson WL: Historical background, in Watson WL (ed): Lung cancer: A study of five thousand Memorial Hospital cases. St. Louis, Mosby, 1968, pp 1–14

Weick JK, Kiely JM, Harrison EG, et al: Pleural effusion in lymphoma. Cancer 31:848–853, 1973

Werf-Messing B van der: Reticulum cell sarcoma and lymphosarcoma: A retrospective study of potential survival in locoregional disease. Eur J Cancer 4:549–557, 1968

Whitcomb ME, Schwarz MI: Pleural effusion complicating intensive mediastinal radiation therapy. Am Rev Respir Dis 103:100–107, 1971

Whitcomb ME, Schwarz MI, Keller AR, et al: Hodgkin's disease of the lung. Am Rev Respir Dis 106:79–85, 1972

Williams A, Heitzman EP, Russell JP: Acute respiratory disease with lymphoma. NY State J Med 72:714–716, 1972

Williams GD, Flanigan WJ, Campbell GS: Surgical management of localized thoracic infections in immunosuppressed patients. Ann Thorac Surg 12:471–482, 1971

Williams KR, Burford TH: The management of chylothorax. Ann Surg 160:131–140, 1964

Williams RD, Andrews NC, Zanes RP: Major surgery in Hodgkin's disease. Surg Gynecol Obstet 93:636–640, 1951

Woolner LB, McConahey WM, Beahrs OH, et al: Primary malignant lymphoma of the thyroid: Review of forty-six cases. Am J Surg 111:502–523, 1966

10
Other Extranodal Malignant Lymphomas

BONE

Osseous Involvement in Lymphoma

Ziegler (1911) apparently was the first one to describe involvement of the osseous system in Hodgkin's disease. Gall and Mallory (1942) recorded that 23 percent of their patients with reticulum cell sarcomas had skeletal involvement. Vieta et al (1942) reviewed the literature and found that the incidence of bony involvement in malignant lymphomas varied from 1 percent to 34 percent. In their own series of 257 Hodgkin's patients, roentgenographic data showed lesions in 14.8 percent; in 213 patients with non-Hodgkin's lymphomas, it was 7 percent. They pointed out that half the lesions in Hodgkin's disease showed a combination of osteoblastic and osteolytic changes, whereas 85 percent of those in lymphosarcomas were osteolytic entirely. The average age of lymphosarcoma patients with bone lesions was considerably below that of the general group, and the patients also appeared to have a longer average survival after diagnosis. However, in 63 percent of the patients, the bone lesions occurred in the final third of the disease span; the authors suggested that development of such lesions was often a terminal event.

In 1269 patients with non-Hodgkin's lymphomas, Rosenberg et al (1961) found 15.6 percent had clinical or postmortem evidence of bone involvement. Bone lesions were the initial manifestation in 48 patients. Five of these were lymphosarcomas; 37, primary reticulum cell sarcomas of the bone; and 6, disseminated reticulum cell sarcomas. Molander and Pack (1963) reported that bone lesions developed in 14 percent of their series of 567 patients with lymphosarcomas; and 5 (1 percent) had primary reticulum cell sarcoma of the bone.

In an autopsy series of 690 patients with malignant lymphomas, Richmond et al (1962) found that 32 percent of the patients with Hodgkin's disease and 25 percent of those with reticulum cell sarcomas had bone and bone-marrow involvement.

Kooreman and Haex (1943) reported that roentgenographic picture of Hodgkin's disease involving the bone could be very confusing and suggested carcinomatosis, Paget's disease, osteomyelitis, etc. In Hodgkin's disease, sternal tumors are occasionally the presenting symptoms and are usually associated with disease in the mediastinum (p. 300). Fisher et al (1962) found by x-ray that 16 percent of 154 patients with Hodgkin's disease had bone lesions. The common sites of involvement, in decreasing frequency, were: the dorsal and lumbar spine (D12 to L4, which accounted for nearly 50 percent of the lesions); pelvis; ribs; femur; and sternum. They suggested that bone lesions could arise from three sources: hematogenous, de novo change of the reticuloendothelial tissue, or by invasion from contiguous diseased lymph nodes.

Musshoff et al (1964) found bone involvement in 14 percent of 470 patients with Hodgkin's disease. They showed that such lesions were usually secondary to diseased neighboring nodes, and rarely from hematogenous spread. As a group, patients with bone lesions demonstrated better survival than a similarly treated group without bone involvement. Stuhlbarg and Ellis (1965) found 19 percent of 158 patients with Hodgkin's disease had osseous involvement, and the average separate areas of bone lesions per patient was 1.5. They also found that patients with bone lesions had a longer survival than those without such manifestations (57 percent versus 16 percent 5 years after biopsy).

However, others found that bone lesions in Hodgkin's disease are not a good prognostic sign. Granger and Whitaker (1967) studied 108 patients with radiological lesions of the bone and found these represented part of the widespread disseminated disease. Over 60 percent of the patients died within 2 years and 80 percent within 3 years. Only about 4 percent survived 5 years, in contrast to the overall survival of 41 percent. But it must be pointed out that in about one-third of their patients the diagnosis was made not on bone changes, but on periosteal reactions, especially those occurring on the lateral border of the vertebrae. Beachley et al (1972)) found 10 of 49 cases of Hodgkin's disease involving the soft tissues had cortical bone lesions. There was no predilection regarding sex, age, or pathologic classification. In these 10 patients, the survival rate was similar to those without bone involvement.

Pack and Molander (1966) found skeletal lesions were the initial manifestations in 1.3 percent of patients with Hodgkin's disease. They commented that surgical therapy for Hodgkin's bone lesions, other than rare pathologic fractures, is seldom employed. Among the 240 patients hospitalized for Hodgkin's disease, 30 patients had major surgical procedures for palliation (Williams et al 1951). There were 3 who had laminectomy for epidural Hodgkin's disease of the spinal cord. Hustu and Pinkel (1967) pointed out that Hodgkin's disease of mediastinal and para-aortic nodes tended to invade vertebrae, resulting in infiltration of dorsal nerve roots, tabetic pain, or causing vertebral collapse and paraplegia. Hoskins (1967) commented that Hodgkin's tissue could provoke new bone formation in some cases; since sclerotic pelvic lesions were uncommon in younger individuals, the presence of abnormal osteoblastic lesions, especially in the iliac wings, should raise the suspicion of Hodgkin's disease when seen.

Newall et al (1968) found bone comprised about half of the extranodal lesions of patients with reticulum cell sarcomas (32 of 69 cases). They found that osseous lesions had a great propensity to spread to another bone (18 of 32 cases), and they might involve as many as 7 different bones in succession. With radiotherapy alone they obtained a 5-year survival rate of 39.8 percent (Newall and Friedman 1970a,b). They emphasized that the natural course of reticulum cell sarcoma in bone was unpredictable; it could metastasize to bone or viscera, regional or remote, occurring soon or years later. However, all manifestations of the disease, no matter how extensive, could and should be irradiated aggressively.

In the EFSCH series, among the 163 patients with Hodgkin's disease, 6 had bone lesions on x-ray at the time of diagnosis and 16 (10 percent) had involvement of the bone during their clinical courses. Six developed paraplegia of the lower extremities. Five of the six died within 8 months, but one (No. 28036) survived 18 months after laminectomy, postoperative radiotherapy, and chemotherapy (p. 387). Among the 364 patients with non-Hodgkin's lymphomas, 4 percent of those had bone lesions at the time of diagnosis and 11 percent after diagnosis. Four patients had laminectomy as one of the initial diagnostic procedures (p. 151). One patient (No. 21667) presented with femur lesions without significant adenopathy. Open bone biopsy established the diagnosis of well-differentiated histiocytic lymphoma (p. 153).

Primary Reticulum Cell Sarcoma of the Bone

Skeletal changes observed on x-rays can antedate splenomegaly and lymphadenopathy; occasionally a lymphoma presents as a primary bone tumor. For this reason, the orthopedist is sometimes in a position to diagnose lymphoma or leukemia before the hematologist, the internist, or the pediatrician.

Apparently, the earliest suggestion that reticulum cell sarcoma could arise from the reticuloendothelial tissues of bone was made by Oberling (1928). Parker and Jackson (1939) were the first to describe primary reticulum cell sarcoma of the bone as a separate entity, although histologically the lesion is identical with reticulum cell sarcoma elsewhere in the body. Coley et al (1950) further defined the disease as "arising in a single focus in bone and is capable of regional and distant metastasis." Hustu and Pinkel (1967) considered reticulum cell sarcoma of the bone as a true bone tumor rather than a disorder of the lymphatic system.

Parker and Jackson (1939) collected 17 cases of primary reticulum cell sarcoma of the bone from their own institution and the files of the Registry of Bone Sarcoma of the American College of Surgeons. Seven of the 17 patients were apparently free of disease for 10 or more years. Three of the 5 patients treated by amputation alone were alive from 3 to 11 years. Eight out of the 9 patients treated by amputation and radiation lived from 6 months to 14 years. Thus, they suggested that the best treatment procedure appeared to be early diagnosis by biopsy followed by immediate amputation and radiation.

Coley et al (1950) reported on 37 cases of primary reticulum cell sarcoma of the bone, representing 5.3 percent of 1091 cases of malignant bone tumors seen during the same period. They found that two-thirds of the patients were male; and the age of three-fourths of the patients were in the second to fourth decades. The long bones, particularly the femur, are the most commonly involved. The 5-year survival rate was 47 percent; and the 10-year rate, 38 percent. The recommended treatment was radiation therapy with a tumor depth dose of 3000–4000 rads. Among those who were treated curatively, there was a 10-year survival rate of 55.5 percent. Three patients developed recurrence and metastases 9 to 11 years after therapy and were further controlled by radiotherapy or surgery. Ivins and Dahlin (1953) reported 49 cases of reticulum cell sarcoma of the bone among 2000 primary osseous tumors. They also emphasized that this lesion was less malignant than other bone tumors.

Copeland (1967) reviewed his experience with 700 cases of primary malignant bone tumors of all types. The overall 5-year survival rates after irradiation appeared to be equivalent to results obtained by surgical ablation, which varied from 32 percent to 38 percent. He said that many patients ultimately underwent delayed amputation because of bone necrosis. Wang and Fleischli (1968) reviewed 21 patients with primary reticulum cell sarcoma of the bone. Of 16 patients who were treated 5 or more years, 8 had no recurrent disease. Of these 8, 5 were treated by radiotherapy and 3 by amputation. This result suggested that local tumors could be controlled by irradiation more favorably than by surgical resection (Wang 1968). Since the tumor is radio-sensitive, they recommended the initial choice of treatment to be aggressive radiotherapy (4500 to 5000 rads in 4 to 5 weeks) to the entire bone and adjacent soft tissue. If it failed to control the local disease, and if the patient still showed no distant metastasis, radical surgery could still be carried out as a back-up procedure for cure.

Shoji and Miller (1971) set up two additional criteria for the diagnosis of primary reticulum cell sarcoma of the bone: (1) metastasis on admission, if present, should be localized only to the regional lymph nodes; (2) there should be a 6-month interval between the onset of symptoms of primary focus and appearance of distant metastases. Among 147 cases of reticulum cell sarcomas involving the bone, 47 met these criteria. They found that age, sex, or duration of symptoms had nothing to do with prognosis; but involvement of the pelvic girdle had a poor prognosis. Of the 47 patients 36 were treated by irradiation, 1 had total excision, and 10 underwent combined therapy. Of the 10, 2 required internal fixation of pathological fractures before radiation therapy and 8 had surgery following irradiation. These 8 included 2 internal fixations for fracture; 2, hemipelvectomies; 1, local excision; and 1 each of forearm, forequarter, and midthigh amputations. The midthigh amputation was done for radiation-induced osteogenic sarcoma of the tibia; other operations were done for radiation failures or complications. In conclusion, the authors recommended administering large amounts of radiation during short periods to the whole bone as the treatment of choice, since patients who had only local irradiation did poorly. Contrary to the findings of others, they did not find any ideal time/dose relationship of radiation therapy in terms of 5-year survivals.

Miller and Nicholson (1971) reviewed 52 patients with reticulum cell sarcomas of the bone who were treated prior to 1956 with bacterial toxin therapy alone or in combination with surgery and/or radiotherapy, or who had concurrent infection. They had a 50 percent better 5-year survival rate than those who had surgery and/or radiotherapy alone (64 percent versus 35–42 percent). After analysis of multiple factors, they found that the most important ones in influencing the success of the toxin therapy were: (1) the stage and extent of the disease when toxins were begun; (2) the timing and dosage of radiotherapy (better if below 4000 rads); (3) the site, dosage, frequency, and duration of toxin therapy. Sufficient toxins should be given to elicit febrile reactions of 101° to 104°F, and 3 to 6 courses given in about 6 to 12 months (each course comprises 12 to 15 injections given in about 3 weeks). For optimal results, injection of microbial toxins should be instituted immediately after diagnosis, before or immediately after surgical procedures, including incisional biopsies. It is well demonstrated in experimental animals that surgical trauma or stress may markedly influence the subsequent establishment of metastases (Lee 1968a,b,c). This suggestion of using bacterial toxin as adjuvant therapy is very challenging. However, it should only be attempted in well-controlled clinical trials carried out in qualified cancer or medical centers.

SKIN AND SOFT TISSUE

Incidence

In patients with non-Hodgkin's lymphomas, Rosenberg et al (1961) reported that 5 percent of their 1269 patients presented with skin tumors. During the course of the disease, an additional 12.1 percent developed skin malignancy. Intracutaneous tumors were about twice as common as subcutaneous lesions. Other nonspecific lesions developed in 20.4 percent, herpes zoster in 4 percent, and pruritus in 10.6 percent. Molander and Pack (1963) found skin was the initial site of involvement in 3.1 percent of their 567 patients. Nearly half had lesions of the scalp. Eventually, skin was involved in 15.8 percent of these patients. In addition, 19.4 percent had nonspecific lesions of urticaria, erythema, and dermatitis. Four percent had herpes zoster and 8 percent, pruritus.

Among the 69 patients with extranodal reticulum cell sarcomas reported by Newall et al (1968), 1 had a tumor of the skin and 10 had tumors of the soft tissue. Of the latter lesions, the breast was affected in 3, left cheek in 1, muscle or fascia in 6. When the disease originates in connective tissue, they said both radio-resistant and radio-sensitive tumors might be encountered. Even when the tumor appears to be radio-sensitive, large fields should be used to encompass wide margins of normal tissues to prevent later satellite recurrences. The required radiation dose should be similar to that for bones (Newall and Friedman 1970a).

In patients with Hodgkin's disease, skin lesions occur in one-fourth to one-half of the cases, but specific lesions appear only in about 10 percent of the cases. The nonspecific lesions are numerous. Fromer and Geokas (1963) listed 10 types, including pruritus, exfoliative and eczematous dermatitis, pigmentation, erythema multiforme, etc. Samman (1967) said that true infiltration of the skin with Hodgkin's disease was rare and occurred in less than 1 percent of the cases. He mentioned 2 patients whose initial presenting features were skin lesions: small nodules restricted to small areas of the body. In a series of 316 cases of Hodgkin's disease, skin lesions have been reported in 4.1 percent of patients with Hodgkin's granuloma and in 12.5 percent of those with Hodgkin's sarcomas (Molander and Pack 1968).

Benninghoff et al (1970) encountered 10 patients with skin invasion among a series of 134 patients with Hodgkin's disease. The mode of invasion of the skin was by retrograde lymphatic spread from the corresponding involved regional lymph nodes. In a later series of 150 patients, skin or subcutaneous lesions appeared in 13 instances (Medina et al 1971). In 12 cases, the corresponding regional lymph nodes demonstrated involvement preceding the skin invasion. The 13th patient presented with simultaneous lesions of the skin and underlying tissues of the right breast as well as lymph nodes of the right axillary, supraclavicular, and cervical regions. Six of the 13 patients did not show evidence of systemic disease at the time that skin involvement appeared. In their series, there was no instance of direct invasion of the skin from underlying lymph nodes.

A benign skin condition easily misdiagnosed as malignant lymphoma was described by Macaulay (1968) and Feuerman and Sandbank (1972). The histopathological picture of this condition, "lymphomatoid papulosis," could be very suggestive of malignant lymphoma. The clinical appearances of the lesions were papulonodular with a strikingly symmetrical arrangement. They became necrotic within several weeks, healing spontaneously, and leaving small, pitted scars. There was a continual coming and going of these lesions lasting over several years.

Other benign skin conditions, even those due to known infectious agents, can occur concomitantly in patients with lymphomas. Haim et al (1971) reported a patient with lymphosarcoma who developed cutaneous tuberculosis during the asymptomatic period of his basic disease. Schein and Vickers (1972) reported a patient who had Hodgkin's disease superimposed on lupus vulgaris. The cutaneous tuberculosis was well controlled by antituberculosis treatment, but it became fulminant and systemic 3 months after therapy was discontinued and coincided with the discovery of extensive Hodgkin's disease. The patient also developed anergy to testing with tuberculin.

In the present EFSCH series, 1 of the 163 patients with Hodgkin's disease presented only with subcutaneous nodules over the midsternum, while 4 other patients had skin and soft tissue lesions as part of their generalized disease. Seven additional patients developed such lesions later. Four of the 364 patients with non-Hodgkin's lymphomas had skin and subcutaneous lesions as the only site of extranodal disease at diagnosis. A total of 8 percent (29 patients) had such lesions initially, and 13 percent (47 patients) had secondary lesions during the course of their disease.

Three non-Hodgkin's patients had special management problems in conjunction with their cutaneous lesions. One patient (No. 17335) had a mass in the left thigh followed by adenopathy in the neck and axilla (p. 184). All three lesions were treated by wide excision without further therapy, and he was alive 17 years later. Two other patients had radiotherapy for skin nodules of the leg. One (No. 22192) developed radiation necrosis after receiving radiotherapy of 3500 rads and required multiple procedures to achieve skin coverage. He finally developed osteomyelitis (p. 346). Another patient (No. 30125) developed recurrent multiple satellite lesions 18 months after receiving radiotherapy of 1800 rads. These were treated by wide excision and skin grafts. Two years after the original lesion, he had a superficial groin dissection in conjunction with an inguinal herniorrhaphy (p. 181). None of the 17 lymph nodes in the surgical specimen showed malignancy. However, 2 years later, he developed multiple satellite lesions again of the buttock and upper thigh. A celiotomy was performed and no intraabdominal malignancy was found. Infusion of chemotherapeutic agent through the iliac arteries was attempted, but the catheter had to be removed because of infection (p. 392). He was treated with systemic chemotherapy and was living with disease 2 years later, 12 years after the initial diagnosis.

Breast

Primary lymphoma of the breast is a rare entity, and Kückens (1929) has been credited with reporting the first observation of isolated Hodgkin's disease of the breast. Adair and Herrmann (1944) studied 5 cases and commented that primary lymphosarcoma of the breast, like that of the stomach, was a distinct entity. Adair et al (1945) found 5 out of 406 cases (1.3 percent) of Hodgkin's disease presented with mammary lesions, and 2 were primary lesions clinically. During the same period, there were 3901 carcinomas of the breast seen.

Hellwig (1947) reported a patient who had radical surgery alone for "lymphocytoma" of the breast. The patient was living and well 7 years later. In a series of 240 patients hospitalized for Hodgkin's disease, Williams et al (1951) reported 1 patient who had massive involvement of the breast. Palliative mastectomy was performed to remove the large painful tumor and also as an adjunct to x-ray therapy.

Lawler and Richie (1971) presented a case of primary reticulum cell sarcoma of the breast. They reviewed the literature and found 60 to 70 such cases reported. The condition occurred in women over a wide age range (9 to 75 years), but was most common in the sixth decade. Malignant lymphoma of the breast could be treated by surgery with or without postoperative irradiation, and the disease could be controlled for extended periods of time. Klopp (1968) commented that surgery should consist only of adequate removal of the tumor rather than a routine standard radical mastectomy.

Newall and Friedman (1970b) described the unusual case of a patient who had a radical mastectomy before the diagnosis of reticulum cell sarcoma was known. One year later, multiple bony and soft tissue lesions developed and she received several separate courses of radiotherapy over 16 months. Then for no detectable reason, the disease became quiescent and the patient was well 5 years after the mastectomy.

In the present EFSCH series, 4 of the 527 non-Hodgkin's patients with malignant lymphomas had radical mastectomies for diagnosis and therapy (p. 183).

Herpes Infection

Herpes infection of the skin appeared to have special importance in patients with malignant lymphomas. Dayan et al (1964) said herpes zoster was recorded in 0.2 percent of the patients with non-neoplastic diseases, but was reported as high as 13 percent in patients with lymphomas. They reported 4 patients who had generalized herpes zoster: 2 had Hodgkin's disease, and 2 had lymphosarcomas. Among 51 Hodgkin's patients who had autopsies, Casazza (1966) found 8 instances of herpes zoster and 1 of adult varicella.

Sokal and Firat (1965) found 8 percent of 600 patients with Hodgkin's disease had one or more episodes of varicella-zoster infections. Fifty-four episodes occurred in 49 patients; 4 infections occurred in patients with regional disease, and 50 in patients with disseminated disease. The location of active Hodgkin's disease appeared to determine the distribution of herpes zoster infection. In their series, corticosteroid therapy did not seem to be an important factor in precipitating varicella-zoster disease or causing dissemination of viral lesions. Localized herpes zoster did not constitute an ominous prognostic sign; but disseminated eruption, which occurred in 25 percent of the patients infected, did. Large doses of pooled human gamma-globulin might exert a favorable effect in some cases, but not in others. Hall et al (1973), Hryniuk et al (1972) found that disseminated herpes zoster infection could be controlled with low doses of cytosine arabinoside (10-40 mg/m^2/day) given intravenously. But Stevens et al (1973) showed that cytosine arabinoside (100 mg/m^2/day) had adverse effect in a controlled trial.

Wilson et al (1972) reported a high incidence (19 percent) of herpes zoster in 163 consecutive patients with Hodgkin's disease. All had irradiation for stages I to III disease. The chance of zoster infection was increased in patients with mixed cellularity histology, advanced disease, and in those patients who were treated with extensive irradiation. The majority of patients developed shingles within 6 months of primary treatment, suggesting immunosuppression by lumphoma and/or irradiation. Such early lesions did not associate with a high incidence of relapse of the Hodgkin's disease. However, in those in whom zoster occurred later than 6 months following primary therapy, a high incidence of lymphomatous recurrence (10 of 13) was noted. This finding suggested that herpes zoster could be an important prognostic factor in selected individuals.

Goffinet et al (1972) found herpes zoster and varicella infections occurring in 11.4 percent of 1130 patients with malignant lymphomas. In the 592 patients with Hodgkin's disease, the incidence was higher (15.4 percent). Although there was a slightly increased percentage of cases in the 30-year and younger age groups, no striking preponderance of infection was noted at any age. There was no seasonal variation of infection incidence. They found that the period of highest risk for zoster-varicella infection after radiotherapy appeared to be within 2 years. Patients with advanced disease, who were receiving multiple palliative chemotherapy for recurrent disease after radiotherapy, were more predisposed to disseminated herpes zoster. In particular, the authors found a significantly increased incidence of zoster-varicella infections in patients with Hodgkin's disease in 1969. One explanation appeared to be the institution, since 1968, of exploratory laparotomy and splenectomy on most of their new patients with Hodgkin's disease.

Twenty-two percent of the patients who had splenectomies developed zoster-varicella infections, in contrast with 13 percent of those without splenectomies (< 0.05). Another possible factor was the administration of combination chemotherapy (MOPP). The latter therapy, with or without splenectomy, had a high viral infection rate of 29 percent, in contrast to 12 percent in those without chemotherapy and without splenectomies.

In a study covering 2 recent years (1969–1971), Schimpff et al (1972) found an even higher incidence (25 percent) of patients with Hodgkin's disease developed varicella-zoster infections. The rate in patients with other lymphomas was only 8.7 percent (less than 2 percent in patients with acute leukemia or solid tumors). However, among the patients with Hodgkin's disease, they found that the incidence of zoster was similar whether or not a splenectomy had been done. Confirming the reports of others, the authors also found that patients with advanced Hodgkin's disease, cutaneous anergy, and recent nodal radiotherapy were inordinately predisposed to zoster. They believed zoster was an exogenously acquired reinfection in many patients, and that hyperimmune plasma could produce both subjective and objective improvement. In addition, strict isolation of infected patients should be carried out, and the exposed patients should be separated to prevent large outbreaks among susceptible individuals.

Stevens and Merigan (1972) found dissemination of herpes zoster infection was associated with concurrent Hodgkin's disease, or the use of immunosuppressive therapy, or both. They also demonstrated that local interferon production and hormonal antibodies were active in preventing or shortening dissemination of any initially localized disease.

Muller et al (1972) showed that patients with hematologic malignancies also were especially vulnerable to the development of herpes simplex infections affecting the skin and mucous membranes. All of these complications suggested that some common factors occurring in the course of patients with malignant lymphomas increased their susceptibility to viral infections. Whether the etiological factor is a disease-related host deterioration or a secondary effect of radiotherapy or chemotherapy, the clinical picture can all be explained on the basis of depressed or loss of immune competence. Thus, when patients with malignant conditions presented with unusual vesicular or ulcerative cutaneous lesions of an acute or chronic nature, they suggested that viral cultures should be obtained in addition to bacterial and fungal tests.

CENTRAL NERVOUS SYSTEM

Overall Incidence

Hunter and Rewcastle (1968) studied 393 patients who had intracranial metastatic neoplasms of various types; 3.5 percent had malignant lymphomas. Lesions of the cerebral hemisphere were demonstrated in 66 percent of the cases, cerebellar lesions in 33 percent, and brain stem involvement in 11.7 percent. The true incidence of malignant lymphomas among all primary tumors of the central nervous system is hard to find. Percy et al (1972) found that the average annual incidence rates per 100,000 general population were 12.5 for primary brain neoplasms; 1.9 for pituitary neoplasms; 1.3 for primary spinal cord; and 11.1 for metastatic lesions of the central nervous system.

Historically, Murchison (1869) was the first to describe a case in which a "lymphoblastoma" (probably Hodgkin's disease) invaded the dura near the foramen magnum. The patient did not have any clinical evidence of neurological disturbance. The first case of malignant lymphoma involving the spinal cord was described by Welch in 1910. Weil, in 1931, reviewed world literature and found 43 cases of central nervous system involvement secondary to Hodgkin's disease and added 3 cases of his own. Forty of the 46 cases had epidural masses. Winkelman and Moore (1941) reported 1 patient with Hodgkin's disease in the spinal dural space and another who had intracerebral lesions and dural plaques. They thought the cerebral lesions indicated a blood-borne metastasis.

Sparling et al (1947) studied a series of patients with lymphomas and leukemias. They reported the overall incidence of involvement of the nervous system at autopsy was 16 percent. There were 7 cases of Hodgkin's disease (1, primary in the brain; 2, questionably primary in the brain; 4, spinal epidural space), 9 cases of reticulum cell sarcoma (3, primary in the brain; 3, extending from cranial bone to meninges and brain; 3, epidural space), and 1 case of lymphosarcoma with spinal cord compression. Whisnant et al (1956) studied 76 cases and summarized that, during the course of the illness, lymphomas involved the central nervous system in 18 percent of those with Hodgkin's disease; 17 percent, lymphosarcoma; and 44 percent, reticulum cell sarcoma. The ratio of intraspinal-to-intracranial involvement is about 2 : 1 or 3 : 1. The most common types of intracranial abnormality in patients with malignant lymphomas were lesions of the skull with extension through the inner table to involve the meninges and cranial nerves. Whisnant et al (1956) cited 7 patients from the literature who had involvement of the basal cranial structures from lymphosarcoma of the nasopharynx or of the cerebellopontine angle. From their own data and a survey of the literature, the authors said the chief clinical syndromes of neurologic involvement were: (1) compression of the spinal cord by a collapsed vertebra or epidural deposit; (2) spinal cord necrosis after occlusion of vascular supply by the tumor; (3) compression of nerves in the abdomen and pelvis by a retroperitoneal tumor; (4) diffuse meningeal involvement with or without cranial or spinal nerve involvement; (5) involvement of basal intracranial structures, including cranial nerves; and (6) intracerebral lymphomas.

Diamond (1957) reported 12.9 percent of 1583 Hodgkin's patients and 13.8 percent of 5778 patients with malignant lymphomas and leukemia had significant neurologic complications. Williams et al (1958) reported that 302 out of 1992 Hodgkin's patients and 196 out of 1773 non-Hodgkin's lymphoma patients had neurological complications (incidence rates of 15.2 percent and 11.1 percent, respectively). The 6 categories of neurological manifestations were: herpes zoster, peripheral nerve palsies, spinal cord compression, cerebral syndromes, cranial nerve palsies, and infections or hemorrhage. Most lymphoma patients manifested cerebral symptoms without histological evidence of involvement of the brain, while leukemia patients, not uncommonly, had asymptomatic cerebral involvement. Cranial and peripheral nerve involvements occurred in 1.1 percent and 2.3 percent, respectively; these usually were due to local compression by the tumor, and about half were cleared with radiotherapy. The third, sixth, and seventh cranial nerves are affected most often. The site of involvement for peripheral nerves was equally divided between a "central" group (recurrent laryngeal, cervical sympathetic, and phrenic nerves) and a "peripheral" group (brachial plexus, cervical through sacral plexuses). The latter group had a 65 percent chance of excellent response compared with 22 percent for the former.

Currie and Henson (1971) found that 26 percent of 774 patients who had "reticulosis" developed malignant and nonmalignant neurological syndromes. Their term "reticulosis" included multiple myeloma, reticulum cell sarcoma, Hodgkin's disease, follicular lymphoma, lymphosarcoma, chronic and acute leukemia, and polycythemia vera. Malignant tumor deposits, most of them involving compression of the spinal cord or nerve roots, accounted for only about half of these. Spinal cord involvement was more common than intracranial lesions in all reticulosis except leukemia. Nonmalignant complications caused about 25 percent of all the neurological manifestations; the most common ones were infection and vascular lesions. Herpes zoster occurred most frequently in those with Hodgkin's disease; hemorrhage in patients with thrombocytopenia and thrombosis in those with polycythemia vera. Nonmetastatic neurological syndromes of obscure origin were detected in 2.5 percent of the whole group. Three patients developed progressive multifocal leucoencephalopathy, which is an uncommon demyelinating disease usually associated with Hodgkin's disease or lymphosarcoma (Richardson 1965; Dolman and Cairns 1961; Deep et al 1964). The etiology is unknown but appears to be related to viral infection or autoimmune disease (Silverman and Rubinstein 1965; Woodhouse 1967).

It was pointed out that meningitis, secondary to bacterial or viral origin, must be considered in every patient with malignant lymphoma and headache, stiff neck, or unexplained fever. The most common organisms are: Cryptococcus neoformans, Listeria monocytogenes, herpes zoster virus, Diplococcus pneumoniae, and Toxoplasma gondii (Williams et al 1959). Vietzke et al (1968) reviewed 20 cases with toxoplasmosis infection, showing that this condition had an unusual predilection for the central nervous system. Eight of the 20 patients had Hodgkin's disease, and 4 had toxoplasmosis encephalitis. Rosenblum and Hadfield (1972) described granulomatous angiitis of the brain and cord with thrombosis of the affected vessels in

2 patients; both had varicella and lymphosarcoma but did not have involvement of the central nervous system.

One aspect of neurological complications of lymphoma and leukemia which is becoming increasingly important is the damage done to the nervous system secondary to modern therapy. Vincristine neuropathy, radiation myelopathy, and cerebral hemorrhage due to thrombocytopenia induced by cytotoxic agents are all beginning to contribute appreciably to the neurological complications seen in these disorders. Similarly, infection of the nervous system will probably increase as immunosuppressive drugs are employed in higher doses and in more potent combinations. The effect of radiation therapy on the central nervous system is discussed in more detail on pp. 369–370.

It has been suggested that intracranial lymphomas may themselves be produced by immunosuppressive therapy, because their prevalence is higher than expected in patients who have received organ transplants (Schneck and Penn 1971). Among 52 known instances of malignant tumors in long-term survivors who received renal transplants, 11 represented lymphomas involving the brain. In 8 of these patients, the brain was the only organ involved. Sharma et al (1972) added a ninth patient who had a localized cerebellar reticulum cell sarcoma probably of leptomeningeal origin.

Brain

Abbott and Adson (1943) reported 2 cases of primary intracranial lymphosarcoma which originated from dura or bone. Sparling and Adams (1946) apparently reported the first case of primary Hodgkin's sarcoma of the brain. They also encountered 2 cases with involvement of the cerebellum.

Troland et al (1950) reported 5 cases of primary reticulum cell sarcoma of the brain and reviewed the literature. They concluded that these lesions and those of Hodgkin's disease and lymphosarcoma probably should be grouped as mesenchymal tumors of the brain (under the category of microglioma) and not as malignant lymphomas. However, Plafker et al (1972) reported a case of neoplasm of the reticuloendothelial tissue involving both the brain and viscera. The viscera lesions were typical of reticulum cell sarcoma. The multiple lesions in the brain appeared to have arisen from similar reticulum cells within the brain. Thus, the microglioma or primary lymphoma in the brain only represented a pattern of morphologic differentiation peculiar to the reticuloendothelial system in the central nervous system.

Schaumburg et al (1972) reviewed 25 cases of primary reticulum cell sarcomas of the nervous system. Twenty-three patients died, 15 of whom were autopsied. The tumors remained confined to the nervous system in all but 1 patient and originated from all areas of the central nervous system except the spinal cord. The lesion appeared to be very radio-sensitive, and several patients had 2 and 3 separate recurrences completely eliminated by radiotherapy.

Most of the malignant lymphomas involving the brain occurred as part of the generalized disease. Sparling et al (1947) said that Hodgkin's disease showed a predilection for the cerebellum and frontal lobes, whereas reticulum cell sarcoma more often invaded the temporal lobes. Fein and Newill (1954) cited 4 patients reported in the literature who had possible invasion of the brain by Hodgkin's disease and added a patient of their own who had invasion of both cerebral hemispheres by Hodgkin's granuloma. John and Nabarro (1955) also reviewed the literature and found 7 other cases of actual invasion of the brain substance in Hodgkin's disease confirmed by postmortem examination. They reported on a patient who had partial removal of the lesion with considerable clinical improvement. In addition, they found 5 patients with generalized lymphosarcoma and 1 with reticulum cell sarcoma who had clinical evidence of intracranial deposits confirmed at autopsy. Schricker and Smith (1955) described a patient with Hodgkin's granuloma of the right temporal lobe who presented with primary intracerebral manifestations. The tumor was removed surgically and radiotherapy (1500 rads) given locally. The patient had no evidence of systemic or recurrent disease for 3 years.

Malignant lymphoma of the posterior pituitary with diabetes insipidus has been reported but is not too common. Melton and McNamara (1946) found 4 cases of "lymphogranuloma" of the hypophysis with 3 showing the symptoms of diabetes insipidus. They added a fourth case. White (1955) reviewed 219 cases with diabetes insipidus and said 43 percent of these were secondary to cerebral and pituitary neoplasms (including few malignant lymphomas). Recommended treatment included administration of exogenous antidiuretic hormone and reduction of urinary solute load. Williams et al (1958) found 32 of 5778 patients with malignant lymphomas had pituitary involvement when autopsied, and only 1 patient manifested clinical diabetes insipidus. Spittle (1966) described a case of inappropriate secretion of antidiuretic hormone in Hodgkin's disease. Miller et al (1971) reported a similar case but with reticulum cell sarcoma. Hadfield et al (1972) described a case of hypoglycemia secondary to invasion of the hypothalamus by lymphosarcoma.

Intracranial malignant lymphomas can have unusual neurological findings, which cause confusion in diagnosis. Hodgkin's disease with involvement of cranial meninges could present as acute meningoencephalitis (Barker 1934). Allison and Gordon (1955) and Clausen et al (1956) presented cases with diffuse lymphosarcomatosis of the central nervous system simulating acute infectious polyneuritis. Lascelles and Burston (1962) reported a case of Hodgkin's disease with involvement of several cranial nerves and diabetes insipidus. Symptoms of the cranial nerve pareses fluctuated because there were periods of ischemia secondary to vascular thrombosis, necrosis, and transient edema. There was no direct infiltration by the tumor. Cerebral Hodgkin's lesions could also cause epileptic seizures and cerebellar symptoms (Haynal and Regli 1964). Kaufman (1965) presented a case diagnosed as Guillain-Barre syndrome and diabetes insipidus. Diffuse Hodgkin's involvement of the meninges, nerve roots, and brain was found at autopsy. Sohn et al (1967) presented a case of Hodgkin's disease originating in the unusual site of the hypothalamus and extending to the optic chiasm and cranial nerves. Clinically, the patient had diabetes insipidus, hallucination, and peripheral neuropathy.

On the other hand, many more cerebral symptoms occurred during the course of malignant lymphoma without corresponding lesions documented by tissue examinations. Williams et al (1958) found 31 percent of those lymphomatous patients with cerebral manifestations had spontaneous remission of symptoms. Of 35 Hodgkin's patients with true cerebral symptoms, only 4 had verified cerebral deposits. Todd (1967) reported that intracranial lesions of Hodgkin's disease probably occurred only in 0.25–0.5 percent of the patients. He suggested that the most common explanations for cerebral manifestations in Hodgkin's disease, in the order of frequency, were: (1) complication of fever, anemia, uremia, steroid therapy, or chemotherapy; (2) local infiltrations of Hodgkin's disease; and (3) complication of multifocal leukoencephalopathy. Currie and Henson (1971) reported that neurological syndromes occurred in 24 percent of 210 patients with Hodgkin's disease, and cranial deposits were found in 1.5 percent. The comparable figures for 136 patients with lymphosarcomas were 25 percent and 3 percent; and for 63 patients with reticulum cell sarcomas, 27 percent and 10 percent.

Marshall et al (1968) reviewed the world literature on invasive Hodgkin's disease of the brain, excluding those cases of secondary pressure changes from bone and meningeal tumors or ischemic changes due to compression of the vessel by the tumor. They found 12 cases of well-documented secondary invasion of brain substance and added 2 cases of their own. However, many reports, such as John and Nabarro (1955), Williams et al (1958), Todd (1967), and Sohn et al (1967) were not included in their review. They commented that Hodgkin's disease could present initially with complaints of the central nervous system, and diffuse meningeal presentation should be distinguished from complicating infectious disease. Two of the 14 patients had microscopical evidence of Hodgkin's disease of the brain without gross abnormality. The preponderance of evidence indicated that brain tissue invasion was accomplished through perivascular spaces as extensions from overlying meningeal tumors.

None of the 14 cases reported by Marshall et al (1968) demonstrated Hodgkin's disease within the spinal cord tissue. However, Todd (1967) reported one case with Hodgkin's granuloma infiltration of the small vessels of the pia and the cord. Parker (1972) reported another case of Hodgkin's disease involving cranial nerves, meninges, and the thoracic spinal cord. He pointed out that the spinal cord was frequently excluded from routine postmortem examination. Thus, the involvement of this structure with malignant tumors could not be evaluated accurately.

Occasionally craniotomy for diagnostic purposes and/or palliative resections has been carried out. Williams et al (1959) reported a patient who developed neurologic symptoms 2.5 years after the initial diagnosis of Hodgkin's disease. At craniotomy, a 3-cm tumor was found in the left frontal region. He was treated with radiotherapy (3900 rads) and was well 6 years later. Craver (1964) mentioned an example of a life-threatening situation that required surgical removal: a bulky mass invading both plates of the skull and extending into the brain.

Thompson and DeNardo (1969) reported a patient who had cerebral symptoms 4 years after the onset of Hodgkin's disease. A radioisotope brain scan established the diagnosis which was confirmed by biopsy. The entire brain was irradiated with 4000 rads, and serial brain scans showed continued diminution of abnormal radioactivity. In another report of 8 patients with intracranial lymphomas (4, Hodgkin's disease; 3, reticulum cell sarcoma; 1, lymphosarcoma), Thompson et al (1972) described three basic patterns of radioisotopic findings: nodular, meningitic, and combinations thereof. Among 7 patients who had examinations of the cerebrospinal fluid, 6 had elevated proteins, 5 had increased white blood cell counts, and 3 had positive malignant cells.

Leeds et al (1971) used direct serial magnification angiography which improved vascular details and detected the changes involving small intracerebral vessels. Two patterns of cerebral lymphoma were described: (1) a localized, but not encapsulated, mass with the gross appearance of a glioma; and (2) a diffuse cellular infiltration with cerebral swelling resembling encephalitis.

Griffin et al (1971) reported 21 patients with lymphomatous infiltration of the leptomeninges diagnosed by cytology of the cerebrospinal fluid during life and confirmed at autopsy. They found this complication particularly common in patients with histiocytic lymphoma, which frequently presented as cranial nerve palsies. They suggested that aggressive therapy, especially with methotraxate, might be worthwhile.

It is apparent that when accurate diagnosis can be made by cytology, radioisotope scan, and/or angiographic examination, and when palliation can be achieved by the administration of radiotherapy and/or chemotherapy, the necessity of utilizing surgical procedures for diagnosis and treatment will be greatly diminished.

Spinal Cord

The first description of compression of the spinal cord resulting from a tumor was by Mongagni in 1769; and the first successful removal of a spinal cord tumor by surgery was achieved by Horsley in 1887 (Rubin et al 1969). Welch (1910) was given the credit for being the first to report a case of malignant lymphoma involving the spinal cord. Smith and Stenstrom (1948) reported 11 cases of cord compression due to Hodgkin's disease.

They suggested that the treatment of choice should be immediate laminectomy followed by deep x-ray treatment.

Lawes and Ham (1953) raised the problem of radiation edema and
favored the initial use of nitrogen mustard. However, Pack and Molander
(1966) commented that, "This contingency seldom occurs unless previous
radiation therapy has been given, or the focus of Hodgkin's disease in the
epidural space is fibrotic and unusually radioresistant. Under these and
certain other circumstances, laminectomy is feasible for quick decompression. Laminectomy is also indicated whenever there is bony compression
of the spinal cord secondary to vertebral fracture due to osteolytic Hodgkin's
disease."

Love et al (1954) presented 39 patients with malignant lymphoma (7
had Hodgkin's disease) in which the primary symptoms were tumors of
the spinal cord without clinical involvement elsewhere in the body. The
diagnosis was made by surgical decompression in all. In the series of 5778
patients reported by Williams et al (1958), symptoms of spinal cord compression were present in about 2 percent of the patients with lymphomas and
leukemia. Spinal cord symptoms were usually caused by epidural lymphomas, and recovery was more frequent in patients who had Hodgkin's
disease, less than complete paraplegia, and in those who received radiotherapy combined with chemotherapy and/or laminectomy. Patients with
Hodgkin's disease had a 66 percent rate of excellent results compared with
a 29 percent rate for those with other lymphomas and leukemia. Excellent
result was achieved only in 16 percent of those with complete paraplegia,
whereas patients with lesser motor symptoms had a 68 percent rate. Seventy-
three percent of the patients who had combination therapy had excellent
results versus 43 percent of those treated with radiotherapy alone. The
optimal therapy for spinal cord lesions recommended by the authors was
to give a course of nitrogen mustard followed by radiotherapy to cover
4 spinal segments above and below the level of neurological lesions.

Botterell and Fitzgerald (1959) found the mean interval from the onset
of pain to physical findings or other symptoms was 3.5 months. In their
29 patients, 25 had thoracic extradural lymphomas; 3, lumbar; and 1, the
cervical spine. Bhagwati and McKissock (1961) also found that the thoracic
spine is the most common site of cord compression in patients with Hodgkin's
disease, reflecting the frequent involvement of mediastinal lymph nodes.
Bansal et al (1967) studied 60 patients with metastatic extramedullary lesions,
and 10 of these had lymphomas or multiple myelomas. Their survival ranged
from 2 months to 4.5 years. They found no neurological recovery in patients
who had sphincteric involvement lasting more than a day.

Rubin et al (1969) reviewed the literature from 1929 to 1967 and questioned the recommended treatment of extradural malignant tumors with
laminectomy and surgical resection with or without the use of radiotherapy
or chemotherapy postoperatively. (Steroids have been used in order to

decrease edema as well as for their lympholytic effect.) Their own experimental data showed that the rate of relieving spinal cord compression was related to the speed of onset, extent of neurological loss, and degree of paralysis. And they found high-dose radiotherapy alone could give prompt relief (Rubin 1969). They administered radiotherapy up to 500 rads daily initially, using large fields to include mediastinal or retroperitoneal nodes and encompassing 2 vertebra above and below the obstructing lesion. They pointed out that lymphoma and metastatic carcinoma, unlike meningioma or neuroma, rarely developed circumferential lesions, and laminectomy might further weaken an already damaged vertebral column. In their experience, 5 patients with Hodgkin's disease and reticulum cell sarcoma recovered with radiotherapy alone, including 1 patient who had treatment to two separate areas.

Silverberg and Jacobs (1971) also felt that laminectomy was not always mandatory. Among their 120 patients with Hodgkin's disease, 5 had secondary spinal cord lesions. Four of these 5 were given alkylating agents intravenously with rapid regression of neurological symptoms. Definitive radiotherapy was then given. In addition to nitrogen mustard, other useful chemotherapeutic agents included cyclophosphamide and vinblastine (Silverberg and Jacobs 1971; Bonadonna 1971).

Currie and Henson (1971) found that the incidence of spinal cord compression was 3 percent for patient with reticulum cell sarcomas, 4.5 percent for Hodgkin's disease, and 6 percent for lymphosarcomas. Mullins et al (1971) gave their corresponding figures as 0.5 percent, 4.3 percent, and 1.3 percent, respectively. They reported on 21 cases and 20 had laminectomy. Mechanical compression of the cord by an epidural tumor was the major factor in producing the neurologic deficit. Tumor growth along the intervertebral foramina appeared to be the most common route of spread to the epidural space. Other factors, such as occlusion of radicular arteries, might also be important in the pathogenesis of spinal cord dysfunction (Verity 1968).

Mullins et al (1971) described the prodromal symptoms of extradural tumors as being characterized by back pain, radicular pain, and, occasionally, the appearance of herpes zoster. Back pain occurred in 85 percent of the cases with a mean duration of 7.4 months. They suggested the possibility of avoiding complete spinal cord compression by earlier use of myelography. The contrast medium should be left in situ to delineate the response of tumor to irradiation. They emphasized that the current trend of management was to use irradiation alone and save laminectomy for patients who were severely affected or who did not show rapid improvement with irradiation. In conclusion, they said that "vigorous management should be undertaken even in the most severe cases, especially in view of instances of useful recovery reported after prolonged and complete paraplegia."

SUMMARY

Involvement of the bone can be demonstrated by x-rays in about 15 percent of the patients with malignant lymphomas; in 1–4 percent of the cases, this was the initial manifestation. The lesions in Hodgkin's disease showed a combination of osteoblastic and osteolytic changes, whereas the predominent tumors of non-Hodgkin's lymphomas are osteolytic. At autopsy, the incidence in Hodgkin's disease is higher than that of the non-Hodgkin's lymphomas. The most common site is the dorsal and lumbar spine, usually secondary to invasion from contiguous lymphadenopathy.

Primary reticulum cell sarcoma of the bone represented about 2–5 percent of all osseous malignant tumors. The prognosis is better than other bone tumors (5 year survival rate about 50 percent). The treatment of choice appears to be aggressive radiotherapy to the whole bone, reserving radical surgery for resistent tumors or radiation failures.

Skin and soft tissues, including breast, can be involved with malignant lymphoma, in about 5 percent of the patients initially and 15 eventually. Herpes zoster and many nonspecific dermatological conditions occurred much more frequently. The chance of developing herpes zoster infection was higher in patients with Hodgkin's disease, especially those with advanced disease or those who were treated with multiple chemotherapy and/or extensive irradiation, and, possibly, those who had splenectomy.

Clinically, about 10–15 percent of the patients with malignant lymphoma had neurological complications. Tumor deposit accounted for about half of the symptoms; and non-malignant lesions caused about 25 percent of all the neurological manifestations. Lesions of the spinal cord are more than twice as common as intracranial involvement. Cranial and peripheral nerve palsies occurred in 1–2 percent of the patients.

Most of the malignant lymphomas of the brain occurred secondary to lesions of the skull and meninges, as part of the generalized disease. However, primary reticulum cell sarcomas of the nervous system have been reported. Most lymphoma patients manifested cerebral symptoms without histological evidence of involvement of the brain by the tumor. On the other hand, intracranial malignant lymphomas often present with unusual neurological findings. Radioisotopic brain scan and cytologic examination of the cerebrospinal fluids can be very useful in the diagnosis of intracranial lymphomas.

Symptoms of spinal cord compression are present in about 5 percent of the patients with malignant lymphomas, especially those with Hodgkin's disease; and lesions of the thoracic spine were most common. Tumor growth along the intervertebral foramina appeared to be the major route of spread to the epidural space. Radiotherapy and/or chemotherapy is the treatment of choice, but occasionally laminectomy is required for diagnosis, for rapid decompression, and for radio-resistant lesions.

REFERENCES

Abbott KH, Adson AW: Primary intracranial lymphosarcoma: Report of 2 cases and review of literature. Arch Surg 47: 147–159, 1943

Adair FE, Craver LF, Herrmann JB: Hodgkin's disease of breast. Surg Gynecol Obstet 80:205–210, 1945

Adair FE, Herrmann JB: Primary lymphosarcoma of breast. Surgery 16:836–853, 1944

Allison RS, Gordon DS: Reticulosis of nervous system simulating acute infective polyneuritis. Lancet 2:120–122, 1955

Bansal S, Brady LW, Olsen A, et al: The treatment of metastatic spinal cord tumors. JAMA 202:686–688, 1967

Barker LF: Severe acute meningoencephalopathy of lymphogranulomatous origin occurring in course of Hodgkin's disease. Arch Neurol Psychiatr 32: 1038–1044, 1934

Beachley MC, Lau BP, King ER: Bone involvement in Hodgkin's disease. Am J Roentgenol Radium Ther Nucl Med 114:559–563, 1972

Benninghoff DL, Medina A, Alexander LL, et al: The mode of spread of Hodgkin's disease to the skin. Cancer 26:1135–1140, 1970

Bhagwati SN, McKissock W: Spinal cord compression in Hodgkin's disease. Br J Surg 48:672–676, 1961

Bonadonna G: Present position of radical and palliative treatment of malignant lymphomas, in Chiappa S, Musumec R, Uslenghi C (eds): Endolymphatic Radiotherapy in Malignant Lymphomas. New York, Springer-Verlag, 1971, pp 1–22

Botterell EH, Fitzgerald GW: Spinal cord compression produced by extradural malignant tumors: Early recognition, treatment and results. Can Med Assoc J 80:791–96, 1959

Casazza AR, Duvall CP, Carbone PP: Summary of infectious complications occurring in patients with Hodgkin's disease. Cancer Res 26:1290–1296, 1966

Clausen RE, Lincoln AF, Silberman HK: Diffuse lymphosarcomatosis of the central nervous system simulating infectious polyneuritis. Am J Med 20:292–300, 1956

Coley BL, Higinbotham NL, Groesbeck HP: Primary reticulum-cell sarcoma of bone. Radiology 55:641–658, 1950

Copeland MM: Primary malignant tumors of bone: Evaluation of current diagnosis and treatment. Cancer 20:738–746, 1967

Craver LF: Treatment of Hodgkin's disease, in Pack GT, Ariel IM (eds): Treatment of Cancer and Allied Diseases (ed 2). New York, Hoeber, 1964, pp 168–191

Currie S, Henson RA: Neurological syndromes in the reticuloses. Brain 94: 307–320, 1971

Dayan AD, Morgan HE, Hope-Stone HF, et al.: Disseminated herpes zoster in the reticuloses. Am J Roentgenol Radium Ther Nucl Med 92:116–123, 1964

Deep WD, Fraumeni JF, Tashima CK, et al: Leukoencephalopathy and dermatomyositis in Hodgkin's disease. Arch Intern Med 113:635–640, 1964

Diamond HD: Hodgkin's disease: Neurologic sequelae. Mo Med 54:945–956, 1957

Dolman CL, Cairns AR: Leukoencephalopathy associated with Hodgkin's disease. Neurology 11:349–353, 1961

Fein SB, Newill VA: Cerebral Hodgkin's disease: Case report of Hodgkin's granuloma with cerebral invasion. Am J Med 17:291–294, 1954

Feuerman EJ, Sandbank M: Lymphomatoid papulosis. Arch Dermatol 105:233–235, 1972

Fisher AM, Kendall B, Van Leuven BD: Hodgkin's disease: A radiological survey. Clin Radiol 13:115–127, 1962

Fromer JL, Geokas MC: Cutaneous manifestations in lymphomas. NY State J Med 63:3222–3228, 1963

Gall EA, Mallory TB: Malignant lymphoma: clinico-pathologic survey of 618 cases. Am J Pathol 18:381–429, 1942

Goffinet DR, Glatstein EJ, Merigan TC: Herpes zoster-varicella infections and lymphoma. Ann Intern Med 76:235–240, 1972

Granger W, Whitaker R: Hodgkin's disease in bone, with special reference to periosteal reaction. Br J Radiol 40: 939–948, 1967

Griffin JW, Thompson RW, Mitchinson MJ, et al: Lymphomatous leptomeningitis. Am J Med 51:200–208, 1971

Hadfield MG, Vennart GP, Rosenblum WI: Hypoglycemia: Invasion of hypothalamus by lymphosarcoma. Arch Pathol 94: 317–321, 1972

Haim S, Friedman-Birnbaum R, Tatarsky I: Lymphosarcoma and cutaneous tuberculosis: Report of a case. Dermatologica 143:221–226, 1971

Hall TC, Douglas RG, Holton C, et al: Cytosine arabinoside treatment of varicella-zoster. Postgrad Med J 49: 429–436, 1973

Haynal A, Regli F: Neurologische Symptome bei Morbus Hodgkin. Schweiz Med Wochenschr 94:1515–1518, 1964

Hellwig CA: Malignant lymphoma: Value of radical surgery in selected cases. Surg Gynecol Obstet 84:950–958, 1947

Hoskins EO: Unusual radiological manifestations of Hodgkin's disease. Proc R Soc Med 60:729–732, 1967

Hryniuk W, Foerster J, Shojania M, et al: Cytarabine for hypesvirus infections. JAMA 219:715–718, 1973

Hunter KM, Rewcastle NB: Metastatic neoplasms of the brain stem. Can Med Assoc J 98:1–7, 1968

Ivins JC, Dahlin DC: Reticulum-cell sarcoma of bone. J Bone Joint Surg 35—A: 835–842, 1953

John HT, Nabarro JD: Intracranial manifestations of malignant lymphoma. Br J Cancer 9:386–400, 1955

Kaufman G: Hodgkin's disease involving the central nervous system. Arch Neurol 13:555–558, 1965

Klopp CT: Surgical treatment of primary lymphoma. Cancer Management: A special graduate course on cancer. Sponsored by American Cancer Society, Inc. Philadelphia, Lippincott, 1968, pp 393–397

Kooreman PJ, Haex AJ: Hodgkin's disease of skeleton. Acta Med Scand 115: 117–196, 1943

Kückens H: Zur Frage der zyklischen Veränderungen der Mamma und des menschlichen Scheidenepithels. z Geburtshilfe Perinatol 93:55–76, 1929

Lascelles RG, Burston J: Hodgkin's disease: Disease presenting with symptoms of cranial nerve involvement. Arch Neurol 7: 359–364, 1962

Lawes FA, Ham HJ: Case of Hodgkin's disease with spinal cord involvement treated by nitrogen mustard. Med J Aust 1: 104–106, 1953

Lawler MR Jr, Richie RE: Reticulum cell sarcoma of the breast. Cancer 20:1438–1446, 1971

Lee YN: Experimental studies of metastases: A review. Part I. Mo Med 65:36–39, 1968a

Lee YN: Experimental studies of metastases: A review. Part II. Mo Med 65:123–128, 1968b

Lee YN: Experimental studies of metastases: A review. Part III. Mo Med 65:205–210, 1968c

Leeds NE, Rosenblatt R, Zimmerman HM: Focal angiographic changes of cerebral lymphoma with pathologic correlation: A report of two cases. Radiology 99:595–599, 1971

Love JG, Miller RH, Kernohan JW: Lymphomas of spinal epidural space. Arch Surg 69:66–76, 1954

Macaulay WL: Lymphomatoid papulosis: A continuing self-healing eruption, clinically benign-histologically malignant. Arch Dermatol 97:23–30, 1968

Marshall G, Roessmann U, Van den Noort S: Invasive Hodgkin's disease of brain: Report of two new cases and review of American and European literature with clinical-pathologic correlations. Cancer 22:621–630, 1968

Medina A, Benninghoff DL, Camiel MR: Extra nodal spread of Hodgkin's disease. Am J Roentgenol Radium Ther Nucl Med 111:368–375, 1971

Melton EI, McNamara WL: Hodgkin's disease involving pituitary gland with diabetes insipidus. Ann Intern Med 25: 525–531, 1946

Miller R, Ashkar FS, Rudzinski DJ: Inappropriate secretion of anti-diuretic hormone in reticulum cell sarcoma. South Med J 64:763–764, 1971

Miller TR, Nicholson JT: End results in reticulum-cell sarcoma of bone treated by bacterial toxin therapy alone or combined with surgery and/or radiotherapy (47 cases) or with concurrent infection (5 cases). Cancer 27:524–548, 1971

Molander DW and Pack GT: Lymphosarcoma: Choice of treatment and end-results in 567 patients. Role of surgical treatment for cure and palliation. Rev Surg 20:3–31, 1963

Molander DW, Pack GT: Review of treatment and results in 316 patients, in Molander DW, Pack GT (eds): Hodgkin's disease. Springfield, Ill, Thomas, 1968, pp 132–205

Muller SA, Herrmann, EC Jr, Winkelmann RK: Herpes simplex infections in hematologic malignancies. Am J Med 52: 102–114, 1972

Mullins GM, Flynn JP, el-Mahdi AM, et al: Malignant lymphoma of the spinal epidural space. Ann Intern Med 74:416–423, 1971

Murchison C: Case of "lymphadenoma" of the lymphatic system, spleen, liver, lungs, heart, diaphragm and dura mater, & c. Trans Pathol Soc London 21:372–389, 1869–1870

Musshoff K, Busch M, Kaminski H: Lymphogranulomatose (Morbus Hodgkin) mit Knochenbefall. Symptomatologie mit besonderer Berucksictigung des Röntgenbildes, Therapie and Prognose. Ein Bericht über 66 Fälle (Freiburger Krankengut 1948–1961). Fortschr Geb Rontgensttr Nuklearmed 101:117–137, 1964

Newall J, Friedman M: Reticulum-cell sarcoma. Part II. Radiation dosage for each type. Radiology 94:643–647, 1970a

Newall J, Friedman M: Reticulum-cell sarcoma. Part III. Prognosis. Radiology 97:99–102, 1970b

Newall J, Friedman M, Narvaez F de: Extra-lymph-node reticulum-cell sarcoma. Radiology 91:708–712, 1968

Oberling C: Les réticulosarcomes et les réticulo-endothélio sarcomes de la moelle ósseuse (sarcomes d'Ewing). Bull Cancer (Paris) 17:259–296, 1928

Pack GT, Molander DW: The surgical treatment of Hodgkin's disease. Cancer Res 26:1254–1263, 1966

Parker F Jr, Jackson H Jr: Primary reticulum-cell sarcoma of bone. Surg Gynecol Obstet 68:45–53, 1939

Parker JC Jr: A typical Hodgkin's disease with intramedullary spinal cord involvement. J Neuropathol Exp Neurol 31:202, 1972 (Abstr)

Percy AK, Elveback LR, Okazaki H, et al: Neoplasms of central nervous system: Epidemiologic considerations. Neurology 22:40–48, 1972

Plafker J, Martinez AJ, Rosenblum WI: A neoplasm of the reticulo-endothelial system involving brain (microglioma) and viscera (reticulum cell sarcoma). South Med J 65:385–389, 1972

Richardson EP Jr: Progressive multifocal leukoencephalopathy: Remote effects of cancer on the nervous system, in Brain L, Norris FH Jr (eds): Contemporary Neurology Symposia, vol 1. New York, Grune & Stratton, 1965, pp 6–16

Richmond J, Sherman RS, Diamond HD, et al: Renal lesions associated with malignant lymphomas. Am J Med 32:184–207, 1962

Rosenberg SA, Diamond HD, Jaslowitz B, et al: Lymphosarcoma: A review of 1269 cases. Medicine 40:31–84, 1961

Rosenblum WI, Hadfield MG: Granulomatous angitis of nervous system in cases of herpes zoster and lymphosarcoma. Neurology 22:348–354, 1972

Rubin P: Extradural spinal cord compression by tumor. I. Experimental production and treatment trials. Radiology 93:1243–1248, 1969

Rubin P, Mayer E, Poulter C: Extradural spinal cord compression by tumor. II. High daily dose experience without laminectomy. Radiology 93:1248–1260, 1969

Samman PD: Hodgkin's disease. Cutaneous manifestations. Proc R Soc Med 60:736–737, 1967

Schaumburg HH, Plank CR, Adams RD: The reticulum cell sarcoma-microglioma group of brain tumors: A consideration of their clinical features and therapy. Neurology 22:396, 1972 (Abstr)

Schein PS, Vickers HR: Lupus vulgaris and Hodgkin's disease. Arch Dermatol 105: 244–246, 1972

Schimpff S, Serpick A, Stoler B, et al.: Varicella-zoster infection in patients with cancer. Ann Intern Med 76:241–254, 1972

Schneck SA, Penn I: De-Novo brain tumours in renal-transplant recipients. Lancet 1: 983–986, 1971

Schricker JL, Smith DE: Primary intracerebral Hodgkin's disease. Cancer 8: 629–633, 1955

Sharma BK, Poticha SM, Oyasu R: Reticulum cell sarcoma involving the cerebellum in a renal transplant recipient. Transplantation 13:52–53 1972

Shoji H, Miller TR: Primary reticulum-cell sarcoma of bone: Significance of clinical features upon the prognosis. Cancer 28: 1234–1244, 1971

Silverberg IJ, Jacobs EM: Treatment of spinal cord compression in Hodgkin's disease. Cancer 27:308–313, 1971

Silverman L, Rubinstein LJ: Electron microscopic observations on a case of progressive multifocal leukoencephalopathy. Acta Neuropathol 5:215–224, 1965

Smith MJ, Stenstrom KW: Compression of spinal cord caused by Hodgkin's disease: Case reports and treatment. Radiology 51:77–84, 1948

Sohn D, Valensi Q, Miller SP: Neurologic manifestations of Hodgkin's disease. Intracerebral Hodgkin's granuloma. Arch Neurol 17:429–436, 1967

Sokal JE, Firat D: Varicella-zoster infection in Hodgkin's disease: Clinical and epidemiological aspects. Am J Med 39: 452–463, 1965

Sparling HJ Jr, Adams RD: Primary Hodgkin's sarcoma of brain. Arch Pathol 42: 338–344, 1946

Sparling HJ Jr, Adams RD, Parker FJ: Involvement of nervous system by malignant lymphoma. Medicine 26:285–332, 1947

Spittle MF: Inappropriate anti-diuretic hormone secretion in Hodgkin's disease. Postgrad Med J 42:423–425, 1966

Stevens DA, Jordan GW, Waddell, et al: Adverse effect of cytosine arabinoside on disseminated zoster in a controlled trial. N Engl J Med 289:873–878, 1973

Stevens DA, Merigan TC: Interferon, antibody, and other host factors in herpes zoster. J Clin Invest 51:1170–1178, 1972

Stuhlbarg J, Ellis FW: Hodgkin's disease of bone: Favorable prognostic significance? Am J Roentgenol Radium Ther Nucl Med 93:568–572, 1965

Thompson RW, DeNardo GL: Therapeutic response of intracranial Hodgkin's disease documented by brain scanning. Cancer 24:981–984, 1969

Thompson RW, DeNardo GL, Kottra JJ: The diagnostic value of brain scanning in intracranial lymphomas. Radiology 102: 111–116, 1972

Todd ID: Intracranial lesions in Hodgkin's disease. Proc R Soc Med 60:734–736, 1967

Troland CE, Sahyoun PF, Mandeville FB: Primary mesenchymal tumors of brain, so-called reticulum cell sarcoma. Report of 5 cases. J Neuropathol Exp Neurol 9:332–334, 1950

Verity GL: Neurologic manifestations and complications of lymphoma. Radiol Clin N Am 6:97–106, 1968

Vieta JO, Friedell HL, Craver LF: Survey of Hodgkin's disease and lymphosarcoma in bone. Radiology 39:1–15, 1942

Vietzke WM, Gelderman AH, Grimley PM, et al: Toxoplasmosis complicating malignancy: Experience at the National Cancer Institute. Cancer 21:816–827, 1968

Wang CC: Treatment of primary reticulum-cell sarcoma of bone by irradiation. N Engl J Med 278:1331–1332, 1968

Wang CC, Fleischli DJ: Primary reticulum-cell sarcoma of bone: With emphasis on radiation therapy. Cancer 22:994–998, 1968

Weil A: Spinal cord changes in lymphogranulomatosis. Arch Neurol Psychiatr 26:1009–1026, 1931

Welch JE: Tumor of the neck showing unusual histological features. Proc NY Pathol Soc 10:161–169, 1910

Whisnant JP, Siekert RG, Sayre GP: Symposium on hematologic disorders: Neurologic manifestations of lymphomas. Med Clin North Am 40:1151–1161, 1956

White AG: Diabetes insipidus: A discussion, including a reexamination of site and mode of action of antidiuretic hormone. Mt Sinai J Med MY 22:15–23, 1955

Williams HM, Diamond HD, Craver LF: The pathogenesis and management of neurological complications in patients with malignant lymphomas and leukemia. Cancer 11:76–82, 1958

Williams HM, Diamond HD, Craver LF, et al: Neurological Complications of Lymphomas and Leukemias. Springfield Ill, Thomas, 1959

Williams RD, Andrews NC, Zanes RP: Major surgery in Hodgkin's disease. Surg Gynecol Obstet 93:636–640, 1951

Wilson JF, Marsa GW, Johnson RE: Herpes zoster in Hodgkin's disease: Clinical, histologic, and immunologic correlations. Cancer 29:461–465, 1972

Winkelman NW, Moore MT: Lymphogranulomatosis (Hodgkin's disease) of nervous system. Arch Neurol Psychiatr 45:304–318, 1941

Woodhouse MA, Dayan AD, Burston J, et al: Progressive multifocal leukoencephalopathy: Electron microscope study of four cases. Brain 90:863–870, 1967

Ziegler K: Die Hodgkinsche Krankheit. Jena, Gustav Fischer, 1911

11

Surgery and Radiobiological Changes

The increasing use of radiation therapy for the treatment of lymphomas of all types has important surgical ramifications. The collaboration of the surgeon with the therapist in staging, biopsies, and the performance of splenectomies is covered elsewhere in the book (pp. 189–228). Our purposes in this section are to review the effect of radiotherapy on the healing of wounds and to review the complications of radiotherapy that have required surgical intervention. Also, unusual conditions for which no really effective intervention exists are discussed since the surgeon must consider these problems in his differential diagnosis, understand the pathophysiology of radiation effect, and appreciate the limits of surgical treatment. The details of surgical technique will be confined to a general consideration of the restrictions radiation injury places on surgery at all sites.

Complications compound the cost and morbidity of any illness, but their occurrence is inconsistently included in the comparative evaluation of treatments. In cancer therapy, the tendency has been to rely almost entirely on the comparison of stage-specific 5-year survival rates. Unfortunately, this parameter tells nothing of the duration of treatment, cost morbidity, quality of survival, and the comparative value of treatment of conditions from which no one survives 5 years. A more concise method of evaluation might be to compare the age-specific and disease-specific proportion of functional man-days preserved by treatment. This comparison would permit an assessment of the accumulative patient downtime that might occur during the course of an illness or its treatment. Common downtime factors are given in Tables 11-1 and 11-2.

These downtime factors can be included in a mathematical model which recognizes the fact that the human life span is limited to about 25,000 days

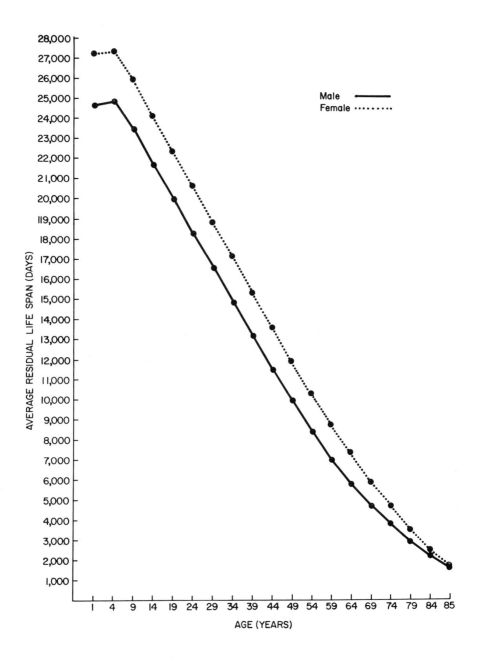

Fig. 11-1. Reprinted from: Spratt, J.S., Jr.: The measurement of the value of the clinical process to individuals by age and income. J Trauma 11:966–973, 1971

Table 11-1
Individual Downtime Factors in the Clinical Process Accruing to the Advantage
of the Individual

Time spent in diagnostic effort leading to discovery and effective treatment of diseases that
could reduce life span or function
Time spent in beneficial treatment
Time spent in beneficial rehabilitation
Time spent in educating and motivating people to remain well
Time spent in educating and motivating people to make logical requests for health services
that will accrue to their benefit
Time spent in educating and motivating people to participate effectively in their own care and
rehabilitation when they do become sick

Source: Spratt JS, Cunningham CJ: Operational Research and Patient Response to Therapy, sponsored
by the Cancer Clinical Investigation Review Committee, Clinical Investigation Branch of the National
Cancer Institute, Atlanta, January 24–25, 1972.

Beneficial treatment is defined as treatment that will alleviate symptoms, preserve a functional attitude
and motivation, restore function or preserve longevity at a cost tolerable to the beneficiary.

Table 11-2
Individual Downtime Factors in the Clinical Process Not Accruing
to the Advantage of the Individual

Time lost for diagnostic effort not leading to beneficial treatment
Treatment not restoring or preserving function
Treatment not preserving maximum longevity
Cost in excess of ultimate value
Time consumed in the coordination of interdisciplinary consultation and treatment that does
not lead to added patient benefit
Time wasted in travel and waiting
Time wasted by avoidable morbidity
Avoidable mortality from elements of the clinical process
Time spent in treatment not preserving longevity or function
Time lost from delay in rehabilitation

Source: Spratt JS, Cunningham CJ: Operation Research and Patient Response to Therapy, sponsored
by the Cancer Clinical Investigation Review Committee, Clinical Investigation Branch of the National
Cancer Institute, Atlanta, Jan. 24–25, 1972

Beneficial treatment is defined as treatment that will alleviate symptoms, restore function or preserve
longevity at a cost tolerable to the beneficiary.

containing an average complement of only 94,000 working hours (Fig. 11-1).
The earning potential also approaches a limit and to avoid economic
morbidity, the cost of treatment must relate on a variable scale to the estate
size and preserved earning power of the treated patient. Insurance can only
partially compensate for this. Insurance also introduces other biases into
the compensation system and supports a very sizable bureaucracy which
contributes in no minor way to the economic morbidity of illness.

    The mathematical models of tumor dose response support the observation that 4000 rads in 4 weeks will control almost 90 percent of the aggregates of 10^6 tumor cells and 99 percent of 10^5 cells. Given 17 days, 2600 rads will kill 10^5 cells. The slope of the dose–response curve is very steep at this 90 percent control point and any gain in cancer cell kill above this point is obtained at the expense of fibrosis. A 10 percent increase in biological kill can bring about disasterous complications. As Fletcher and Jesse (1971) so correctly state, "The surgeon and radiotherapist, as members of the team, must be aware of the role each will play in the patient's treatment when the patient is first seen." They were referring to the management of epidermoid cancers of the head and neck, but the same assertion applies to lymphomas. By protraction of time and dose and attention to the uniform distribution of radiation throughout the tissues, the radiotherapist strives to take advantage of the differential tendency of normal tissue to exhibit a greater capacity to recover from irradiational injury than does cancer. No extant technique completely protects normal tissue.

    In the EFSCH series, 143 out of 163 with Hodgkin's disease (88 percent) and 285 out of 364 (78 percent) patients with non-Hodgkin's lymphomas had radiotherapy. The survival rates of these patients at the end of one year were about 70 percent for those with Hodgkin's disease and 60 percent for the non-Hodgkin's group. Various radiotherapists were in charge from 1940 to 1971 and the equipment, philosophy and technique of radiotherapy have changed over the years (Table 11-3). In 1957 the cobalt 60 machine was installed and subsequently more patients received radiotherapy to the adjacent nonpalpable nodal areas. The administration of high-dose multifield radiotherapy for lymphomas has only recently been implemented at the EFSCH and very few complications attributable to radiobiological effects on normal tissue have accumulated. Only 3 patients summarized in Table 11-4, have required surgical intervention. Another patient (No. 26738) had radiotherapy for coexisting carcinoma of the cervix. Five years later, ileal resection was required for bowel infarction (p. 388).

    To review the nature of complications attributable to the radiotherapy of lymphomas, it is necessary to rely upon the literature. These complications are divisible into 2 large groups. The first group is due to the general effect of irradiation upon the healing of surgical wounds. The second group consists of organ specific irradiational injuries that require recognition by the surgeon and often specialized surgical management. The latter group is secondary to the direct effects of irradiation on normal vascular and parenchymatous structures. The literature contains numerous case reports and special site studies but little information exists on the incidence of these complications. The real incidence of complications with various treatment methods is often very difficult to ascertain for the following reasons:

1. Differentiation between radiation and neoplastic complications can often

Table 11-3

Analysis of First Radiotherapy Given at EFSCH*

	Hodgkin's disease					Other lymphomas				
		Radiation Therapy to next lymph node		Given dose (× 100 rads)*			Radiation therapy to next lymph node		Given dose (× 100 rads)	
Year	No. of Patients	No.	%	Range	Mean	No. of Patients	No.	%	Range	Mean
1940–1945	20	2	10	10–27	18.7	15			10–30	19.4
1946–1950	16	1	6	12–40	26.8	11			10–33	25.3
1951–1955	22	3	14	10–50	26.9	42			10–52	25.2
1956–1960	20	3	15	10–28	20.1	58			10–60	24.5
1961–1965	17	5	29	11–50	35.1	27	5	18	10–42	25.3
1966–1970	21	7	33	10–50	37.4	40	9	23	10–68	39.7
1971	6	3	50	31–44	39.2	9	3	33	19–54	38.8
Total	122	24	20			202	17	8		

Listed dose is higher dose given to an area, excluding total body radiation and incomplete therapy. Radiation therapy machine used: 1940–1950, 200 ky and 218 kv; 1950–1957, majority of the patients were treated with 250 kv; since 1957, most were treated with cobalt 60 apparatus.

*From Lee YN, Say C, Hori JM, et al: Clinical courses of Hodgkin's disease and other malignant lymphomas. Am J Roentgenol Radium Ther Nucl Med 117:19–29, 1973.

Table 11-4
Operation for Radiotherapy Complications

Patient No.	Age	Sex	Date	Diagnosis	Radiotherapy (rads)	Primary Lesion			Complication	Operation	Findings	Survival (months) * = alive	Lymphoma at follow-up
						Site	Interval to Op.	Active					
37422	61	F	11-71	HWD	2650	AP para-aortic nodes	40 M	+	Leg swelling, hydronephrosis	Exploration	Retro-peritoneal fibrosis	3*	+
37779	51	M	3-71	LPD	2250 4750	AP pelvis Testes, groin	136 M	–	Tender mass left testes	Orchiectomy	Chronic orchi-epididymitis, interstitial fibrosis	9*	+ –
22192	54	M	10-56 12-56 1-57 2-57 2-57 11-57	Und	3500	R-legs soft tissue	5 M	+	Leg Ulcer Graft necrosis Tendon exposed Osteomylitis Testes enlarged	Excision, STSG Debridement Postage graft BK-amputation Left orchiectomy Right orchiectomy	Radiation necrosis	20	+

346

be made only when very complete autopsies are performed on all patients dying after radiotherapy.

2. The latent period between radiotherapy and the appearance of a major complication may be several decades, necessitating the lifelong follow-up and terminal autopsy of all treated cases.

Obviously, the attainment of such completeness may exceed the life span of the radiotherapist, and the performance of adequate terminal autopsies is frustrated by many factors including refusal of permission and death at a facility not having access to anatomical pathologists who will perform the autopsies with the necessary detail.

Consequently, the best that can be done is to summarize some of the better case reports that have appeared in the literature since supervoltage treatment of lymphomas by multifield therapy has become rather generally available and accepted. The earlier literature of radiation complications to orthovoltage therapy is unbelievably large but is not very relevant to current treatment methods. Also, it is irrelevant to review the irradiational complications of organ-specific treatment such as for cancers of the cervix uteri. The surgical problems in these situations are specific to the anatomical region and its function and require special consideration (Spratt et al 1972).

Because of the latent period between treatment and the appearance of complications, the surgeon will continue for some years to see complications in patients originally treated by orthovoltage. The frequency of these late complications is unquestionably reduced by the fact that many cancer patients die of their disease or other causes before they have lived long enough to experience the late complications of radiotherapy.

As examples of older studies, Denny-Brown and Foley (1953) mentioned that radiation necrosis of the cerebral hemispheres may occur after excessive irradiation. Slaughter (1965) mentioned that tumor doses in the order of 3000 to 4500 rads are not innocuous, and 10 to 20 year survivors will have serious changes in lung, larynx, and pharyngeal mucosa, aside from the fibrosis of soft tissues themselves. In addition, disastrous late results may occur even after treatment by expert radiotherapists; his group had to ligate a carotid artery on one patient and do an emergency hindquarter amputation on another for radionecrosis of the femoral artery and subsequent hemorrhage. Copeland (1967) mentioned that radiotherapy is preferred as a form of treatment for primary reticulum cell sarcoma of the bone. However, "many cases ultimately undergo delayed amputation because of bone necrosis."

RADIATION AND THE HEALING OF SURGICAL WOUNDS

The peculiarities of the healing of wounds within irradiated tissue are pertinent to the surgery of all lymphomas. The biologic effects of irradiation within a mass of tissue are distributed randomly to all cell types and the cells of normal tissue are affected as well as the cells of a neoplasm (Spratt and Sala 1962). The purpose of this section is to discuss some of the alterations in the healing of wounds secondary to the effects of radiation on the noncancerous cells and tissues.

The retardation of wound healing by irradiation is dependent upon the amount of radiation, its physical qualities, and the length of time over which that dose is administered. In 1931 Pohle et al demonstrated that in rats 1000 rads in a single dose given 1 to 30 days before wounding exerted no demonstrable influence on wound healing as measured by the strength and morphology on the scar although more refined measurements have shown that as little as 500 rads, single dose, preoperatively, will reduce the rate of wound contraction (Grillo and Potsaid 1961). Any tissue receiving in excess of 1300 rads from a single dose is subject to spontaneous necrosis (Pohle et al 1931).

Van den Brenk (1956, 1957) demonstrated that no budding or proliferation of either lymph or blood capillaries occurs after the irradiation of mammalian tissue with 2000 rads in a single dose. However, capillary regeneration takes place normally in tissues irradiated with single doses of 1000 rads or less. Following single doses of from 1000 to 2000 rads, capillary regeneration occurs irregularly and the flow of red blood cells through these capillaries is slow. In addition, the capillaries in tissue receiving over 1000 rads tend to rupture. Extensive lymph and blood capillary budding normally follows injury and infection in nonirradiated tissue, and the inhibition of capillary budding by irradiation may contribute to necrosis and nonhealing wounds within irradiated tissues. When the capillary permeation of heavily irradiated tissues occurs, it proceeds from the adjacent nonirradiated tissues (Spratt et al 1961). Such revascularization is a slow and incomplete process; a relatively avascular scar persists. By protracting the administration of the total dose over many days, the tolerance of tissue to radiation can be increased with some preservation of the ability of wounds to heal. Protraction permits sublethally irradiated cells a chance to regenerate (Lockart et al 1961).

A clear knowledge of the correlation of the time–dose factors of preoperative irradiation with the ability of wounds to heal is necessary if increased mortality and morbidity from surgical procedures are to be avoided, but concise data correlating the frequency of postsurgical complications with various time–dose factors in irradiated human tissue are not abundant. A midpelvic dose of 4000 rads given by protracted therapy (3 to 4 weeks) seems compatible with postirradiation hysterectomy (Sala and del Regato 1962) and lymphadenectomy (Chau et al 1962), but when the surgery is performed in pelves that have received 6000 rads or more (5 to 6 weeks), the frequency of complications rises percipitously (Chau et al 1962). The most thorough clinical report on a single region (the neck) was cited earlier and is relevant to this problem (Fletcher and Jesse 1971).

Difficulty with wound healing can be expected in any tissue that has been irradiated to "tolerance" since treatment to tolerance implies less capacity to regenerate after injury and a reduction in the number of blood and lymph vascular conduits with resulting ischemia. Tolerance is dependent upon time of administration, dose, and tissue-specific factors. Thus, no "rule of thumb" is available to define tolerance. In a specific patient, the surgeon must rely on the therapist's opinion as to whether tissue tolerance to radiotherapy has been reached or exceeded.

Resections in tissue irradiated to tolerance are possible, provided that no vital reconstruction such as anastomosis of irradiated intestine or ureters is attempted since these anastomoses are subject to spontaneous dissolution (Spratt and Butcher, unpublished; Spratt et al 1973). Resection of a total mass of heavily irradiated tissue is feasible in certain instances leaving wound margins of nonirradiated tissue and, if a tensionless approximation of the nonirradiated tissues can be effected, healing may occur. Unfortunately, primary healing does not always occur and irradiated structures such as ureters, intestines, and/or arteries may be subject to exposure, fistula formation, and hemorrhage.

Recent radiobiological studies in vitro suggest that surprisingly small doses of radiation may impair the reproductive viability of a large percentage of the cells within a cancer, while a large dose beyond tissue tolerance might be requisite for complete tumor sterilization. These reproductively dead cells may appear morphologically normal for a while though they may enlarge (Puck 1960). Cell death may not actually occur until the cells have undergone one or several attempts at cell division. This observation may have a practical application if one assumes that the use of a small dose of preoperative irradiation may reduce the chances of local implantation and the growth of colonies of cells scattered during the surgery. If cumulative survival data establish that these moderate doses of preoperative irradiation ranging from 1500 rads in 1 week to 4500 rads in 4 weeks can achieve a reduction in the frequency of implantation and dissemination of cancer without additional surgical morbidity, then the more frequent use of preoperative irradiation for such tumors as carcinoma of the lung, rectum, bladder, breast, and uterus may be justified (Bloedorn and Cowley 1960; Leaming et al 1961; and Sala and del Regato 1962). As Fletcher and Jesse (1971) noted, preoperative radiotherapy is more effective in eradicating small well-oxygenated foci of cancer in lymph nodes or at the periphery of large cancers than it is in eradicating large masses of cancer with poorly oxygenated centers.

Important considerations before undertaking surgery in any irradiated tissue should include: (1) the exact location and size of all external ports, (2) the direction of the beam traversing these ports, (3) the location of and tissue dose at all exit ports (linear accelerator), and (4) the approximate time–dose factors and physical characteristics of radiation received by the skin at each port and the dosage received by all organs and tissues traversed by the beam or its penumbra that might be included in the area of contemplated surgery.

Higher-energy radiation has an effect upon tissues similar to that achieved by lower-energy irradiation, but the effect is more deceptive. The higher-energy sources of cobalt 60 teletherapy and betatron produce maximum ionization well below skin surface, and a greater dose to the deeper tissues can be delivered without effecting detectable changes in the skin at the port of entry. Also, a considerable percentage of the incident beam from these high-energy sources may traverse the entire body, particularly in thin individuals, and leave through a cutaneous exit port. To this exit port is added the forward scatter of the secondary radiation produced in the tissues. The exit ports can receive a significant irradiation effect and the location of these exit ports should also be considered before surgery. Gross appearance is not an infallible index of irradiation effect, and the surgeon must know what has been irradiated and how much irradiation it received. With these various radiobiological observations and radiotherapeutic factors in mind, specific surgical restrictions still exist:

1. Closed-space abscesses in tissues that have been irradiated have to be drained promptly and by the shortest appropriate route in order to prevent extensive necrosis of the irradiated tissues.
2. Anastomoses of irradiated bowel heal slowly and often will not heal at all unless proximal diversion of feces is effected for a period of months. The anastomoses will tolerate no traction and no sutures that are tied too tightly.
3. Pedicle flaps that are to cover irradiation ulcers should be sewn to nonirradiated tissues bridging the irradiated area when possible.
4. Tissue whose vascularity has been reduced by radiation should not be included in the base or body of a pedicle flap.
5. Colostomies, ileostomies, or ureterostomies should not be constructed through skin or abdominal wall situated in fields of previous external roentgenotherapy.
6. Surgical incisions should be planned to avoid fields of irradiation and should never be angulated in and around irradiated areas.
7. Necrotic tissue in fields of irradiation will not hold sutures and the control of hemorrhage in these areas frequently necessitates the ligation of vessels afferent to the irradiated bleeding points.
8. Abdominal incisions through fields of irradiation heal slowly and are subject to necrotizing infections and wound evisceration. Such incisions should not be made when other alternatives exist and under no circumstances should an incision be angulated in or near a radiation port.
9. Fractured irradiated bones heal poorly and secondary infection yields a progressive osteomyelitis that is difficult to manage.
10. Simple biopsies in heavily irradiated tissue may be followed by extensive necrosis. Endoscopic biopsy of a heavily irradiated area in the anterior rectal wall followed by necrosis of the rectovaginal septum and the development of a rectovaginal fistula is a typical example.

All restrictions placed on surgery in irradiated tissue are attributable to the decreased vascularity of irradiated tissue, reduced ability of irradiated tissue to exhibit the normal regenerative response to injury, and the susceptibility of irradiated tissue to spontaneous necrosis in the presence of trauma or infection.

In spite of present enthusiasm for the possible chemotherapeutic and immunological eradication of cancer, surgery and radiotherapy remain the only effective modalities for the treatment of most forms of human cancer. The awareness of the poor healing of wounds within irradiated tissue and a close degree of cooperation in the planning of cancer therapy are important to both the surgeon and the radiotherapist if the best level of cancer therapy with a minimum of complications is to be achieved.

ORGAN-SPECIFIC IRRADIATIONAL INJURIES

With the increasing availability of high-energy radiotherapy for the delivery of large doses of irradiation to structures in the mediastinal, lumbar, and para-aortic regions for the treatment of lymphomas, it is natural to assume that late effects might arise in the normal anatomical structures. Specific organs in the path of the irradiation include the pericardium, heart, great vessels, spinal cord, intestines, and bone as well as surrounding tissues, skin, and muscle. Basically, radiation affects all tissues the same, accelerating aging, killing normal cells as well as neoplastic, and damaging small blood and lymph vessels with resulting sclerosis. Healing occurs by absorption of the dead tissue, contracture, ingrowth of fibroblasts, and incomplete revascularization. Ultimately all areas receiving therapeutic doses of irradiation develop characteristics in common—incomplete regeneration of original structure, fine to gross scar formation, reduced vascularity, and reduced capacity to tolerate injury or infection with a tendency to develop acute necrosis or late spontaneous necrosis.

Though the goal for radiation therapy to the mediastinum and para-aortic areas is generally to control suspected or radiographically visible foci of neoplasms in lymph nodes, these nodes constitute a very small volume of the total tissue mass that must be irradiated in order to deliver tumoricidal doses to the nodes. The integral dose of irradiation to a very large volume of *normal* tissue is equally as great. With orthovoltage the effect on the skin at the port of entry of the irradiation was very great, and this skin effect tended to limit the dose of irradiation that could be given to deeper tissues. With high-energy sources such as from a cobalt unit or betatron, the incident energy is so great that the high-energy photons may be driven completely through the skin at the port of entry producing little effect on the skin. As the photons slow or begin to hit the components of cells, they or their forward scatter produces tracts of intracellular ionization that causes the tissue damage characteristically leading to irradiation effect. What used to occur on the skin where it could be seen now occurs in the deeper tissues where it cannot be seen. With high-energy irradiation, the skin effect, paradoxically, may be greater where the irradiation leaves the body (exit port) than at the entrance port. The only manifestations of deeper tissue injury will be the later symptoms associated with the progressive tissue damage that succeeds the irradiation. That such late manifestations of serious damage would develop was quite predictable from the beginning of many current treatment programs, and scattered case reports are now confirming these predictions. Very likely, some of these manifestations of irradiation damage are being attributed incorrectly to the progression of the neoplasm. The unfortunate aspect of these cases is that many persons have been irradiated unnecessarily in the interest of "prophylaxis." Our purpose is to call attention to some of the types of damage that are being reported and to encourage an effort to differentiate—pathologically where possible- —between the problems caused by neoplasm and the problems caused by irradiation.

General

Ackerman (1972) has provided us with a history of the anatomical pathologist's evolving insight into the pathophysiology of radiation injury and describes the early awareness of radiation injury. He also documents how this injury pattern has changed as the radiotherapist has acquired different types of radiation sources. As the pathologist has perceived the extent of injury in various tissues, he has labeled various tissues "radio-resistant" or "radio-sensitive." The pathologist has been asked to provide from static morphological data answers that had to await the evolution of mammalian cell radiobiology with its assessment of the interrelation between radiation and cellular kinetics (Mendelsohn and Shackney 1970; Anderson 1971).

Abscopal Effects

Abscopal effects of irradiation are those occurring in tumor tissue situated outside the treated area. These effects unquestionably occur under a variety of circumstances though no general hypothesis has been tested that would establish cause (Jansen et al 1964). Looney and Chang (1967) hypothesized that abscopal effects may be due to one systemic factor affecting DNA synthesis and another affecting mitotic activity.

A recent review of the literature by Nobler (1969) failed to demonstrate a single well-documented case for any neoplasm other than chronic leukemia. He reported an abscopal response in a patient with malignant lymphoma and attributed this to the reduction of recirculating lymphocytes by depleting excessive and often abnormal lymphocytes as they circulated through lymph nodes under treatment. Secondarily, the reduction in the number of lymphocytes clogging the lymphatic system may have improved lymphatic circulation.

Radiation sickness is a systemic effect of local radiation but is dose dependent and should be seen infrequently at low incremental doses. Rarely, a surgeon might have to differentiate between surgical and irradiational causes of nausea and vomiting.

Skin

Nearly all external beam radiation must traverse the skin. Von Essen (1969) has provided a current review on skin effect entitled "Radiation Tolerance of the Skin." He concludes that the response to radiation injury to the skin is determined by dynamic process of cellular recovery, proliferation, and migration. The accelerated proliferation rates of surviving epidermal and dermal cells in addition to the migration of unirradiated cells may be of importance in differentiating the restitution of normal skin during the treatment of skin tumors. Repair of normal skin is favored by small dose increments. The skin is subject to damage from supervoltage radiation by subcutaneous overdosage. He points out that the dose required to produce a given skin reaction varies with the cube root of the exposure time (in days) and inversely with the cube root of the diameter of the irradiated field.

Cell kinetics are important in the skin because the skin is a cell renewal system with a normal turnover time of 13 to 18 days. Acute doses of 1000–4000 rads produce a drop in the mitotic activity in this cell renewal system within 12 hr. Approximately 10 surviving epithelial cells are necessary to repopulate 1 cm^2 of denuded skin in 10 days after irradiation, approaching a reepithelization rate of 0.5 mm/day.

Survival of these epidermal cells is dependent upon blood vessels in the dermis. When sufficient radiation is given to sterilize these blood vessels, they are incapable of regeneration. This necessary regeneration proceeding through granulation tissue formation and revascularization can occur only in ulcers not heavily infected by bacteria. Thus, when a radiation ulcer is either imminent or has already occurred, there is reason to believe that treatment should follow the same course used for a thermal burn to prevent aggravation of the burn by bacterial action (Order and Moncrief 1965).

Supervoltage therapy is more likely to spare the epidermis and to affect the dermis. The dermis develops fibrosis and endarteritis, and may in time exhibit atrophy, depression, and loss of hair follicles and other skin appendages. Telangiectasia may develop over time and the overlying epidermis permanently retains an increased capacity to ulcerate.

Herpes Zoster

Herpes zoster occurs with all forms of lymphoma and particularly with Hodgkin's disease. It is a problem that may develop anytime during the course of the illness with or without previous radiation therapy (pp. 000–000). In the report by Wilson et al (1972), the majority of patients developed shingles within 6 months after primary treatment suggesting that immunosuppression by either the lymphoma or irradiation might be a precipitating factor. Herpes zoster also developed frequently when the lymphomatous process recurred. The development of herpes zoster was a bad prognostic sign in that it frequently antedated the recurrence of the lymphoma itself. This was true in 10 of 13 patients and only 4 of these patients survived following additional treatment by chemotherapy or irradiation therapy. If the herpes zoster developed within the first 6 months after the initial treatment then no additional morbidity from the lymphoma itself was noted. The authors speculated that two separate situations existed. In the first 6 months the development of shingles might have been associated with alteration in the immune mechanisms from the radiation therapy. When it developed 6 to 12 months after therapy it is possible that neural tissue was involved by the lymphoma or the lymphoma was responsible for the immunosuppression. In contrast, patients who developed shingles at a time closer to radiation therapy reflected the cumulative immunosuppression of active disease and radical irradiation.

Thyroid

Whenever a considerable portion of the thyroid gland is included in the field of irradiation, the gland is subject to parenchymatous injury with reduction in function.

Hypothyroidism can develop gradually over a number of months. Initially these patients complain only of some lethargy; both fatigue and weight gain have been observed. The laboratory findings characteristic of hypothyroidism all develop in these cases. Prager et al (1972) reported 23 consecutive Hodgkin's patients who received cobalt 60 irradiation that included the thyroid gland without protection. All patients received over 3900 rads, but under 4600 rads over a similar treatment time of 4 weeks. Five of these 23 patients (22 percent) developed overt hypothyroidism within 1 year after treatment. Their symptoms consisted of weight gain, lethargy, and various manifestations of leg and periorbital edema. The remaining 18 patients were clinically euthyroid at the end of the year and the T4 determinations were within normal limits. All responded satisfactorily to treatment with T4.

Glatstein et al (1971) reported five cases of myxedema in a 3-year period during which 124 patients with malignant lymphoma received 4400 rads to the thyroid gland after lymphangiography. Twenty-three patients had laboratory evidence of hypothyroidism. A control group of 50 patients with other neoplasms who received 4000 to 6000 rads to the neck without lymphangiography did not develop myxedema over the similar period. These suggested that the prolonged high iodide level resulting from iodine in the lymphangiogram material might stimulate thyroid hyperplasia and thereby enhance radiation sensitivity.

In the preoperative evaluation of any patient who has received radiotherapy to parts of the neck that could include a portion of the thyroid gland, latent hypothyroidism should be ruled out. Hypothyroidism must be corrected before the patient is subjected to general anesthesia or major surgery of any type (Cope 1965). Hypothyroid patients may become unduly sensitive to all depressant drugs. Morphine particularly is poorly tolerated. Barbiturates, though given in normal doses, may have an exaggerated effect. Consequently, all doses of depressants should be reduced in patients who have any degree of hypothyroidism (Pallin 1959).

As a preoperative precaution, these patients should also be evaluated for hypoparathyroidism though no case reports of hypoparathyroidism caused exclusively by radiotherapy of lymphomas were encountered. The parathyroid glands seem somewhat more resistant to radiation effect. However, the effect on any endocrine gland is dose dependent and all can be destroyed by the nonspecific microcirculatory and parenchymatous injury of larger doses of radiation (Rubin and Casarett 1972). Consequently, whenever any endocrine gland has been in the field of radiotherapy for a lymphoma, it would be wise to evaluate its function preoperatively or in the presence of any symptoms that could be attributable to hypofunctioning endocrine glands.

Heart

Cohn et al (1967) noted an instance of radiation cardiac disease of 3.4 percent after treatment of carcinoma of the breast, 5.8 percent after the treatment of lymphomas, and 6.7 percent after the treatment of Hodgkin's disease. They observed that the Hodgkin's patients live longer and, therefore, have more time to develop these radiation complications. In reviewing the literature, they observed that myocardial necrosis, degeneration inflammation, and fibrosis have all been observed in both experimental animals and man having higher doses of ionizing radiation. As with other forms of irradiation injury, the time lag may be very long.

Rubin et al (1963) described the development of widespread myocardial fibrosis, hyalinized vessels, cardiac murmurs, left bundle branch block, and Stokes-Adams episodes with periods of prolonged asystole in a 44-year-old woman. This was about 23 years after radiation therapy following a radical mastectomy. They reported a second patient with massive irradiation to the heart who developed a ruptured myocardium probably due to vascular occlusion and myocardial ischemia. The postmortem examination on this patient showed widespread myocardial fibrosis and atrophy with interstitial histiocytes and giant cells and a thick fibrotic pericardium.

The literature documents that radiation is predisposed to or can accelerate the development of atherosclerosis. This may occur in the coronary artery system producing myocardial infarction in very young people. Radiation may produce tissue injury indirectly or it may do so secondarily to this vascular damage. Dollinger et al (1966) reported a case of myocardial infarction associated with postirradiation fibrosis of the coronary arteries. The pathological process observed in the coronary artery was similar to the process observed clinically and experimentally in medium and small arteries exposed to radiation.

Cohn et al (1967) reported a detailed experience with 21 patients who developed significant heart or pericardial disease following supervoltage radiotherapy of the chest for malignant neoplasms. All of the affected patients had received at least 4000 rads to the area of the heart. Nineteen patients predominantly had pericardial disease. Cases were classified as acute pericarditis, chronic pericardial effusion, chronic constrictive pericarditis with or without inflammation and effusion, myocardial disease with mitral insufficiency, and myocardial infarction due to coronary artery disease. Most of these patients developed acute pericarditis early during the course of the radiation and later developed the symptoms of chronic pericardial effusion. This effusion was followed by constrictive pericarditis and finally a severe pancarditic fibrotic reaction including myocardial fibrosis and endocardial fibroelastosis.

In the differential diagnosis of patients with pericardial effusion who have also received radiation to the thyroid, it is necessary that myxedema be excluded in the differential diagnosis. Actually the significance of the radiation effect on the heart is variable, and the outlook can be improved by recognition and management of the various forms of radiation heart disease. Cohn observed that the signs and symptoms attributable to this problem have frequently been blamed in the past on malignant disease or the direct complications of tumors. The differential diagnosis and management is not, however, simple and often requires a great number of elaborate studies including echocardiogram, RISA scan, carbon dioxide contrast study, or angiocardiography. Even these studies do not always differentiate between effusion and constriction. Cohn considered that cardiac catheterization combined with pericardiocentesis was most useful in establishing a differential diagnosis. The significance of cardiac tamponade can be determined by measuring the pressure in the pericardial space before and after removal. Through the cardiac catheter, measurement of the right atrial space before and after removal of the pericardial fluid will help to give an indication of the degree of the cardiac tamponade in any pressure elevation. The residual venous pressure elevations may be due to restrictive disease of the pericardium, myocardium, or endocardium, and not to the effusion.

A later paper on radiation-induced heart disease from the Stanford group described experience with 25 patients and correlated the cardiac problems with techniques of radiation therapy. Once again, they observed that it is important to differentiate between cardiac complications and manifestations of advancing neoplasm. Thirteen of the patients who developed pericarditis did so within 48 months of the completion of the radiation therapy.

One 15-year old boy died of myocardial infarction 16 months after receiving 4000 rads to the "mantle" for Hodgkin's disease. This child had no known familial or metabolic predisposition to atherosclerosis and the autopsy showed minimal proliferation and atheromatous deposits in the coronary artery with a fresh myocardial infarction. Mitral insufficiency and left bundle branch block developed in a 20-year-old male 8 years after he received 4700 rads to the left thorax for a round cell tumor of the ribs. It was concluded from the work-up that myocardial fibrosis accounted for the left bundle branch block and that dysfunction of the papillary muscles produced the mitral insufficiency. Among the 155 patients who were at risk for at least 1 year, 9 cases of heart disease had developed with an incidence of about 0.6 percent. In the majority of patients, the detectable heart disease developed after a delay of several months and nearly all affected cases had received an excess of 4000 rads.

Aortic and Elastic Arterial Injury

The aorta has been subjected to extensive radiation with supervoltage therapy in efforts to sterilize both mediastinal and abdominal periaortic lymph nodes. A variety of iatrogenic complications have been reported as a result of this irradiation. Thomas and Forbus (1959) reported a 29-year-old man whose death was secondary to splenic and renal infarctions from thrombi dislodged at the site of aortic injury. Whitaker et al (1964) discussed the death of a 16-year-old boy with vascular insufficiency of the upper limbs. He had received radiation therapy 8 years previously. This was associated with a chronic fibrosing arteritis affecting the entire aorta and its branches including the lower abdominal segment. A portion of these vessels was not directly included in the field of irradiation. In the case cited by Fraumeni et al (1967), the aortitis was associated with dilatation in the development of aortic valve incompetence.

Poon et al (1968) reported the rupture of an aorta after radiation therapy; however, this case was associated with an empyema. Abscesses of adjacent major arteries can be associated with rupture, with or without the presence of radiotherapy, and this case does not establish a cause-and-effect relationship. However, they did describe the electron microscopic observations of the site of rupture and noted the complete breakdown of the elastic fibers in the region with minimal cellular reaction. "Slitlike spaces" were present in the elastic fibers. Disruption of these elastic fibers had been previously described by light microscopy (Warren 1942; Hutchison 1953).

Marcial-Rojas and Castro (1962) provided a review of radiation injury to elastic arteries in the course of treatment of neoplastic diseases. In the course of their review, they described 11 cases in which large elastic arteries had ruptured spontaneously after radiation. Latarjet mentioned that thiosulfate had been used for selective protection of the arterial wall against the effects of irradiation, but no details or references were given (Zubrod 1966).

The literature is very sparse in defining effective treatment of these aortic and arterial complications. The incidence of thromboembolic catastrophies from the clots that form on the damaged aortic intima is not known and whether the incidence could be reduced by anticoagulants is also uncertain.

Any surgical intervention to correct vascular rupture would require attention to the general principles of wound healing in irradiated tissue. Arterial grafts would have to be placed to bridge between nonirradiated arteries leaving no irradiated artery or aorta behind that might have intimal damage, elastic tissue fragmentation, or restricted healing capacity. Attempts to repair ruptures with primary suturing might lead to further arterial necrosis and rupture and would have to be used on a temporary basis. The vascular prosthesis would usually be lying in a bed of irradiated tissue and it would certainly have to be free from infection.

The greatest surgical experience in the management of ruptures occurring in irradiated arteries has accumulated with the carotids. These ruptures have occurred most frequently after combinations of cancericidal irradiation and resective surgery that exposes the arteries. These problems are not very analogous to radiation injury that might occur with lymphomas since there are few indications for associated surgery that would expose the carotids in the management of lymphomas. The key to avoiding rupture and restoring continuity is coverage of the artery with an uninfecting, well-vascularized skin and muscle flap. Even emergency coverage by a split-thickness skin graft may help prevent rupture of exposed arteries.

Lung

Varying volumes of lung may be included in the fields of irradiation. Just how much depends upon the field size and integral dose which are further determined by location and size of the lymphoma under treatment, either prophylactic or definitive therapy. If extensive enough, radiation pneumonitis can produce fatal pulmonary insufficiency (Fried and Goldberg 1940; Stone et al 1956).

Vickery, commenting on a case with marked bilateral radiation pneumonitis, describes this condition well:

"Radiation pneumonitis is a curious disease for several reasons. Dyspnea may occur rather suddenly, with functional impairment of the alveolar-capillary-block type. It is most often seen, of course, in patients who have received radiotherapy for breast or lung cancer, but it also occurs with malignant lymphoma. The precise frequency of this complication is not known, and various figures are given by different observers. In a recent report of 72 autopsies of postradiation patients, radiation pneumonitis was found in 7 patients, or 10 percent (Bennett et al 1969). This lesion has occurred with a wide range of radiation doses and time intervals after radiation. It has been described as a complication in patients receiving less than 500 rads and at postradiation intervals of less than 2 weeks (Jennings and Arden 1962; Whitfield et al 1963). There is ample precedent for the low dosage and short time interval associated with the occurrence of this complication in the case under discussion. As was brought out in the discussion of a similar case earlier this year (Case Records of the Massachusetts General Hospital, Case 31–1970), the pathogenesis of radiation pneumonitis is unclear. Its random occurrence and poor correlation with dose and time has [sic] suggested a sensitivity mechanism to some observers" (Case Records of the Massachusetts General Hospital, Case 11–1971).

The above discussion has made it clear that variations in the pattern preclude concise definition, and it is possible that two basic patterns exist, associated with (1) sensitivity to small doses and (2) delayed reactions to the radiobiological effects of fibrosis, sclerosis of small vessels, reduction in pulmonary function commensurate with the volume of lung affected, and susceptibility to infection much as is described in the presupervoltage era.

Landberg et al (1971) found that radiation pneumonitis appeared on x-rays in 9 of 11 patients. Pneumonitis was first diagnosed 3 to 5 months after the first mantle field treatment and lasted as long as 15 months. Durkovský and Krajci (1972) described 2 Hodgkin's patients who died of severe postradiation pneumonitis.

Coulter et al (1972) reviewed the problem of pulmonary complications in 89 patients with stage I to III Hodgkin's disease who received mantle field radiotherapy. Eighteen patients (20 percent) developed respiratory symptoms of dyspnea and/or nonproductive cough within 8 to 12 weeks of treatment. Total lung capacity, determined by chest roentgenograms and helium dilution test, and diffusion capacity all decreased. Pathologic changes of radiation fibrosis and pneumonitis were present in all lungs studied at autopsy or biopsy. The symptoms and functional abnormalities persisted in some patients for 5 to 20 months. Two patients died of pulmonary insufficiency and cor pulmonale. Other pulmonary complications were tracheoesophageal fistula, pneumothorax, and atelectasis. They commented that further study of adequacy of current shielding method and possible pharmacological prevention of radiation injury to the lung was needed.

The group at Stanford said the incidence of radiation pneumonitis used to be about 33 percent. Thus, Palos et al (1971) described a new technique employing a thinner shield to deliver limited whole-lung irradiation during mantle field treatment of Hodgkin's disease. They said this simplified procedure has dropped the incidence of radiation pneumonitis to zero.

Libshitz et al (1973) studied radiation changes in the thorax following extended field radiation therapy using cobalt-60 machine. Of over 200 patients treated for Hodgkin's disease, 20 met the strict critera of no previous radiotherapy, chemotherapy, evidence of pulmonary parenchymal disease, or inadequate radiographic follow-up. Among these 20, 13 had evidence of radiation pneumonitis and 19 showed evidence of radiation fibrosis or loss of volume. Radiation pneumonitis appeared more frequently at 8–12 weeks following the completion of therapy. Radiation fibrosis was generally established by the ninth to twelfth month following the completion of therapy. There appears to be a time-dose relationship, since 3 of the 6 patients who received less than 4000 rads to the mediastinum showed evidence of fibrosis, while 13 of 14 who received over 4000 rads showed radiation fibrosis.

The lung is subject to a form of secondary damage from roentgen diagnostic studies used in lymphomas. When lymphangiography has been performed in the staging of lymphomas, pulmonary complications can occur which include thromboembolic phenomena, infarction, and lipoid pneumonia. These conditions all produce a transient decrease in pulmonary function which can be serious in patients exhibiting borderline pulmonary function beforehand (pp. 66–67). Pulmonary function studies and arterial gas determinations can help determine the degree of interstitial pulmonary injury which could be of significance in the preoperative evaluation of patients who might require major surgery (Case Records of the Massachusetts General Hospital, Case 16–1971).

Guts

The human gut is quite susceptible to injury by radiation and the effects have been reported by innumerable articles in the medical literature since Walsh first reported in 1897 "deep tissue traumatism from roentgen ray exposure." The earlier literature on trial-and-error learning about the cause, incidence, natural history, and successful and unsuccessful treatment of intestinal injury from radiation is enormous. Much of this literature deals with injuries secondary to high-dose local therapy, and the injury pattern with supervoltage radiation is somewhat different (Localio et al 1969). Localio has helpfully correlated the various types of injury seen in the stomach, transverse colon, and small intestine with the tissue dose (Figs. 11-2, 11-3 and 11-4). He observed that the injury may not become symptomatic until many years have elapsed after treatment.

The pattern of intestinal injury in an irradiated abdomen is subject to great variation; unfortunately, many of the variables are neither measurable nor controllable. Consequently, intestinal injury will never be completely prevented. Roswit et al (1972) tabulated nine different technical factors and nine different clinical factors which can influence the risk of radiation injury. To his list, several additional variables have been added and others of less importance have been deleted or modified (Table 11-5). Tumor grade, for example, affects the chances that the tumor will respond favorably to radiotherapy but probably does not affect intestinal susceptibility.

Roswit favored the risk definition offered by Rubin and Casarett (1968, 1972). This classification defines a minimal tolerance dose (TD 5/5) as being that dose that will be associated with a 5 percent chance of manifesting intestinal injury within 5 years of treatment. The maximal tolerable dose

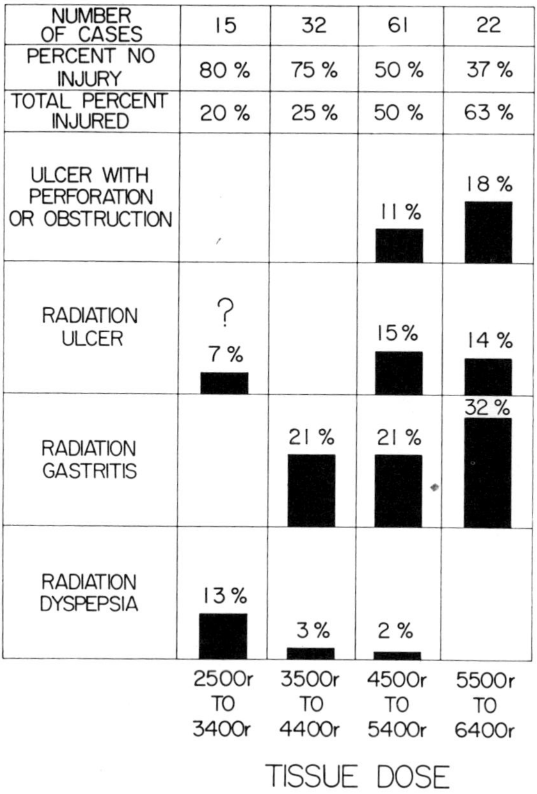

NUMBER OF CASES	15	32	61	22
PERCENT NO INJURY	80 %	75 %	50 %	37 %
TOTAL PERCENT INJURED	20 %	25 %	50 %	63 %
ULCER WITH PERFORATION OR OBSTRUCTION			11 %	18 %
RADIATION ULCER	? 7 %		15 %	14 %
RADIATION GASTRITIS		21 %	21 %	32 %
RADIATION DYSPEPSIA	13 %	3 %	2 %	
	2500r TO 3400r	3500r TO 4400r	4500r TO 5400r	5500r TO 6400r

TISSUE DOSE

Fig. 11-2. Various types of stomach injuries and their incidence in relation to tissue dose. (Reprinted from Localio et al 1969, with permission from the author and Surg. Gynecol. Obstet.)

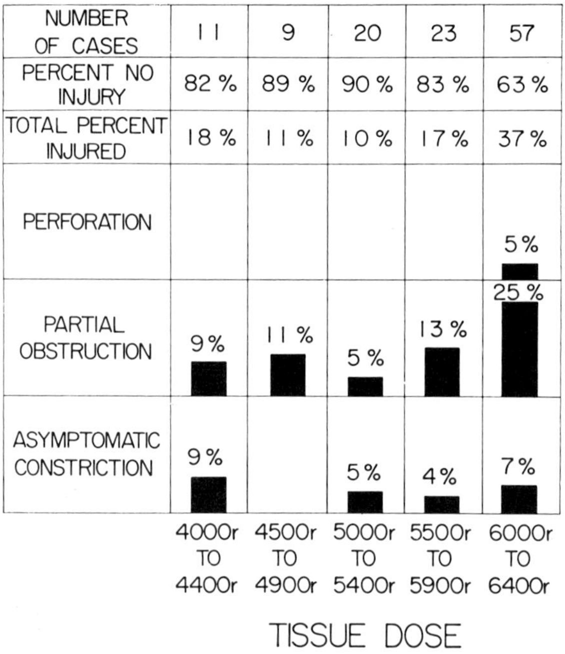

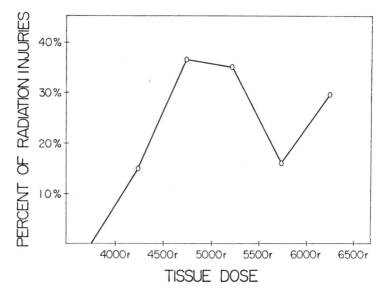

NUMBER OF CASES	11	9	20	23	57
PERCENT NO INJURY	82 %	89 %	90 %	83 %	63 %
TOTAL PERCENT INJURED	18 %	11 %	10 %	17 %	37 %
PERFORATION					5 %
PARTIAL OBSTRUCTION	9 %	11 %	5 %	13 %	25 %
ASYMPTOMATIC CONSTRICTION	9 %		5 %	4 %	7 %
	4000r TO 4400r	4500r TO 4900r	5000r TO 5400r	5500r TO 5900r	6000r TO 6400r

TISSUE DOSE

Fig. 11-3. Various types of transverse colon injuries and their incidence in relation to tissue dose. (Reprinted from Localio et al 1969, with permission from the author and Surg. Gynecol. Obstet.)

Fig. 11-4. Incidence of all types of radiation injuries to the small intestine in relation to tissue dose. (Reprinted from Localio et al 1969, with permission from the author and Surg. Gynecol. Obstet.)

362

Table 11-5

Variables that Affect the Risk of Radiation Injury to the Intestines

Technical	Clinical
1. Total dose	1. Location of the neoplasm
2. Overall treatment time	2. Size of the neoplasm
3. Number of fractions	3. Previous surgery or peritonitis that would
4. Individual dose	fix intestines in field
5. Treatment volume	4. Anatomic location and extent of neoplasm
6. Physical characteristics of the	(stage)
beam	5. Height, weight and physical configuration
7. Field size	of the host
8. Integral dose	6. Infection or abcess in or near intestines in
9. Quality of technique (physics,	treatment field
dosimetry, localization, and	7. Previous radiotherapy to same region
administration)	8. Other diseases
	9. Nutritional status
	10. Oxygenation of tissues
	11. Immeasurable variation in host susceptibility
	12. Age

Modified from: Lacalio SA, Stone A, Friedman M: Surgical aspects of radiation enteritis. Surg Gynecol Obstet 129:1163–1172, 1969.

(TD 50/5) was defined as that dose associated with a 50 percent chance of risk within 5 years of treatment. They determined that the minimal tolerance dose for the stomach was 4500 rads; for the small bowel, 4000 rads; for the transverse colon, 5500 rads; and, for the sigmoid rectum, 5000 rads. This dose should rarely be exceeded for lymphomas but could develop from overlapping fields and other variations. These tolerance dosages are defined statistically, which indicates that they are only a point in a larger frequency distribution where individual patient sensitivity is a significant and uncontrollable variable.

The pathogenesis of high incremental dose injury to small intestine was evaluated in dogs by Spratt et al (1961). Intense segmental injury is marked by rapid ulceration followed by progressive blood vascular and lymphatic occlusion. The submucosa and muscle retain their continuity in most cases, but undergo fragmentation and disappearance by absorption, probably through adjacent lymphatics. The result is a longitudinal contracture of the bowel that proceeds exponentially. The ulcerated segments reduce their length by half every 54 days and after 8 months segments originally 5 cm. in length are reduced to narrow bands. For larger segments (15 cm.), the envelopment of the segment by omentum from which capillaries and fibroblasts grow into the infarcted segment is necessary for survival.

This study gave some insight into the sequence of changes that occur over time. Many individual case reports in the literature describe individual phases of a continuous process determined by the initial injury and subsequent healing. This study as well as clinical observations (Localio et al

1969) established that radiation ulcers of the intestine can and may heal without incident. Consequently, the mere presence of an ulcer is not an indication for resection. Healing proceeds very slowly over many months and may ultimately end in permanent ulcers or stenotic segments of intestine. In clinical situations these segments may be difficult to demonstrate radiographically and have to be suspected on the basis of intermittent abdominal cramps and other signs of partial intestinal obstruction. These segments may also entrap bezoars producing acute intestinal obstruction. The types of stenoses remaining in man are demonstrated in Fig. 11-5.

When the abdomen is irradiated rather diffusely and to a dose that will not actually infarct intestine, the extent of mucosal atrophy and fibrotic changes in the gut wall may be adequate to produce significant disability from malabsorption syndrome.

When the surgeon has to explore an abdomen for partial or complete intestinal obstruction due to irradiation injury of the intestine, many of his usual rules do not apply. First, the location of his surgical incision may be affected by the location of radiation ports as described on p. 350. Second, the irradiated intestine presents some unique surgical problems if it is extensively matted together or is extensively adherent to some portion of the abdominal wall or pelvis. These adhesions are much more dense than those usually encountered and vascular bridging that occurs between the unirradiated and relatively devascular irradiated tissue eliminates tissue planes. Attempts to take down or separate irradiated intestines that have become extensively adherent may actually be physiologically undesirable from the standpoint of destroying anastomotic vascularity on which the healing intestines may be dependent. Such dissection is certainly tedious, time consuming, and fraught with the risk of unnecessary bleeding, intestinal perforation, and sepsis. Most surgeons with experience in this problem have found it better to bypass these matted intestines by anastomosing proximal and distal nonirradiated intestine. When this matting occurs in the presence of perforation or fistula, enteroenterostomy must divert the fecal stream completely away from the fistula. This usually requires that the afferent and efferent loops of the fistula be brought to the skin as decompressing enterostomies.

When extensive matting is not present and radiation injury is suspected, the entire length of small intestine should be examined by palpation and observation. Early after treatment, intensely irradiated segments have a thick red sausagelike appearance which later can become reduced to narrow rings or may heal without ring formation. All persistent narrow rings have to be resected by segmental intestinal resection with anastomosis of proximal and distal nonirradiated intestine. If there is any question about the degree of irradiation effect in the ends of the intestines to be anastomosed, a specimen of the intestinal end should be submitted to the pathologist for frozen section examination.

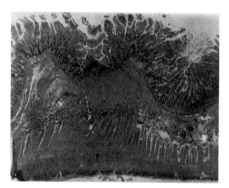
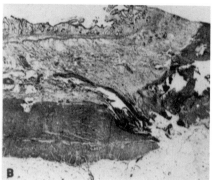
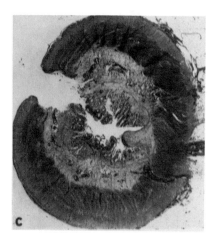

Fig. 11-5. Annular stenoses in human ileums resected because they obstructed the intestine 8, 8, and 14 years, respectively, after intracavitary radium and external roentgen therapy for cervical carcinoma. In all 3 cases the mucosa is atrophic and focally ulcerated within the narrowed intestine. Stenosing cicatrices were located beneath the atrophic and focally ulcerated mucosa. These cicatrices were composed of mature hyalinized scars having no peculiarities. The muscle surrounding the submucosa cicatrices is traversed by strands of this scar tissue. *A*, ileum resected 8 years after therapy (W.U. ill. 60-4375). *B*, ileum resected 8 years after therapy. The serosal mesothelium is absent, and the omentum is adherent to the stenotic segment (W.U. ill. 60-4374A). *C*, ileum resected 14 years after therapy (U.W. ill. 60-4373). From: Spratt JS Jr, Heinbecker P, Saltzstein SL: The influence of succinylsulfathiazole (sulfasuxidine) upon the response of canine small intestine to irradiation. *Cancer* 14:862–874, 1961.

Liver

Ingold et al (1965) evaluated the response of the liver to supervoltage radiotherapy and ascertained that its previously believed radio-resistance is only relative. The individual can obviously tolerate high doses of radiation to a portion of his liver without deleterious effect to himself just as he can tolerate resection of a large portion of the organ. However, the maximum dose that the entire liver can tolerate is between 3000 and 3500 rads over 3 to 4 weeks. The authors were uncertain about the capacity of this dose to sterilize intrahepatic lymphomas. In greater amounts, radiation hepatitis develops with hepatomegaly, ascites, and jaundice. Liver functions deteriorate. Supportive therapy, as with other forms of hepatitis, may lead to recovery or may not affect the progression of the radiation injury with eventual host death from hepatic insufficiency.

The microscopically observed effects include centrolobular hemorrhage, sinusoidal congestion, and minimal hepatic cellular atrophy. Later changes are described as showing still more hepatic cellular damage and changes in the central vein wall. Histological observations varied according to the length of time elapsing after treatment.

Late effects of radiation hepatitis have really not been fully evaluated by this report since the period of observation was still too short. At less than 60 days, the effects were acute and by the time 100 days had passed after treatment, hyalin thickening of the endothelium, with complete occlusion of some vessels, and atrophy were developing. When the radiation dose was in excess of 5000 rads to the left lobe, frank necrosis occasionally developed.

Kidney

The kidney is susceptible to radiation effects that can produce arteriolonephrosclerosis and hypertension (Asscher et al 1961; Wachholz and Casarett, 1970; Wilson et al 1958). All skilled therapists attempt to shield the kidney whenever tumor and treatment characteristics permit, but this is not always feasible. As Wachholz and Casarett have shown, the initiation of hypertension can occur with little renal damage demonstrable by light microscopic examination. They observed that the nephrosclerosis progressed after the hypertension had developed. Shielding the kidney was not entirely effective and they did not exclude the possibility that some extrarenal effects of the radiation might also contribute to the hypertension–nephrosclerosis cycle. The latent period between irradiation and the development of hypertension may be many months. In total body irradiation without shielding of the kidneys, nephrosclerosis is a significant problem (Lamson et al 1959).

As a result of this risk, all potential surgical candidates who have had irradiation should be evaluated for the possible development of the hypertension–nephrosclerosis cycle. How this would affect surgical decisions would have to be ascertained on an individual case basis according to the severity of the hypertension and altered renal function, and the response to medical management.

Bone

The surgeon gets involved at several different levels with the secondary effect of irradiation upon bone. When children who have not completed their bone growth receive irradiation to bones, further growth may be arrested. If the child survives and continues to grow, skeletal distortions and disproportions evolve. The resulting deformities may present specialized problems in rehabilitation, prostheses, and cosmetic surgery. The therapist has developed numerous techniques to reduce risk. Since the distortion or contracture is progressive over such a long period of time and the underlying tissue injury so permanent and irreversible, the deformities cannot be totally stopped once the process has been initiated. All of these processes are so varied and infrequent that they must be individually evaluated by an expert who is also familiar with the nature of the underlying irradiation injury and the limitations it places on reconstructive surgical intervention, bone growth arrest techniques, and corrective braces (Rubin and Casarett 1968).

Any time a fracture occurs in a bone that has had previous radiotherapy involving the fracture site, the possibility exists that the fracture is due to the irradiation, metastatic neoplasm, or trauma.

The method of fracture management is site specific and will be determined by the specific orthopedic problem. Even after high doses or irradiation for carinoma of the cervix, spontaneous fractures of the femoral neck heal after pinning. Such high-dose local radiation is infrequent in the treatment of lymphomas. Whenever an open reduction is performed for any fracture occurring in a cancer patient or in a patient who has had previous radiotherapy, the fracture site should be biopsied to exclude the presence of cancer. The presence of cancer is no contraindication to internal reduction and stabilization since the stabilization relieves pain and permits earlier mobility of the patient. Also, if the fracture is due to the presence of neoplasm, further radiotherapy may be indicated and the internal fixation of the fracture will facilitate treatment (Spratt and Donegan 1967).

Collapse of vertebra is occasionally seen after radiotherapy for lymphomas. In the rare instance when this problem might be anticipated, an appropriate back or cervical brace may reduce pain and help prevent spinal cord injury. Of emergency significance is the vertebral collapse that produces acute spinal cord injury. Surgical intervention in these cases requires good neurological as well as roentgen evaluation since multiple sites may be involved. It is not our philosophy to engage in heroic surgical exercises to prevent quadriplegia or paraplegia in these cases unless the prognosis with respect to the neoplasm is good. The cost and morbidity of the intervention may be greater than the human salvage justifies. Again, when surgical intervention is undertaken, a biopsy of the affected bone should always be obtained to be examined for the presence of neoplasm and/or the extent of the radiation effect. These cases must be differentiated from the direct effect of radiation on the spinal cord itself (see myelitis).

The radiobiological effect upon bone and cartilage is dependent upon time–dose factors and the physical characteristics of the radiation. Lower kilovoltage is associated with greater effect upon bone. Though megavoltage has a theoretical bone-sparing effect, statistical proof of this differential effect in clinical radiotherapy is negligible. The bone itself is most easily affected when it is undergoing growth. Radiation's capacity to arrest growth in growing bones is precipitated by intracartilaginous ossification (Moss 1965). Localized radiation is infrequently used with lymphomas to a dose that will produce bone necrosis with secondary osteomyelitis and bone dissolution, as occurs at other sites (Serna 1967; Guerra 1971; Slaughter 1942; Paul and Pohle 1942).

Marrow

Abrams and Kaplan (1951) showed in experimental animals that shielding of different parts of the body conferred various degrees of protection when exposed to whole-body irradiation. Abdominal shielding offered the highest degree of protection, but significant benefit was also observed when the chest, skull, or thighs were shielded. This suggested that shielding even a small portion of the bone marrow might be important in allowing recovery of the depleted marrow.

Widespread radiotherapy may profoundly affect the granulocyte reserves. At least 40 percent of the marrow must be irradiated with an excess of 1500 rads to develop abnormal granulocyte response to bacterial endotoxin (Hellman and Fink 1965). Vogel et al (1968) said this effect is generally transient and normal marrow activity seems to be restored within several months.

Vogel et al 1968 estimated that the cases in their series received irradiation to approximately 40 percent of the marrow to an excess of 3000 rads. Patients receiving extended radiotherapy for lymphomas may have in excess of 60 percent of their bone marrow irradiated. Immediately after the completion of contiguous radiotherapy, normal granulocytic response to stimulation was depressed to borderline levels. Extended radiotherapy suppressed the marrow response and reduced the number of circulating granulocytes. Over 5 months were required for recovery, but granulocyte release mechanisms remained significantly changed in patients who went into relapse.

This suppression of the marrow after extended radiotherapy has a threshold beyond which there must be increased susceptibility to bacterial infections. Exactly where this threshold is is not always known in a specific patient. As a general surgical principle, patients who have had marrow-suppressive radiation should probably receive prophylactic antibiotics pre- and postoperatively. The Halsteadean principles of asepsis, hemostasis, and gentleness should be even more significant during surgery in such cases since their capacity to ward off an invasive bacterial infection may be reduced.

Central Nervous System

No element of the central nervous system is immune from the injury of supervoltage radiation. The underlying process of parenchymatous damage, vascular sclerosis, and actual necrosis which develop gradually over many months following radiotherapy is similar to that in other tissues. McDonald and Hayes (1967) consider that ultimate failure of the vascular supply with secondary ischemic necrosis may be more significant than primary damage of the parenchyma of nervous tissue. They observed electron microscopically that capillary injury is limited to the irradiated area and that capillary basal lamina thickening was found primarily in areas adjacent frank necrosis.

However, the spinal cord has been subject to more frequent radiation resulting in myelitis (Dynes and Smedal 1960; Coy et al 1969; Henry et al 1971). Early after or during treatment paresthesias may develop leading to a Brown-Sequard syndrome, consisting of paraplegia, hyperesthesia, loss of joint and muscle sense on the most affected side, and hemianesthesia of the opposite side. These can progress to a complete transection of the cord.

In the study by Dynes and Smedal (1960), radiation myelitis was rarely a major problem before the seventh post-treatment month, but was still developing in at-risk patients as late as the 50th post-treatment month. All cases in their series had probably received in excess of 5000 rads. Only 1 of their 10 cases occurred in a patient with lymphoma.

Coy et al (1969) reported 3 cases of progressive myelopathy. They considered that this problem could only be avoided by keeping radiation to the cord under 3750 rads in 3 to 4 weeks. Henry et al (1971) described their experience with this demyelinating process. In 7 cases the evolution was gradual; this can lead to quadriplegia and death in the absence of residual neoplasms.

Glicksman and Nickson (1973) said that transverse myelitis is one of the most serious consequences of radiotherapy, and it has been reported especially when two fields have been abutted (mantle technique and inverted Y inadvertently overlap directly on the spinal cord). However, when long segments of the spinal cord are irradiated by the dose necessary to be given in Hodgkin's disease, a rare case of transverse myelitis can occur without a breach of technique. Fortunately, this complication does not occur often, and in more than 300 patients at risk, only two had progressive myelitis. They believed it is important to use a posterior cervical spine shield when treating mantle field. Hoogstraten et al (1973) reported the development of transverse myelitis in three patients among 58 patients who had total nodal radiotherapy with or without added chemotherapy; and in two of these, "special" treatment techniques led to radiation pericarditis and severe pulmonary fibrosis as well.

The surgeon has nothing to offer for this problem and has to be certain that he does not become the executioner by precipitating terminal episodes through injudicious intervention. The size of most radiation fields usually encompasses a significant distance of cord and paracordal tissues. Of 5 deaths reported by Dynes and Smedal (1960), 2 were probably precipitated by surgical intervention from which the patient could have accrued no potential advantage. One patient died from meningitis subsequent to surgical exploration of the cord, in keeping with the poor tolerance of irradiated tissue to infection elsewhere in the body. The second patient died from aggravation of his myelitis by surgery.

Thomas and Colby (1972) studied 14 patients with presumed radiation plexopathy and 11 patients with metastatic involvement of the brachial plexus. In 22 patients the cancer had arisen from the breast. In both groups, plexopathy began after a mean interval of six years, the initial symptom usually being sensory. Almost half of the patients with radiation damage had no significant pain; metastatic plexopathy characteristically was very painful. Sensation, muscle power, and stretch reflexes were affected similarly in both groups. Thus no single clinical symptom or sign permitted distinction between the two groups.

New Primary Cancers

The literature contains scattered case reports of new primary cancers appearing in patients who have been previously irradiated. However, the latent period between irradiation and the appearance of additional cancer is long and the incidence remains low enough to require more cases and man-years of follow-up than are available in most reported series to establish that the additional cancers do not occur as a matter of chance (Doll 1971; Spratt and Hoag 1966). From the practical standpoint, the risk of additional primary cancers is too low to merit more detailed follow-up than is accorded the general population of the same age (Spratt 1971). When a new cancer is diagnosed in a patient who has had a previous cancer treated and controlled, then the new cancer should be treated according to its specific requirements and the characteristics of the host. However, if the new cancer occurs in or near a previously irradiated body site, then the amount of additional radiotherapy that could be tolerated is a matter that must be carefully evaluated by the therapist to avoid tissue overdose from the accumulative radiobiological effects. Also, the surgeon must ascertain the extent of the residual radiobiological effects in planning surgical operations that might be required to treat the new primary cancer. All past treatment records should be obtained and reviewed, and the tissue should be inspected for fibrosis, atrophy, telangiectasia, ulceration, or necrosis.

Late malignant changes in irradiated skin have been reported for over 60 years following radiation therapy. Traenkle (1963) concluded that these skin cancers were largely restricted to people who exhibited severe radiation damage to the skin that had been present from 5 years to several decades. Even in these cases, the incidence has remained low. In the same time frame, supervoltage therapy may not have been available long enough for a significant number of patients to develop late cancer.

FINAL COMMENTS

Radiation can produce a variety of vital organ injuries secondary to the treatment of lymphomas. The clinical surgeon must be aware of the possibility of these injuries in any patient who has had radiotherapy any time in the past. As an integral part of the preoperative evaluation, the location of previous radiation ports and time, dose and physical variables must be ascertained as completely as possible. Abscopal effects remote from the sites of treatment are rarely of surgical significance. The surgeon must, however, consider all organs in the path of radiation as potentially injured. The severity of the injury varies with numerous factors and is never absolutely predictable. Consequently, all possibilities must be considered and any surgical approach to solution must consider the unique radiobiological effects which determine natural history and often dictate the method of management. The possibilities considered here are those sometimes encountered with the treatment of lymphomas. The list is not intended to include all types of radiation injury that have been reported. The radiobiological processes are, however, quite similar at all sites and any further consideration would be determined by the functional injuries in the affected organs.

Judging by the numerous case reports in the literature, the prevalence of significant radiation injury may be much greater than is generally appreciated. It could produce iatrogenic illness far greater than the original neoplasm, particularly when used prophylactically.

The plethora of individual case reports contains few series followed by the primary therapist and suggests that he may not have a full appreciation of the number of complications that accumulate over time, the total patient morbidity or downtime, the cost to the patient and his family, or even the treatment-specific mortality rate. When these problems continue to collect over 5, 10, 15, 20, or 25 years or longer, the accumulated morbidity can become enormous. The morbidity of the iatrogenic problems may exceed the morbidity of the neoplasm and when the added cost of treating the iatrogenic problems is considered, the pattern of medical practice can become expensive beyond potential return to either the individual or society. It is for this reason that a more useful method of measurement than the 5-year survival rate is needed. It tells nothing of the duration of treatment, patient downtime from diagnostic studies, complications, and premature lethality as a result of treatment. It certainly tells nothing of the accumulative costs to the patient and society (Spratt 1971).

SUMMARY

The increasing use of radiation therapy for the treatment of lymphomas of all types has important surgical ramifications. Complications of radiotherapy can be divided into two groups: one due to the general effect of irradiation upon the healing of surgical wounds and the other due to organ-specific irradiational injuries.

The retardation of wound healing by irradiation is due to inhibition of capillary budding. And this effect is dependent upon the amount of radiation, its physical qualities, and the length of time over which that dose is administered. Important information before undertaking surgery in any irradiated tissue should include: (1) the exact location and size of all external ports, (2) the direction of the beam traversing these ports, (3) the location of and tissue at all exit ports for linear accelerator, and (4) the approximate time–dose factors and physical characteristics of radiation received by all organs and tissues traversed by the beam or its pneumbra that might be included in the area of contemplated surgery.

Basically, radiation affects all tissues in the same way: it accelerates aging, kills normal cells as well as neoplastic, and damages the endothelium of fine blood and lymph vessels with resulting sclerosis. Ultimately all areas receiving therapeutic doses of irradiation develop the following characteristics: incomplete regeneration of original structure, fine to gross scar formation, reduced vascularity, and reduced capacity to tolerate injury or infection with a tendency to develop acute necrosis or late spontaneous necrosis. Specific organ sites discussed in detail included skin, thyroid, heart, aorta and elastic arteries, lung, guts, liver, kidney, bone, marrow, and central nervous system. Judging by the numerous case reports in the literature, the prevalence of significant radiation injury may be much greater than is generally appreciated. It could produce iatrogenic illness far more grave than the original neoplasm, particularly when used prophylactically.

REFERENCES

Abrams HL, Kaplan HS: Effect of shielding on mortality following irradiation. Stanford Med Bull 9:165–166, 1951

Ackerman LV: The pathology of radiation effect of normal and neoplastic tissue. Am J Roentgenol Radium Ther Nucl Med 114:447–459, 1972

Anderson LD: Fractures, in Crenshaw AH (ed): Campbell's Operative Orthopaedics, vol 1 (ed 5). Louis, Mosby, 1971, pp 477–691

Asscher AW, Wilson C, Anson SG: Sensitisation of blood vessels to hypertensive damage by x-irradiation. Lancet 1:580–583, 1961

Bennett DE, Million RR, Ackerman LV: Bilateral radiation pneumonitis: A complication of the radiotherapy of bronchogenic carcinoma: Report and analysis of seven cases with autopsy. Cancer 23:1001–1018, 1969

Bloedorn FG, Cowley RA: Irradiation and surgery in the treatment of brochogenic carcinoma. Surg Gynecol Obstet 111:141–146, 1960

Brenk HA van den: The effect of ionizing radiations on the regeneration and behavior of mammalian lymphatics: *In vivo* studies in Sandison Clark chambers. Am J Roentgenol Radium Ther Nucl Med 78:837–849, 1957

Brenk HA van den: Studies in restorative growth processes in mammalian wound healing. Br J Surg 43:525–550, 1956

Case Records of the Massachusetts General Hospital: Weekly clinicopathological exercises, case 31–1970. N Engl J Med 283:191–201, 1970

Case Records of the Massachusetts General Hospital: Weekly clinicopathological exercises, case 11–1971. N Engl J Med 284:603–610, 1971

Case Records of the Massachusetts General Hospital: Weekly clinicopathological exercises, case 16–1971. N Engl J Med 284:899–910, 1971

Chau PM, Fletcher GH, Rutledge FN, et al: Complications in high dose whole pelvis irradiation in female pelvic cancer. Am J Roentgenol Radium Ther Nucl Med 87:22–40, 1962

Cohn KE, Stewart JR, Fajardo LF, et al: Heart disease following radiation. Medicine 46:281–298, 1967

Cope O: Thyroid, thymus and parathyroids, in Moyer CA, Rhoads JE, Allen JG, et al (eds): Surgery: Principles and Practice (ed 3). Philadelphia, Lippincott, 1965, pp 662–696

Copeland M: Primary malignant tumors of bone: Evaluation of current diagnosis and treatment. Cancer 20:738–746, 1967

Coulter JW, Ruth WE, Kerby GR: Pulmonary complications in mantle field irradiation of Hodgkin's disease. Am Rev Respir Dis 105:1005–1006, 1972 (Abstr)

Coy P, Baker S, Dolman CL: Progressive myelopathy due to radiation. Can Med Assoc J 100:1129–1133, 1969

Denny-Brown D, Foley JM: Clinical pathologic conference. Neurology 3:615–620, 1953

Doll R: Cancer following therapeutic external irradiation, in Clark RL, Cumley RW, McCay JE, et al (eds): Oncology 1970, vol 5. Chicago, Year Book, 1971, pp 96–102

Dollinger MR, Lavine DM, Foye LV Jr: Myocardial infarction due to postirradiation fibrosis of the coronary arteries. JAMA 195:316–319, 1966

Durkovský J. Krajci M: Complications after radiation treatment in Hodgkin's disease. Neoplasma 19:227–233, 1972

Dynes JB, Smedal MI: Radiation myelitis. Am J Roentgenol Radium Ther Nucl Med 83:78–87, 1960

Essen CF von: Radiation tolerance of the skin. Acta Radiol [Ther] (Stockh) 8:311–330, 1969

Fletcher GH, Jesse RH: Interaction of surgery and irradiation in head and neck cancers. Curr Probl Radiol 1:2–39, Jul-Aug 1971

Fraumeni JF Jr, Herweg JC, Kissane JM: Panaortitis complicating Hodgkin's disease. Ann Intern Med 67:1242–1248, 1967

Freid JR, Goldberg H: Post-irradiation changes in lungs and thorax: Clinical, roentgenological and pathological study, with emphasis on late and terminal stages. Am J Roentgenol Radium Ther Nucl Med 43:877–895, 1940

Glatstein E, McHardy-Young S, Brast N, et al: Alterations in serum thyrotropin (TSH) and thyroid functions following radiotherapy in patients with malignant lymphoma. J Clin Endocrinol Metab 32:833–841, 1971

Glicksman AS, Nickson JJ: Acute and late reactions to irradiation in the treatment of Hodgkin's disease. Arch Intern Med 131:369–373, 1973

Grillo HC, Potsaid MS: Studies in wound healing. IV. Retardation of contraction by local x-irradiation, and observations relating to the origin of fibroblasts in repair. Ann Surg 154:741–750, 1961

Guerra ON: Maxillofacial prosthetics. Mo Med 68:928–931, 1971

Hellman S, Fink ME: Granulocyte reserve following radiation therapy as studied by the response to a bacterial endotoxin. Blood 25:310–324, 1965

Henry P, Castaigns G, Hoerni B, et al: La Myélopathie progressive post-radiothérapeutique tardive. J Neurol Sci 14:325–340, 1971

Hoogstraten B, Holland JF, Kramer S, et al: Combination chemotherapy-radiotherapy for stage III Hodgkin's disease: An Acute Leukemia Group B study. Arch Intern Med 131:424–428, 1973

Hutchison HE: Irradiation pneumonitis: Report of a case with description of histological findings. Glasgow Med J 34:299–307, 1953

Ingold JA, Reed GB, Kaplan HS, et al: Radiation hepatitis. Am J Roentgenol Radium Ther Nucl Med 93:200–208, 1965

Jansen CR, Bond VP, Rai KR, et al: Abscopal effects of localized irradiation by accelerator beams. Ann NY Acad Sci 114:302–315, 1964

Jennings FL, Arden A: Development of radiation pneumonitis: Time and dose factors. Arch Pathol 74:351–360, 1962

Lamson BG, Billings MS, Bennett LR: Late effects of total-body roentgen irradiation. V. Longevity and incidence of nephrosclerosis as influenced by partial-body shielding. J Natl Cancer Inst 22:1059–1075, 1959

Landberg T, Svahn-Tapper G, Wintzell K: Mantle treatment of Hodgkin's disease: Preliminary report of side effects and early results. Acta Radiol [Ther] (Stockh) 10:174–186, 1971

Leaming RH, Stearns MW, Deddish MR: Preoperative irradiation in rectal carcinoma. Radiology 77:257–263, 1961

Lee YN, Say C, Hori JM, et al: Clinical Courses of Hodgkin's disease and other malignant lymphomas. Am J Roentgenol Radium Ther Nucl Med 117:19–29, 1973

Localio SA, Stone A, Friedman M: Surgical aspects of radiation enteritis. Surg Gynecol Obstet 129:1163–1172, 1969

Lockart RZ Jr, Elkind MM, Moses WB: Radiation response of mammalian cells grown in culture. II. Survival and recovery characteristics of several subcultures of Hela S3 cells after x-irradiation. J Natl Cancer Inst 27:1393–1404, 1961

Looney WB, Chang LO: Local and generalized effects of local radiation. Part I. Effects of local radiation to the liver and upper intestines in partially hepatectomized, sham-operated, and normal rats. Radiology 89:906–918, 1967

Libshitz HI, Brosof AB, Southard ME: Radiographic appearance of the chest following extended field radiation therapy for Hodgkin's disease: A consideration of time—dose relationships. Cancer 32:206–215, 1973

McDonald LW, Hayes TL: The role of capillaries in the pathogenesis of delayed radionecrosis of brain. Am J Pathol 50:745–764, 1967

Marcial-Rojas RA, Castro JR: Irradiation injury to elastic arteries in the course of treatment for neoplastic disease. Ann Otol 71:945–958, 1962

Mendelsohn ML, Shackney SE: The growth kinetics of solid tumors: Summary report of meeting. Cell Tissue Kinet 3:405–414, 1970

Moss WT: Therapeutic Radiology: Rationale, Technique, Results (ed 2). St. Louis, Mosby, 1965

Nobler MP: The abscopal effect in malignant lymphoma and its relationship to lymphocyte circulation. Radiology 93:410–412, 1969

Order SE, Moncrief JA: Burn Wound. Springfield, Ill, Thomas, 1965

Pallin I, Collins VJ, Foldes FF, et al: Symposium and panel discussion on "Management of patients requiring operations." NY State J Med 59:4359–4376, 1959

Palos B, Kaplan HS, Karzmark CJ: The use of thin lung shields to deliver limited whole-lung irradiation during mantle-field treatment of Hodgkin's disease. Radiology 101:441–442, 1971

Paul LW, Pohle EA: Radiation osteitis of the ribs. Radiology 38:543–549, 1942

Pohle EA, Ritchie G, Wright CS: Studies of effect of roentgen rays on healing of wounds. I. The behavior of skin wounds in rats under pre- or postoperative irradiation. Radiology 16:445–460, 1931

Poon RP, Kanshepolsky J, Tchertkoff V: Rupture of the aorta due to radiation injury: Report of a case and electron microscopic study. JAMA 205:875–878, 1968

Prager D, Sembrot JT, Southard M: Cobalt-60 therapy of Hodgkin's disease and the subsequent development of hypothyroidism. Cancer 29:458–460, 1972

Puck TT: Radiation and the human cell. Sci Am 202:142–153, 1960

Roswit B, Malsky SF, Reid CB: Severe radiation injuries of the stomach, small intestine, colon and rectum, Am J Roentgenol Radium Ther Nucl Med 114:460–475, 1972

Rubin E, Camara J, Grayzel DM, et al: Radiation-induced cardiac fibrosis. Am J Med 34:71–75, 1963

Rubin P, Casarett GW: Clinical Radiation Pathology, 2 vols. Philadelphia, Saunders, 1968

Rubin P, Casarett G: A direction for clinical radiation pathology: The tolerance dose. Frontiers Radiation Ther Oncol 6:1–16, 1972

Sala JM, del Regato JA: Treatment of carcinoma of endometrium. Radiology 79:12–17, 1962

Serna, GM: Osteoradionecrosis. Mo Med 64:997–1000, 1967

Slaughter DP: Current concepts in cancer: 2. Hodgkin's disease, radical surgery. JAMA 191:26–27, 1965

Slaughter DP: Radiation osteitis and fractures following irradiation, with report of 5 cases of fractured clavicle. Am J Roentgenol Radium Ther Nucl Med 48:201–212, 1942

Spratt JS Jr: The measurement of the value of the clinical process to individuals by age and income. J Trauma 11:966–973, 1971

Spratt JS Jr, Butcher HR Jr: Abdominal visceral irradiation injuries at Barnes and Allied Hospitals. Unpublished data.

Spratt JS Jr, Butcher HR Jr, Bricker EM: Exenterative Surgery of the Pelvis. Philadelphia, Saunders, 1973

Spratt JS Jr, Donegan WL: Cancer of the Breast. Philadelphia, Saunders, 1967

Spratt JS Jr, Heinbecker P, Saltzstein SL: The influence of succinylsulfathiazole (Sulfasuxidine) upon the response of canine small intestine to irradiation. Cancer 14:862–874, 1961

Spratt JS Jr, Hoag MG: Incidence of multiple primary cancers per man-year of followup: 20-year review from the Ellis Fischel State Cancer Hospital. Ann Surg 164:775–784, 1966

Spratt JS Jr, Sala JM: The healing of wounds within irradiated tissue. Mo Med 59:409–411, 1962

Stone DJ, Schwartz MJ, Green RA: Fatal pulmonary insufficiency due to radiation effect upon the lung. Am J Med 21:211–226, 1956

Thomas E, Forbus WD: Irradiation injury to the aorta and the lung. Arch Pathol 67:256–263, 1959

Thomas JE, Colby MY: Radiation-induced or metastatic brachial plexopathy? A diagnostic dilemma. JAMA 222:1392–1395, 1972

Traenkle HL: X-ray-induced skin cancer in man. Natl Cancer Inst Monogr 10:423–432, 1963

Vogel JM, Kimball HR, Foley HT, et al: Effect of extensive radiotherapy on the marrow granulocyte reserves of patients with Hodgkin's disease. Cancer 21:798–804, 1968

Wachholz BW, Casarett GW: Radiation hypertension and nephrosclerosis. Radiat Res 41:39–56, 1970

Walsh D: Deep tissue traumatism from roentgen ray exposure. Br Med J 2:272–273, 1897

Warren S: Effects of radiation on normal tissues. Arch Pathol 34:917–931, 1942

Wilson C, Ledingham JM, Cohen M: Hypertension following x-irradiation of the kidneys. Lancet 1:9–16, 1958

Wilson JF, Marsa GW, Johnson RE: Herpes zoster in Hodgkin's disease: Clinical, histologic, and immunologic correlations. Cancer 29:461–465, 1972

Whitfield AG, Bond WH, Kunkler PB: Radiation damage to thoracic tissues. Thorax 18:371–380, 1963

Whitaker W, Brewer D, Fitzgerald M, et al: Clinical pathologic conference. Am Heart J 68:549–555, 1964

Zubrod CG: Summary of informal discussion on radiation therapy for Hodgkin's disease. Cancer Res 26:1264–1267, 1966

12

Surgery for Complications and New Conditions

SPLENECTOMY FOR HYPERSPLENISM

Apparently Billroth performed the first splenectomy for malignant lymphoma in 1866 (von Hacker 1884). About the same time, Fioravanti performed a splenectomy on a patient suffering from leukemia. Up to that time 46 splenectomies had been performed for various diseases; only 10 patients survived the operation (Strumia et al 1966), Mayo (1928) reviewed 500 splenectomies including 54 cases done for leukemia, lymphoma, and Hodgkin's disease. He believed that worthwhile palliation was attained in a number of instances.

Since then, there has been an ongoing argument regarding the applicability of splenectomy for hypersplenism in patients with Hodgkin's disease, lymphosarcoma, and reticulum cell sarcoma. Hypersplenism, a complication of splenomegaly, is defined as any detrimental increase of splenic activity affecting the hematologic components (Crosby 1962). For all practical purposes, it could be classified etiologically as primary or secondary. In 1939, Wiseman and Doan described the condition of primary hypersplenism which consisted of splenomegaly and leukopenia for which splenectomy was curative. Often there was increased susceptibility to infection and variable degrees of hemolytic anemia and thrombocytopenia, but the bone marrow was normal or somewhat hyperplastic. This primary hypersplenism is diagnosed by the absence of known disease involving the spleen directly. In contrast, secondary hypersplenism is caused by or associated with another pathologic state.

Among 240 patients hospitalized for Hodgkin's disease, Williams et al (1951) reported 31 who had one or more major surgical procedures. Eleven patients had splenectomy for hypersplenism and 9 had improvement of their hematologic patterns. Zollinger et al (1952) reported 54 splenectomies performed for secondary hypersplenism. They found the results in secondary lesions did not approach those obtained in primary hypersplenism. Fisher et al (1952) studied the results of splenectomy performed for 18 patients with leukemia and lymphomas; 2 had Hodgkin's disease and 5 had other malignant lymphomas. Eleven of these 18 received some degree of palliation and perhaps prolongation of life. For cases of splenomegaly, the patients must have a great deal of discomfort before operation is recommended. In cases of acquired hemolytic anemia, they recommended a trial with adrenal corticotropin hormone first.

Zollinger and Williams (1959) reported a series of 696 splenectomies with a mortality of 1.9 percent for those patients with primary hypersplenism and 13.6 percent for those with secondary hypersplenism. They found that the use of corticotropin and cortisone in hypersplenism did not remove or reduce the need for splenectomy. They also emphasized that at the completion of splenectomy "A careful repeated search for accessory spleens should be carried out. And biopsies are routinely taken of the retroperitoneal lymph nodes, liver, and mesenteric lymph nodes." These biopsies established the correct diagnosis in 22 percent of the cases of secondary hypersplenism. Such additional biopsies suggested by them are widely practiced as part of the pretreatment staging exploration and splenectomy for malignant lymphoma now.

Thus, Doan et al (1958) found that splenectomy was valuable in treating secondary as well as primary hypersplenism. They felt "Splenectomy in our hands has given: (a) more prompt remissions, (b) more permanent recoveries, with (c) fewer complications, and (d) less minor sequelae than any other treatment yet suggested and tried." Corticosteroid treatment should be reserved for selected patients, since the risks of treatment with corticotropin or cortisone analogs were appreciable, especially in elderly individuals and in those requiring prolonged therapy (Sloane et al 1962).

Acquired hemolytic anemia as a manifestation of hypersplenism secondary to malignant lymphoma deserves a special discussion, since Kyle et al (1959) and Bowdler and Glick (1966) reported that this problem could be the initial symptom which led to the diagnosis. In 11 patients with lymphoma, survival time after the onset of hemolytic process averaged 7.2 years in those with Hodgkin's disease (7 patients) and 1.6 years in those with follicular lymphoma (3 patients). Direct Coomb's tests were positive in only 50 percent of the cases and probably it is not helpful in determining either the diagnosis or the response to treatment.

Eisner et al (1967) reported that only 3 percent of patients with Hodgkin's disease developed Coomb's-positive hemolytic anemia. They reviewed a series of 10 patients and found that autoimmune hemolytic anemia responded well to various forms of management and did not exert an unfavorable influence upon survival. In a series of 80 patients with reticulum cell sarcoma, Cooper (1970) reported that 5 percent of them had associated Coomb's-positive hemolytic anemia. In one patient, 7 years elapsed between the presentation with hemolytic anemia and the development of reticulum cell sarcoma.

Whether the spleen contained lymphoma or not did not correlate with the presence or absence of hemolytic anemia. In a combined necropsy and surgical series of 14 cases of symptomatic hemolytic anemia and malignant lymphoma, Rappaport and Crosby (1957) found involvement of the spleen in all but one patient. However, Rosenthal et al (1955) reported 3 of 12 spleens and Kyle et al (1959) said 3 of 8 spleens examined afforded no evidence of malignant lymphomatous disease.

Regarding treatment of acquired hemolytic anemia, Welch and Dameshek (1950) felt that "the results in Hodgkin's disease have not been sufficiently good to warrant recommending splenectomy." Scott (1958) mentioned a patient with Hodgkin's disease who presented as hemolytic anemia and splenomegaly. The patient had complete remission lasting nearly 4 years after splenectomy. Wilson, while discussing the paper of Slaughter et al (1958), reported the case of a 17-year-old girl who had complete excision of a large cervical mass of Hodgkin's disease without other therapy. Three years later she developed jaundice and hemolytic anemia. A splenectomy relieved her problem completely and she lived 6 more years without other evidence of Hodgkin's disease. Kyle et al (1959) said splenectomy benefited 4 of their 8 patients. Bouroncle et al (1962) found hemolytic amenia caused jaundice in 11.8 percent of the patients with Hodgkin's disease and splenectomy gave good results in the 4 patients so treated. Ashby and Ballinger (1962) commented that splenectomy in selected patients with hemolytic anemia or thrombocytopenia complicating chronic leukemia, lymphosarcoma and Hodgkin's disease, can result in very worthwhile improvement with reduction in the transfusion needs in about 50 percent of cases.

In 24 patients with malignant reticuloendothelial disease who had splenectomy for hemolytic anemia, Schultz (1964) found that the preoperative trial of corticosteroid did not ensure the selection of patients who would or would not respond to splenectomy. Among 10 cases of Hodgkin's disease and 3 cases of other lymphoma, splenectomy produced hematologic benefit in 6 with a mean duration of 4.7 months. However, this benefit was of doubtful value because serious complication such as subphrenic abscess, pneumonia, or septicemia occurred in 38 percent of the patients and death due to bacterial infection, in 53 percent.

The results of late splenectomy for patients with Hodgkin's disease appear to be poorer than those for other lymphomas. Sykes et al (1954) reviewed 30 cases from the literature of splenectomy in Hodgkin's disease and reported no improvement in 8 patients, slight or temporary improvement in 10, and a significant improvement in 12. They added 7 cases, 5 of which were in an advanced stage; none had benefit from splenectomy. Cole et al (1955) stated categorically that splenectomy was contraindicated in Hodgkin's disease.

Sedgwick and Hume (1960) reported splenectomy for secondary hypersplenism in 11 patients with leukemia and lymphoma. Eight patients died within 1 year, and they concluded that splenectomy earlier in the course of the disease would probably offer greater benefit. Strawitz et al (1961) reported splenectomy in 36 patients (including 1 reticulum cell sarcoma, 9 Hodgkin's disease, and 13 lymphosarcoma). The overall mortality was 8 percent and the postoperative complication rate was 19 percent. They found 80 percent showed a favorable postoperative hematologic response and one-third of the group had survived over a year. Patients with lymphosarcoma and myeloid metaplasia had the longest survival, whereas those with leukemia and Hodgkin's disease, the shortest.

Crosby (1962) said secondary hypersplenic thrombocytopenia in association with Hodgkin's disease or giant follicle lymphoma could get prompt and complete results from splenectomy. Rousselot et al (1962) reported 4 percent of 347 patients with Hodgkin's disease required splenectomy, mainly for unresponsive anemia, and occasionally for severe purpura and marked splenomegaly. Their operative mortality was 7 percent, and the average survival was about 6 months, but 2 patients were alive over 7 and 11 years after splenectomy. They felt that "When the syndrome of hypersplenism occurs early in the disease, splenectomy improves the prognosis; when the disease is advanced, it affects the clinical course only to the extent that fewer transfusions are necessary. However, the patient is made more comfortable and is spared the expense of repeated hospitalization for transfusion."

Duckett (1963) reported on the results of splenectomy in 118 patients with secondary hypersplenism. There were 5 cases of Hodgkin's disease and 4 of other malignant lymphomas included. All except one had good to excellent hematologic response which was defined as return to near normal blood counts with rare transfusions or none. Four of the 5 patients with Hodgkin's disease lived from 2 to 3.5 years. On the other hand, Sandusky et al (1964) reported 4 cases of Hodgkin's disease and 2 of lymphosarcoma among 94 patients who had splenectomy for hematologic disorders. The results in this group were uniformly poor, except for 1 case of lymphosarcoma.

Strumia et al (1966) said splenectomy was frequently effective in chronic lymphatic leukemia and in myelofibrosis, but it was only occasionally effective in reticuloendotheliosis (including Hodgkin's disease). Holt and Witts (1966) also found that the best result of splenectomy was in patients with chronic lymphatic leukemia and cases of follicular lymphoma confined to the spleen. They said splenectomy was rarely indicated or helpful in Hodgkin's disease, although one of their patients had control of the hemolytic anemia and another had improvement of leukopenia to the extent that nitrogen mustard could be given. Grace and Mittelman (1966) reported 20 patients with advanced Hodgkin's disease who had splenectomy for hypersplenism. Seven died in the postoperative period. Uncontrollable hemorrhage and infection were the cause of this high operative mortality. Eight of the 13 survivors showed a beneficial hematologic response but only 1 out of the 13 lived longer than 12 months.

Despite these reports, Crosby et al (1966) commented that they learned "once hypersplenism manifests itself it remains a complication. While it may improve temporarily with treatment of the malignant lymphoma, relapse is inevitable and the hypersplenism seems to become more severe as the patient's condition deteriorates and his marrow is injured by chemotherapy, x-irradiation and the disease itself." Thus, "When hypersplenism is a complication of a permanent or progressive disease, there is usally nothing to be gained by deferring splenectomy once the diagnosis has been established. Especially in the aged, if one waits until the indications for splenectomy are urgent, the patient may have become an almost unacceptable surgical risk." In competent hands, splenectomy carried little risk and no problem was encountered in a series of 20 patients who were 60 years or older (Crosby 1967). One alternative would be the use of splenic irradiation. Sokal used it occasionally, but found it difficult to achieve improvement similar to splenectomy (Zubrod 1966).

Pack and Molander (1966) commented that "There are circumstances which compel the therapist seriously to consider splenectomy in certain patients with generalized Hodgkin's disease. An example is a massive splenic infarction with attendant pain and other acute symptoms. Another example is a spleen which remains large and provocative of discomfort subsequent to proper antecedent irradiation and chemotherapy." And "Patients with Hodgkin's disease that is not accelerating, whose life is in danger from cytopenia and/or hemolysis and who are recalcitrant to steroid therapy, should accept splenectomy as a necessary surgical expedient."

Meeker et al (1967) reviewed 89 splenectomies in patients with malignant lymphoma and chronic leukemia, including 28 patients with Hodgkin's disease, 25 lymphosarcoma, and 8 reticulum cell sarcoma. They proposed a quantitative system to evaluate the hematologic response to splenectomy. Only 1 out of 21 Hodgkin's patients who survived the operation lived longer than 14 months, because the operation was usually performed late in the course of the disease. In contrast, 13 of the 25 patients with lymphosarcoma had excellent response and 15 of the 21 patients were alive after 2 years. They found that the types of operative complications were different between those who had Hodgkin's disease and those with other lymphomas. Pulmonary embolism, hepatic vein thrombosis, hemorrhage, and pulmonary insufficiency were the causes of operative mortality in patients with lymphosarcoma, whereas subphrenic abscess and sepsis were an important cause of operative death in those with Hodgkin's disease. In patients with reticulum cell sarcoma, the response to splenectomy was generally good, but the survival period was short. Rambo and Richardson (1968) reported 35 splenectomies. Two patients with Hodgkin's disease (one had hypersplenism, one had hemolytic anemia) died of primary disease within 7 months.

Gomes et al (1969) did an extensive review of indications for splenectomy in hematologic disease. They concluded that the role of splenectomy in lymphoproliferative disorders was less well defined than that of hereditary spherocytosis, aplastic anemia, and idiopathic thrombocytopenic purpura, but there were indications for splenectomy in selected patients with these disorders.

Schwartz et al (1970) reviewed 200 splenectomies performed for hematologic disorders. Twenty-six of these patients had so-called "malignant hemopathy," including 3 cases of Hodgkin's disease, 6 reticulum cell sarcoma, and 11 lymphosarcoma. In 6 patients, the preoperative diagnosis was primary hypersplenism, but splenectomy and biopsy of the liver and lymph nodes changed the diagnosis. Among the 5 hospital deaths, 2 patients had reticulum cell sarcoma, and 3 had leukemia. There were 7 postoperative mortalities: 3 pulmonary complications, 2 wound infections, 1 wound dehiscence, and 1 pancreatic fistula. Of the 21 survivors, 16 had improvement of the hematologic abnormality for at least 2 months and improvement was sustained for 15 to 70 months in the majority of cases.

Among 1000 patients admitted with the diagnosis of malignant lymphoma, O'Brien et al (1970) reported 18 underwent splenectomy for hypersplenism. Their overall operative mortality was a high figure of 39 percent (especially high in patients with Hodgkin's disease since 6 out of 8 died within 1 month). Splenectomy did favorably influence the course of patients with lymphosarcoma (7 out of 9 had excellent hematologic response and 1 patient was alive at 5 years). Hyatt et al (1970) reported that all of 7 patients with lymphosarcoma who had spenectomy for hypersplenism had hematologic and clinical response. In particular, 6 of the 7 patients were well from 6 months to 10.5 years without another therapy.

Mittelman et al (1970) reviewed all of the splenectomies for patients with malignant lymphoma and chronic leukemia from Roswell Park Memorial Institute, including cases reported by Strawitz et al (1961), Grace and Mittelman (1966), and 44 new cases. The operative mortality for the 124 patients was 16 percent. Twenty of the 21 operative deaths occurred before 1964 and there was only 1 death among the 38 patients operated on between 1965 and 1969. In conclusion, they said splenectomy had a beneficial effect in many patients with lymphocytic lymphosarcoma and chronic lymphatic leukemia but had little or no favorable effect on the course of advanced Hodgkin's disease. Readily demonstrable bone marrow invasion in Hodgkin's disease should be a contraindication for splenectomy.

A new role of splenectomy in advanced malignant lymphoma was suggested by Nies and Creger (1967), who presented a series of 11 patients with malignant lymphomà or chronic lymphocytic leukemia who had severe leukopenia or thrombocytopenia preventing necessary chemotherapy. The white blood cell count rose to at least 5000 after splenectomy in all 8 patients who previously had been leukopenic and the platelet count rose to at least 140,000 in 9 of the 11 who had been thrombocytopenic. These white cell and platelet responses were seen despite the presence of proven bone marrow involvement with malignant cells in 7 of the 11 patients. Lowenbraun et al (1971) reported splenectomy in 10 patients with advanced Hodgkin's disease, 8 had bone or marrow involvement and poor tolerance to myelosuppressive drugs. They found good amelioration of the cytopenia after splenectomy and excellent tolerance to chemotherapy. But De Vita (1971) questioned the role of splenectomy in these cases because in 140 patients treated with the combination chemotherapy (MOPP), he found 12 patients whose pancytopenia improved rather than deteriorated when full dose of drugs was given.

Papp and Penner (1971) reported 3 patients with spontaneous rupture of the spleen without history of trauma; 2 had lymphosarcoma and 1 reticulum cell sarcoma. This association was rather unusual because of 134 cases of splenic rupture seen in their hospital from 1936 to 1969, only 8 cases were of nontraumatic origin. They pointed out that extensive infiltration of the spleen and adjacent organs by malignant lymphoma could result in fatal exsanguination. Such catastrophies should be kept in mind as lives of patients with lymphomatous disorders are being prolonged by the use of chemotherapy and radiotherapy.

Rudders et al (1972) described 3 patients with Hodgkin's disease who presented with a clinical picture indistinguishable from classic thrombocytopenic purpura. Marrow biopsy showed no evidence of tumor or fibrosis, but increased number of megakarocytes. In 2, isologous platelet survival was less than 2 hours. Spleens were not palpable, and splenectomy resulted in one partial and one complete remission.

An old surgical procedure has been utilized in the palliation of hypersplenism in malignant lymphoma recently. Everson and Cole (1948) used ligation of the splenic artery as a treatment in 3 patients with advanced portal hypertension and splenomegaly. Moore et al (1950) ligated splenic artery in 6 patients with advanced cirrhosis, splenomegaly, and marked ascites, and had spectacular improvement in 3 patients. Nuland et al (1970) reported a case of Hodgkin's disease with pancytopenia in which splenectomy was unfeasible because of tumor involvement of the pedicle. Ligation of the splenic artery produced diminution in splenic size and marked improvement in the "hypersplenic" blood picture.

In the EFSCH series, about 18 percent of the patients had splenomegaly at diagnosis. Among the 364 patients with non-Hodgkin's lymphoma, 2 patients presented with splenohepatomegaly and required celiotomy, splenectomy and other tissue biopsy for diagnosis (p. 272). One patient (No. 24711) had late splenectomy for splenomegaly or hypersplenism (p. 392). Among the 164 patients with Hodgkin's disease, 4 had late splenectomy (Table 12-1). One patient died postoperatively. The one patient (No. 30118) who had excellent hematologic response also lived the longest (34 months).

Schwartz et al (1971) defined the current overall therapeutic role of splenectomy in patients with malignant lymphoma as follows: "It is useful in patients whose disease is still responsive to irradiation or chemotherapy, when there is symptomatic splenomegaly, hypersplenism or autoimmune complication. Anemia and thrombocytopenia, and occasionally leukopenia, are not attributed to increased splenic destruction of the blood cells unless there is a cellular or hypercellular marrow with an increase in the respective precursor cells, and unless there is splenomegaly. The demonstration of increased splenic uptake of chromium-51 labeled red cells is associated with a more predictable response to splenectomy." An ongoing dialogue among surgeons, chemotherapists, and radiotherapists is essential. Also, it is apparent that if pretreatment staging exploration and splenectomy would be performed for patients with early malignant lymphoma, the problems of splenomegaly and hypersplenism would be greatly diminished in the future.

SURGERY FOR OTHER COMPLICATIONS

It is important to know that both nonmalignant lesions and malignant complications can occur in patients with Hodgkin's disease and other lymphomas. With the prolongation of survival resulting from improved radiotherapy and chemotherapy, it is to be expected that a higher percentage of patients will have time to develop new problems, either associated or unassociated with malignant lymphoma, secondary to complications of their treatment, or due to the changed natural course of the lymphomatous process.

There are very few reports dealing with the surgical treatment of complications in patients with malignant lymphoma. Williams et al (1951) reported 31 of 240 (12.9 percent) Hodgkin's disease patients hospitalized needed 35 surgical procedures. Other than 1 patient who had curative surgery and 11 who required major surgery for diagnosis, 16 surgical procedures were done for the treatment of complications arising from the disease and 7 for unrelated conditions. Among the complications related to Hodgkin's disease, there were hypersplenism (11), spinal cord compression (4), and massive involvement of the breast (1). They commented that surgery followed by x-ray therapy might also give good palliation for tracheal, gastrointestinal, and genitourinary tract compressions. It was pointed out that major surgery did not accelerate the course of Hodgkin's disease and such patients tolerated major surgical procedures well. A relatively normal postoperative recovery is to be expected except in those cases in which the Hodgkin's disease is generalized or terminal.

Table 12-1
Late Splenectomy for Hodgkin's Disease (EFSCH series)

Patient No.	Age	Sex	Date	Diag-nosis	Primary lesion		Stage at op.	Indication	Spleen		Survival	Postoperative		
					Site	Interval (months)			Wt (g)	HD		Radio-therapy	Chemo-therapy	Hematologic response
03922	38	M	6-46	LP	Neck	51	III	Spleno-megaly	—	+	5 mo	+	–	no change
24728	18	M	2-58	MC	Neck	10	IV	Hyper-splenism	980	+	8 days	–	–	
23964	17	M	8-63	LP	Neck	73	III	Hemolytic anemia	970	+	8 mo	+	+	no change
30118	32	M	7-65	MC	Neck, axilla, mediastinum	48	III	Hyper-splenism	1700	+	34 mo	+	+	excellent

Jelliffe and Thompson (1955) reviewed a series of 227 patients with histologically documented Hodgkin's disease. They mentioned specifically that 3 patients developed a perforation of the duodenal ulcer. Two had the diagnosis established at postmortem examination; one case was recognized and successfully dealt with. In addition, proven peptic ulcer occurred in another 7 patients and was a constant source of difficulty in diagnosis, the pain being confused with that found with retroperitoneal gland involvement. They commented that this high incidence might be attributed to the constant nervous tension experienced by the majority of these patients.

Rosenberg et al (1961) reported a series of 1269 patients with non-Hodgkin's lymphoma. Seventy-six patients underwent radical operations for possible cure with 13.1 percent developing postoperative complications. They did not report the incidence of palliative surgery for malignant lymphomas, but commented that "Intestinal or tracheal obstruction, perforation of an abdominal viscus, or gastrointestinal hemorrhage may demand emergency surgical intervention. Rarely, obstructive jaundice has been temporarily relieved by the removal of extrahepatic tumor and the insertion of a common duct T-tube." They did report that, among the 1102 patients who received radiation therapy, 21 (1.9 percent) developed relatively severe complications. Examples: "Radiation osteitis occurred in 5 patients. Persistent and severe radiation pneumonitis and fibrosis developed in 4 patients, and in some of these was probably the major cause of death. Severe skin ulcerations were seen 3 times and were managed satisfactorily with plastic surgical techniques. Two patients developed severe iritis and glaucoma requiring enucleation after radiation therapy to the orbit. In two instances, radiation therapy appeared to hasten the demise of patients with tracheal and superior vena caval obstruction."

Pack and Molander (1966) reported a series of 316 patients with Hodgkin's disease; 12 patients (4 percent) had curative surgery for unifocal disease and 12 patients had palliative surgical procedures, apparently all related with malignancy (7 intestinal obstruction, 2 gastric hemorrhage, 2 retroperitoneal bulky mass, and 1 hemolytic anemia). Among 567 patients with non-Hodgkin's lymphoma also reported by Molander and Pack (1963), 42 patients (7.4 percent) had curative surgical resection and 10 patients had palliative surgery. These latter groups included by-pass and decompression for intestinal obstruction (4), operation for gastric hemorrhage (2), removal of retroperitoneal mass (2), portacaval shunt and splenectomy (1 each).

In the present EFSCH series, among 163 patients with Hodgkin's disease, 12 (7.4 percent) required surgical procedures for complications. Four of these 12 had splenectomy for hypersplenism and are discussed on p. 384. Three had operations for nonmalignant complications (appendicitis, perforated duodenal ulcer, and pregnancy requiring caesarean section), and 5 had complications secondary to Hodgkin's disease (Table 12-2).

Among the 364 patients with non-Hodgkin's lymphomas, 36 (10 percent)

Table 12-2
Operation for Other Complications of Hodgkin's Disease (EFSCH series)

Patient No.	Age	Sex	Date	Diagnosis	Primary lesion Sites	Interval to op.	Indication	Operation	Survival (* = alive)	Lymphoma at follow-up
Nonmalignant										
08968	16	M	9-46	LP	Axilla	5 days	Appendicitis	Appendectomy	25 mo	+
31344	56	F	9-67	NS	Neck, axilla, mediastinum, para-aortic	65 mo	Perforated duodenal ulcer	Vagotomy, antrectomy	48 mo	+
40366	20	F	12-69	MC	Neck	1 mo	Normal pregnancy	Cesarean section	25 mo*	+
Malignant										
18934	23	F	2-57	NS	Mediastinum, neck, axilla, bone, skin	40 mo	Perforated ileum	Ileal resection	14 days	+
29308	71	M	7-61	UC	Groin	6 mo	Jaundice	Liver and retroperitoneal biopsy	4 days	+
35450	55	F	7-67	NS	Neck, axilla, mediastinum	25 mo	Abscess over thyroid cartilage, respiratory distress	I and D abscess, tracheostomy	8 mo	+
28036	37	F	3-69	MC	Mediastinum, aortic, lung	108 mo	Paraplegia	Laminectomy (T 6-10)	18 mo	+
39646	20	M	2-71	LD	Axilla, hilar, liver	1 mo	Chylothorax	Thoracostomy, tracheostomy	2 mo	− (radiation pneumonitis)

Table 12-3
Operation for Non-Malignant Complications of Non-Hodgkin's Lymphoma (EFSCH series)

Patient No.	Age	Sex	Date	Diagnosis	Site	Interval (months) to op	Active	Complication	Operation	Survival (months) * = alive	Lymphoma at follow-up
					Primary lesion						
15243	69	M	7-51	LWD	Neck, groin	2	+	Bowel obstruction	Paracolostomy hernia repair and bowel resection	14	? (Ca rectum)
19749	52	M	11-54	MCN	Neck, axilla mediastinum	37	+	Appendicitis	Appendectomy	6	+
18935	59	M	12-56	LWN	Neck, mesentery	33	+	Inguinal hernia	Inguinal herniorrhaphy	58	+
21848	72	M	5-56	UC	Stomach	3	+	Incarcerated hernia	Inguinal herniorrhaphy	177	– (heart attack)
			1-56	UC	Stomach	107	–	Recurrent hernia	Inguinal herniorrhaphy	73	–
24711	37	F	9-59	Mix	Ileum	21	–	Small bowel obstruction	Resect congenital jejunal stricture	107	
			4-60	Mix	Ileum	28	–	Small bowel obstruction	Adehesionolysis		
12818	70	M	11-64	Mix	Ileum	83	+	Cervicitis	Cold cone cervix	3	+
29936	59	M	5-61	HWN	Mesentery	10	+	GI Obstruction	Adehesinolysis	6	? (trauma)
			10-62	LWN	Groin	8	+	Aortic aneurysm	Resection aneurysm		
04031	81	F	11-63	Und	Stomach	69	–	Cholelithiasis	Cholecystectomy, CBDE	35	– (old age)
26738	66	F	12-64	LWD	Thigh, abdomen (RT to Ca cervix)	65	–	Infarction, ileum	Ileal resection	19	– (stroke)

28276	69	M	2-65	LWD	Neck, groin	65	?	Duodenal ulcer	Vagotomy and antrectomy	85	–
37788	54	M	8-67	LWD	Neck, groin	95	?	Umbilical hernia	Herniorrhaphy	1	+
			9-70	LWD	Forehead	132	+	Recurrent hernia	Herniorrhaphy		
			11-68	HPD	Cecum	1	+	Pelvic abscess, bowel obstruction	I and D, adehesinolysis		
39025	46	F	9-70	LWD	Axilla, neck, aortic, pelvis	5	+	Cholecyctitis	Cholecystectomy	14	+
39296	50	F	11-70	LWD	Axilla, groin	3	+	Thrombophlebitis, pulmonary embolism	IVC clipping	18*	?
38567	71	M	3-71	LWD	Neck, tonsil	53	+	Inguinal hernia	Inguinal herniorrhaphy	8*	?
39644	43	M	4-71	LWD	Neck, axilla	2	+	Cholecystitis	Cholecystectomy	6	+

required 48 surgical procedures for various complications. Fifteen patients had 20 operations for nonmalignant lesions including gastrointestinal obstruction (6), abdominal hernia (6), cholecystitis (3), aortic aneurysm, appendicitis, cervicitis, duodenal ulcer, and pulmonary embolism (1 each) (Table 12-3). Ten patients had 11 operations for various gastrointestinal complications secondary to non-Hodgkin's lymphoma (p. 255). Eight patients had 9 operations for malignant complications not related to the gastrointestinal tract (Table 12-4).

Three patients who had surgery for lesions related to radiotherapy were discussed on p. 346. The problem of palliative surgery for malignant lymphomas of the gastrointestinal tract was discussed on pp. 234–250; for bone lesions, pp. 317–319; for spinal cord compression, pp. 332–334; for pleural effusion and chylothorax, pp. 305–308; for hypersplenism, pp. 377–384; and for obstructive jaundice, pp. 139–141.

It is evident that palliative surgery performed for malignant complications usually was carried out when patients had advanced or generalized disease (pp. 255, 385, 387, 392). All 27 patients in the EFSCH series died within 8 months except 3; one (No. 28036) lived 18 months after laminectomy for spinal cord compression, one (No. 30118) lived 34 months after splenectomy for hypersplenism, and another (No. 30125) had multiple operations for subcutaneous lesions and is still living 12 years after initial diagnosis. The result of surgical treatment for nonmalignant conditions was much better (Tables 12-2, 12-3). Among the 18 patients, 4 are still living at 8, 18, 25, and 85 months after operation. Among the 14 who died, 5 died within 6 months, 3 died within 1.5 years and 6 died more than 2 years postoperatively (4 of the 14 patients had no evidence of malignant lymphoma at death).

SURGERY FOR ADDITIONAL CANCERS

The coexistence of secondary neoplasms (excluding leukemia) with malignant lymphoma could be just an incidental finding. In 1940, Craver and Sunderland reported a case of Hodgkin's disease of the stomach with carcinoma of the colon. Jackson and Parker (1947) reported the coexistence of Hodgkin's disease, mycosis fungoides, and carcinoma. Tillman (1965) recorded a case of Hodgkin's disease of the neck node and gingiva. Two years later the patient had an adenocarcinoma arising from a salivary gland of the hard palate.

In the series of 1269 patients with non-Hodgkin's lymphoma, Rosenberg et al (1961) found that additional cancers were diagnosed during life in 3.4 percent of the series, and 6.1 percent of those that had autopsy had separate second cancers. Among the 56 known lesions, 21 were skin cancers. Dawson et al (1961) found 4 of their 37 cases of primary intestinal lymphomas had associated carcinomas. In 3, primary adenocarcinoma of the colorectum appeared within 2 years; the fourth patient died of lung cancer 16 years after resection of multiple lymphosarcoma of the jejunum and ileum.

In the 249 patients with lymphoma of the head and neck regions, Catlin (1968) recorded 7 patients who presented with a second cancer; 2 breast, 2 colon, 1 cervix uteri, 1 kidney and 1 case of chronic lymphatic leukemia. All except the last case were controlled by surgery. Gellhorn (1968) mentioned that a second neoplastic disease, most often a gastrointestinal carcinoma, was present in many cases with lymphocytic lymphosarcoma, suggesting that it might be one of the manifestations of defects in immune mechanisms. Among 265 patients with histologically verified reticulum cell sarcoma, Hansen (1969) found a second malignancy developing during life in 4.5 percent of the patients. Lipton and Lee (1971) reported 26 patients with stage I non-Hodgkin's lymphoma, documented by negative lymphangiogram. Two patients were treated by surgery alone; one, who had lymphosarcoma of the parotid gland, was free of disease for 54 months when he died of adenocarcinoma of the stomach. Munnell (1971) mentioned 1 patient who had reticulum cell sarcoma with mediastinal mass. Rhabdomyosarcoma was found and confirmed at mediastinoscopy.

In a series of 402 patients with Hodgkin's disease, Lacher (1969) reported 90 patients survived more than 10 years (an incidence rate of 22 percent). He pointed out that extensive initial and repeated radiotherapy was responsible for such long survival. But many patients had local radiation skin necrosis, and 1 patient died with radiation-induced spindle cell sarcoma. He commented: "Only time will tell to what extent complications of this type of therapy will influence our future course of action." Strum and Rappaport (1971) reported that 40 percent of their 280 Hodgkin's patients (14 percent) survived 10 years or more. Twenty-nine of the 40 patients have died, and in 21 the cause of death was known. In 7 patients the cause of death could not be directly attributed to Hodgkin's disease but to conditions such as disseminated breast carcinoma, malignant melanoma; coronary occlusion; enteritis, nephritis, hepatitis, and pulmonary fibrosis secondary to radiation; pneumonia and systemic coccidioidomycosis.

Sherwood et al (1967) extracted a parathormone-like substance from a spleen involved with reticulum cell sarcoma. Klion (1972) discussed an unusual case of hypercalcemia and reticulum cell sarcoma involving multiple organs. At autopsy, an adenocarcinoma of the lung was found with additional multiple endocrine adenomatous syndrome which consisted of parathyroid hyperplasia, non-beta islet cell tumor of the pancreas, and adenomatous goiter. Brincker (1972) studied 19 cases showing sarcoid reactions in biopsy, selected from a series of 1500 cases with malignant lymphoma. Among the 19 patients, 5 had systemic sarcoidosis, 4 had associated malignancies (adenocarcinoma of the colon, 1; uterine cervix, 2; and squamous cancer of the lip, 1) and one had an autoimmune disease. He felt that "This remarkable association of sarcoid reactions or sarcoidosis with malignant lymphoma

Table 12-4
Operation for Malignant and Nongastrointestinal Complications of Non-Hodgkin's Lymphoma (EFSCH series)

Patient No.	Age	Sex	Date	Diagnosis	Primary lesions			Interval to op. (months)	Indication	Operation	Survival (* = alive)	Lymphoma at follow-up
					Radiotherapy	Chemotherapy	Sites					
19430	37	M	12-54	LPD	+	–	Mesentery	6	Ureter obstruction	Ureterostomy	1 mo	+
27893	45	F	2-62	Und	+	+	All nodes, bone	45	Pathologic fracture (femur)	Intramedullary nail fixation	2 mo	+
30125	67	M	12-65	HPD	+	+	Leg subcutaneous nodules	47	Recurrent satellosis	Celiotomy, insertion of iliac artery catheter	71 mo *	+
34837	17	F	2-66	Uc	+	+	Neck, mediastinum	6	Pancytopenia	Iliac bone biopsy	14 days	+
36654	35	F	8-67	HPD	–	–	Neck, mediastinum leg edema, viscera	1	Respiratory distress	Tracheostomy	7 days	+
24711	46	F	7-68	MC	+	+	Mesentery	127	Jaundice, hepatosplenomegaly	Liver biopsy, splenectomy, insertion of hepatic artery catheter	1 mo	+
36830	43	F	1-68	Und	+	–	Neck, bone	4	Jaundice	Exploration	1 mo	+
39025	47	F	7-71	LWD	+	–	Axilla, neck, pelvis, aortic	15	Chylothorax	Left thoracostomy	5 mo	+
			11-71	LWD	+	–	Axilla, neck, pelvis, aortic	19	Chylothorax	Right thoracostomy		

and associated malignancies seems to justify speculation on the possibility of a common etiological factor, e.g. in the form of an altered immune reaction.''

Rigby et al (1965) studied 63 patients with biopsy-proven leukemia and lymphoma and their closely related family members. Fifty-seven of the 63 patients had one or more blood relatives with malignant disease. The incidence of cancer was definitely increased in these particular families, since 161 of the 940 family members studied had neoplasms.

Berg (1967) conducted a prospective study of the incidence of multiple primary cancers among 1561 patients with leukemia, 1871 with lymphosarcoma, 1028 with Hodgkin's disease, and 207 with myeloma. In all, 95 further cancers were found during the 9840 patient-years of observation when only 45.4 were expected from the incidence rates for a population with similar sex and age distribution. Prostate, bladder, endometrial, and breast cancers were somewhat more frequent than expected. The greatest increase was in skin cancers: 6 were expected, whereas 43 patients developed over 60 asynchronous carcinomas. The minimum increases were ninefold in patients with leukemia, fourfold in lymphatic leukemia, 2½-fold in lymphosarcoma, and twofold in Hodgkin's disease. Among the patients with Hodgkin's disease, the incidence of previous cancer was 1.4 percent, of later clinical cancers 1.1 percent, and of cancers found at autopsy 0.3 percent. The comparable figures for those with lymphosarcoma and reticulum cell sarcoma were: 3.7 percent, 2.3 percent, and 0.7 percent.

Among the 56 second cancers coexisting with non-Hodgkin's lymphoma, Rosenberg et al (1961) found 4 cases of breast cancers. Herrmann (1971) reported that lymphoma might occur with a higher than usual incidence in patients who had breast cancer. Among his personal series of 387 women with carcinoma of the breast, there were 4 with associated diagnosis of lymphoma and 2 with leukemia (an incidence rate of 1.5 percent). The lymphoproliferative disease appeared subsequent to the breast cancer, 0 to 20 years later, and mimicked recurrent or metastatic breast cancer. From the literature, he found an incidence of 1 percent with associated breast cancer among 1744 reported patients with multiple malignant cancers and among 4648 cases of leukemia or lymphoma. All 6 patients had blood type A and were Rh positive. Hyman et al (1963) also found an apparent increase of blood type A among 21 patients with carcinoma of the colon associated with leukemia or lymphoma (65 percent with type A versus 35 percent type A in normal population or 38.7 percent of patients with colon-cancer alone).

There are many other papers reporting the increased frequency of certain blood groups in patients with various cancer and premalignant conditions, although so far the only statistically significant association was that of blood type A and stomach cancer. Several studies on the association of breast cancer and blood groups revealed conflicting results (Lee 1971a).

There were reports showing that the blood group distribution in patients with leukemia and Hodgkin's disease was the same as normal population (Buckwalter et al 1956; Tubiana 1971). De George (1970) found no difference in the distribution of ABO blood groups between age category or chronicity of leukemia in 581 patients with leukemia. However, he found higher Rh-negative frequencies among patients who were younger than 4 years old and more than 50 years old as compared with those between age 5 and 50.

The study of leucocyte histocompatibility antigens of the HL-A system has shown an increase of antigens of the 4C region in patients with Hodgkin's disease (Amiel 1967). However, it was later found that the associated specificities included in the 4C region were the factors HL-A5, W5, CM, or group 5 system with antigens 5a and 5b. Van Rood et al (1968), Zervas et al (1970), Morris and Forbes (1971), and Thorsby et al (1971) confirmed the increased frequency of leucocyte phenotype HL-A5. Other disturbances of HL-A frequencies in Hodgkin's disease were: significant excess of 5a but not of 5b, and decreased incidence of 4a (van Rood and van Leeuwen 1971); reduced frequency of HL-A3 (Coukell et al 1971); surplus of phenotype HL-A1, HL-A8 (Kissmeyer-Nielsen et al 1971; Falk and Osoba 1971), W15 (Jeannet et al 1971), and W18 (Bertrams et al 1972).

Apparently different histological subtypes of Hodgkin's disease might have different distribution of HL-A antigens. There is a frequent association of A1 and A8 with the mixed cellularity and lymphocyte predominance types of disease. In contrast, the frequencies of these specificities are not increased in patients with nodular sclerosis. Thus, Falk and Osoba (1971) stated that "the excess frequencies of A1 and A8 present in the whole Hodgkin's disease population are accounted for entirely by patients having the mixed cellularity or lymphocytic predominance patterns. Patients with nodular sclerosis have an increased frequency of A5 only."

In 127 patients with Hodgkin's disease and in relatives of 40 of these patients, very significant association was found between Hodgkin's disease and 2 antigens: HL-A11 and W5 (Morris and Forbes 1971, Forbes and Morris 1972). Antigen W5 was far more common in the male patients, especially those with lymphocyte predominance, whereas in female patients the increased frequency of HL-A11 was more marked with nodular sclerosis. A normal mendelian segregation of the relevant antigen was found in all 12 families of positive HL-A11 patients and in 6 of 8 families of W5-positive patients. These findings suggested that certain Hodgkin's patients not only had a genetically determined susceptibility to their disease, but the particular nature of their pathology might also have been predetermined.

Regarding the study of HL-A antigens in patients with non-Hodgkin's lymphoma, Jeannet and Magnin (1971) found an excess of W18 in such patients. Morris and Forbes (1971) and Forbes and Morris (1971) found that HL-A12 was markedly increased in patients with follicular lymphoma and reticulum cell sarcoma, whereas HL-A7 was significantly increased in patients with lymphosarcoma. Sybesma et al (1972) found that the frequency of HL-A7 and HL-A8 was higher among patients with Hodgkin's disease and other lymphomas than among control subjects. Rege et al (1972) found that the positive association of leucocyte antigens HL-A5 or W5 with Hodgkin's disease also might be extended to other types of lymphoma. This finding suggests that individuals with the leucocyte antigen HL-A5 or W5 on their tissue cells may have an increased tendency to develop one or another type of lymphoma. This poses the question of viral etiology of human lymphomas, since susceptibility of viral leukomogenesis in mice is associated with certain alleles of the H-2 locus; H-2 being analogous to the HL-A locus in man (Lilly 1966).

It is apparent that the association between malignant lymphoma with its heterogenous pathological types and subgroups and HL-A antigens is a complex one. Presently the terminology of different antigens in the HL-A system is not standardized. An interesting link of antigenic pattern and prognosis of patients with Hodgkin's disease was suggested by the report of Falk and Osoba (1971). They found an increased frequency of HL-antigens A1, A5, and A8 in 112 Hodgkin's patients as compared with 122 controls. In particular, A8 increased in frequency only· in those having the disease for more than 5 years, whereas the frequencies of A1 and A5 were high regardless of the duration of disease.

Garriga and Ghossein (1963) published the first report relating the radiation response of tissue to the ABO blood groups. Their results suggested that patients with type O blood as well as stages I and II carcinoma of the uterine cervix had a 20 percent higher 3-year survival rate than did patients with types A and B. Cook and Watson (1968) found that men with blood type AB and prostatic carcinoma had a more favorable prognosis. Among patients who had therapeutic castration for advanced carcinoma of the breast, Lee (1971b) found that patients with blood types B and AB had a higher objective response rate, even when all the factors known to effect the objective remission rate were considered. Patients with blood type O had the lowest response rate to therapeutic castration and the poorest prognosis. Among 1198 patients who had radical mastectomy for breast cancers, Donegan (1972) found that patients with the AB blood type had an exceptionally good survival rate, and those with blood type B, the poorest. The 5-year relative survival rates were 70.0 percent and 47.7 percent respectively, and the 10-year rates, 66.2 percent and 27 percent. Thus, it appears that investigations of therapeutic results and natural histories of cancer in human beings should not disregard the blood group factors and leucocyte antigens.

Spratt and Hoag (1966) studied the incidence of multiple primary cancers of 4318 patients with various neoplasms and 1000 consecutive persons with no cancer on first examination. All patients were seen from 1940 to 1961 at EFSCH and followed through 1964. Among the patients with neoplasms, 1130 had colorectal cancer, 1853 had cancer of the cervix uteri, 710 had breast cancer, 458 had lymphoma, and 167 had chronic leukemia. The results showed that prior cancer at these sites neither increased nor decreased the risk for developing additional neoplasms. The prevalence rate of simultaneous cancer was 3.77 percent and the average annual incidence of developing new cancer during follow-up was 1.06/100 patients. For patients who were 90 or over, the chance of having cancer was 51 percent; 17.5 percent would have 2 cancers, and 6.0 percent, 3 cancers.

In the present EFSCH series of 163 patients with histologically confirmed Hodgkin's disease and 364 patients with other malignant lymphoma seen from 1940 to 1971, 11 patients (2 percent) had neoplasms diagnosed simultaneously, or within 1 year, as lymphoma and 28 new tumors (6 percent) were diagnosed after the first year of follow-up (details are listed in Table 12-5). It needs to be pointed out that about 35 percent of the patients died during the first year after diagnosis of malignant lymphoma. In this series of 527 patients, 31 patients (5.9 percent) had 40 other malignancies diagnosed and treated at EFSCH before the diagnosis of malignant lymphoma.

From the surgical point of view, it is important to realize that a high proportion of the additional neoplasms needed surgical procedure for diagnosis and treatment (Table 12-6). Excluding skin cancers, out of the 7 malignant lesions diagnosed simultaneously as malignant lymphoma, 5 required radical surgical treatment for the coexisting neoplasms (cancers of the rectum, lip, pyriform sinus, lung, and breast) and one needed cold conization of the uterine cervix. Among the 6 nonskin cancers diagnosed during life, 2 had surgical treatment (radical mastectomy for breast cancer and hysterectomy for carcinoma of the uterine cervix) and 2 had endoscopic procedures (for cancer of the lung and bladder). All benign lesions diagnosed during life were excised surgically (4 rectal polyps, 3 benign breast tumors, and 1 thyroid adenoma).

SUMMARY

Hypersplenism is defined as any detrimental increase of splenic activity affecting the hematologic components. The result of splenectomy for hypersplenism secondary to malignant lymphoma is not as good as that for primary hypersplenism. The mortality for secondary hypersplenism is also higher than that for primary disorders (about 10 percent versus 2 percent). In patients with acquired hemolytic anemia or thrombocytopenia secondary to lymphomas, very worthwhile improvement with prolonged reduction in the need of transfusions have been reported in about 50 percent of the cases.

Table 12-5

Second Neoplasms in Patients with Malignant Lymphoma (EFSCH series)

I. 364 patients with non-Hodgkin's lymphoma

   A. Tumor diagnosed at EFSCH before diagnosis of non-Hodgkin's lymphoma.
      26   patients with 35 malignant lesions
           25   skin cancer
           9   other lesions
                3   colon (1, 6, 12 years before)
                2   breast (6, 7 years before)
                2   prostate (7, 11 years before)
                2   endometrium (5, 6 years before)
                1   uterine cervix (7 years before)*
      4   patients with benign lesions
           1   fibrous dysplasia of skull
           1   schwannoma of leg
           1   leiomyoma of uterus
           1   mixed tumor of parotid gland

   B. Cancer diagnosed simultaneously with non-Hodgkin's lymphoma
      8   patients with 10 malignant lesions
           4   skin cancer
           1   pyriform sinus squamous cancer
           1   lung cancer (7 years after pelvic exenteration for cancer of cervix)*
           1   breast cancer
           1   lip cancer
           1   uterine cervix cancer
           1   rectal cancer

   C. Second tumor diagnosed after diagnosis of non-Hodgkin's lymphoma
      16   patients with malignant lesions
          11   skin cancer
          5   other lesions
               1   endometrium (5 years later)
              1   breast (11 years later)
              1   carcinoma in situ of cervix (5 years later)
              1   bladder transitional cell cancer (2 years later)
              1   lung cancer (3.5 years later)
      7   patients with benign lesions
          4   rectal polyps
          2   breast papilloma
          1   thyroid adenoma
      8   patients had tumors diagnosed at autopsy
          1   endometrium cancer
          1   sigmoid colon cancer
          1   lung cancer
          2   prostate cancer
          1   leiomyoma-stomach
          1   leiomyoma-uterus
          1   Brenner's tumor—ovary

Table 12-5 *(continued)*

II.	163 patients with Hodgkin's disease		
	5	tumors diagnosed before Hodgkin's disease at EFSCH	
		3	skin cancer
		1	hemartoma of gall bladder (2 years before)
		1	breast cancer (11 years before)
	3	cancers diagnosed simultaneously	
		2	skin cancer
		1	carcinoma in situ of cervix
	5	tumors diagnosed afterwards	
		3	skin cancer
		1	breast fibroadenoma
		1	cervix cancer

It is reported that about 4 percent of all patients with Hodgkin's disease required splenectomy for splenomegaly and hypersplenism. When hypersplenism occurs early in the course of the disease, splenectomy improves the prognosis. When the disease is advanced, the operative mortality and postoperative complication rates become too high (about 30 percent). Patients with lymphosarcoma appear to have better results after splenectomy than those with Hodgkin's disease. It is apparent that if pretreatment staging laparotomy and splenectomy become routine practice for patients with malignant lymphoma, the problem of splenomegaly and hypersplenism would automatically disappear in the future.

With the prolongation of survival resulting from improved radiotherapy and chemotherapy, it is to be expected that a higher percentage of patients may have time to develop new problems, either associated or unassociated with malignant lymphoma. In addition to hypersplenism, malignant complications that require surgical intervention include gastrointestinal and genitourinary involvement, perforation of abdominal viscus, massive hemorrhage, obstructive jaundice, tracheal obstruction, chylothorax, and spinal cord compressions. Complications secondary to radiation therapy that require surgical corrections include enteritis pericarditis, osteonecrosis, soft tissue fibrosis, and skin ulcerations. Patients with nonmalignant conditions should be treated just like patients without malignant lymphoma.

In a large series of patients with non-Hodgkin's lymphoma, additional cancers were diagnosed during life in 3.4 percent of the cases, and at autopsy in 6.1 percent (Rosenberg et al 1961). Among patients with Hodgkin's disease, the figures were lower (about 1.1 percent and 0.3 percent, respectively). Berg (1967) found that patients with malignant lymphoma had a more than twofold increase in the incidence of skin cancers when compared to a control population. There has been a higher frequency of patients with blood type A among those who had malignant lymphoma and carcinoma of the colon or breast. In the EFSCH series of 527 patients with malignant lymphoma,

Table 12-6
Operations for Second Cancer (EFSCH series)

Patient No.	Age	Sex	Date	Diagnosis	Radiotherapy (rads)	Chemotherapy	Sites	Interval (months)	Activity	Site	Diagnosis	Operation	Survival (months) * = alive	Lymphoma at follow-up
					Primary lymphoma					Second cancer				
15243	69	M	7-51	LWD	2100	–	Groin, axilla	2	+	Rectum	Adenoca	A-P resection Noble plication	14	?
18935	57	M	3-54	LWN		–	Neck	0	+	Lip	Squamous	Radical neck dissection	91	+
26842	34	F	8-59	HD (NS)		–	Neck, axilla	0	+	Cervix	Carcinoma in situ	Cold conization	59	+
31826	60	M	9-63	MC		–	Neck	0	+	Pyriform sinus	Squamous	Laryngectomy and radical neck dissection	9	+
21257	61	F	5-66	Und	2100	–	Mesentery	130	–	Breast	Adenoca	Radical mastectomy	65	–
24861	72	F	6-67	LPD		–	Groin	9	–	Lung	Squamous	Pneumonectomy	29	–
36548	71	F	6-67	UC		–	Axilla	0	+	Breast	Ductal carcinoma	Radical mastectomy	2	+
36319	43	F	10-68	HPD	4000	+	Mesentery	42	–	Lung	Squamous	Bronchoscopy and biopsy	1	–
36677	66	M	9-69	HWD	4500	–	Neck, mediastinum	25	–	Bladder	Transitional cell carcinoma	Cystoscopy and resection	23*	?
39463	45	F	10-70	LWN	3000	+	Groin	65	+	Cervix	Carcinoma in situ	Hysterectomy	11	+

2 percent had a second cancer diagnosed simultaneously and another 6 percent developed additional cancers subsequently. Excluding skin cancers, more than two-thirds of the additional cancers required major surgical procedures for diagnosis and treatment.

REFERENCES

Amiel JL: Study of the leukocyte phenotypes in Hodgkin's disease, in Curton ES, Mattiuz PL, Tosi MR (eds): Histocompatibility Testing, 1967. Copenhagen, Munksgaard, 1967, pp 79–81

Ashby WB, Ballinger WF II: Indications for splenectomy: Changing concepts as a result of advances in hematology. Arch Surg 85:913–927, 1962

Berg JW: The incidence of multiple primary cancers. I. Development of further cancers in patients with lymphomas, leukemias, and myeloma. J Natl Cancer Inst 38:741–752, 1967

Bertrams J, Kuwert E, Böhme U, et al: HL-A antigens in Hodgkin's disease and multiple myeloma: Increased frequency of W18 in both diseases. Tissue Antigens 2:41–46, 1972

Bouroncle BA, Old JW Jr, Vazques AG: Pathogenesis of jaundice in Hodgkin's disease. Arch Intern Med 110:872–883, 1962

Bowdler AJ, Glick IW: Autoimmune hemolytic anemia as the herald state of Hodgkin's disease. Ann Intern Med 65:761–767, 1966

Brincker H: Sarcoid reactions and sarcoidosis in Hodgkin's disease and other malignant lymphomata. Br J Cancer 26:120–128, 1972

Buckwalter JA, Wohlwend EB, Colter DC, et al: ABO blood groups and disease. JAMA 162:1210–1215, 1956

Catlin D: Surgery for head and neck lymphomas. Surgery 60:1160–1166, 1966

Cole WH, Majarakis JD, Limarzi LR: Surgical aspects of splenic disease. Arch Surg 71:33–46, 1955

Cook GB, Watson FR: Events in the natural history of prostate cancer: Using salvage curves, mean age distributions and contingency coefficients. J Urol 99:87–96, 1968

Cooper IA: Clinical presentation of reticulum-cell sarcoma: A disease with many faces. Med J Aust 1:697–704, 1970

Coukell A, Bodmer JG, Bodmer WF: HL-A types of 44 Hodgkin's patients. Transplant Proc 3:1291–1293, 1971

Craver LF, Sunderland DA: Hodgkin's disease and carcinoma of colon: Mistaken diagnosis of carcinoma of stomach. JAMA 114:1623–1625, 1940

Crosby WH: Hypersplenism. Ann Rev Med 13:127–146, 1962

Crosby WH: Indications for splenectomy. Hosp Pract 2:28–33, Aug 2967

Crosby WH, Whelan TJ, Heaton LD: Splenectomy in the elderly. Med Clin North Am 50:1533–1558, 1966

DeVita VT: Hodgkin's disease. Lancet 2: 46–47, 1971

Dawson IM, Cornes JS, Morson BC: Primary malignant lymphoid tumours of the intestinal tract: Report of 37 cases with a study of factors influencing prognosis. Br J Surg 49:80–89, 1961

Doan CA, Bruce MD, Wiseman BK: Hypersplenic cytopenic syndromes: A 25 year experience with special reference to splenectomy. Proceedings of the Sixth International Congress of the International Society of Hematology, 1956. New York, Grune and Stratton, 1958, pp 429–442

Donegan WL: Mastectomy in the primary management of invasive mammary carcinoma, in Hardy JD (ed): Advances in Surgery, vol 6. Chicago, Year Book, 1972, pp 1–101

Duckett JW: Splenectomy in treatment of secondary hypersplenism. Ann Surg 157: 737–746, 1963

Eisner E, Ley AB, Mayer K: Coombs'-positive hemolytic anemia in Hodgkin's disease. Ann Intern Med 66:258–273, 1967

Everson TC, Cole WH: Ligation of splenic artery in patients with portal hypertension. Arch Surg 56:153–160, 1948

Falk J, Osoba D: HL-A antigens and survival in Hodgkin's disease. Lancet 2:1118–1120, 1971

Fisher JH, Welch CS, Dameshek W: Splenectomy in leukemia and leukosarcoma. N Engl J Med 246:477–484, 1952

Forbes JF, Morris PJ: Analysis of HL-A antigens in patients with Hodgkin's disease and their families. J Clin Invest 51:1156–1163, 1972

Forbes JF, Morris PJ: Transplantation antigens and malignant lymphomas in man: Follicular lymphoma, reticulum cell sarcoma and lymphosarcoma. Tissue Antigens 1:265–269, 1971

Garriga R, Ghossein NA: The ABO blood groups and their relation to the radiation response in carcinoma of the cervix. Cancer 16:170–172, 1963

Gellhorn A: A new look at lymphomas. Postgrad Med 43:136–141, 1968

George FV de: Differences in Rh type between age groups of leukemia patients. Nature 228:168–169, 1970

Gomes MM, Silverstein MN, ReMine WH: Indications for splenectomy in hematologic diseases. Surg Gynecol Obstet 129:129–139, 1969

Grace JT Jr, Mittelman A: Surgery in the management of Hodgkin's disease. Cancer 19:351–355, 1966

Hacker, V von: Demonstration eines milztumors (primares Sarkom), welces von prof. Billroth, am. 20. Marz. d. J. mit glucklichen Erfalge durch laparotomic entfernt wurd. Verh Dtsch Ges Pathol 13:30, 1884

Hansen HS: Reticulum cell sarcoma treated by radiotherapy. Acta Radiol [Ther] (Stockh) 8:439–458, 1969

Herrmann JB: Lymphoproliferative disease secondary to breast cancer. NY State J Med 71:1108–1111, 1971

Holt JM, Witts LJ: Splenectomy in leukaemia and the reticuloses. Q J Med 35:369–384, 1966

Hyman GA, Ultmann JE, Slanetz CA Jr: Chronic lymphocytic leukemia or lymphoma and carcinoma of the colon: Correlation with blood type A. JAMA 186:1053–1056, 1963

Hyatt DF, Skarin AT, Moloney WC, et al: Splenectomy for lymphosarcoma. Surg Gynecol Obstet 131:928–932, 1970

Jackson H Jr, Parker F Jr: Hodgkin's disease and Allied Disorders. New York, Oxford University Press, 1947

Jeannet M, Alberto P, Wyss M: Antigènes HL-A et affections hematologiques malignes. Schweiz Med Wochenschr 101:1798–1800, 1971

Jeannet M, Magnin C: HL-A antigens in malignant diseases. Trans Proc 3:1301–1303, 1971

Jelliffe AM, Thomson AD: Prognosis in Hodgkin's disease. Br J Cancer 9:21–36, 1955

Kissmeyer-Nielsen F, Jensen KB, Ferrara GB, et al: HL-A phenotypes in Hodgkin's disease: Preliminary report. Trans Proc 3:1287–1289, 1971

Klion FM: Reticulum cell sarcoma and hypercalcemia in an elderly woman. Mt Sinai J Med NY 39:202–212, 1972

Kyle RA, Kiely JM, Stickney JM: Acquired hemolytic anemia in chronic lymphocytic leukemia and the lymphomas. Arch Intern Med 104:61–67, 1959

Lacher MJ: Long survival in Hodgkin's disease. Ann Intern Med 70:7–17, 1969

Lee YN: The ABO blood groups and cancer. Surg Gynecol Obstet 132:1093–1097, 1971a

Lee YN: The ABO blood groups and results of therapeutic oophorectomy for advanced carcinoma of the breast. Surg Gynecol Obstet 132:871–875, 1971b

Lilly F: The histocompatibility-2 locus and susceptibility to tumor induction. Natl Cancer Inst Monograph 22:631–641, 1966

Lipton A, Lee BJ: Prognosis of Stage I lymphosarcoma and reticulum-cell sarcoma. N Engl J Med 284:230–233, 1971

Lowenbraun S, Ramsey HE, Serpick AA: Splenectomy in Hodgkin's disease for splenomegaly, cytopenias and intolerance to myelosuppressive chemotherapy. Am J Med 50:49–55, 1971

Mayo WJ: Review of 500 splenectomies with special reference to mortality and end results. Ann Surg 88:409–415, 1928

Meeker WR J dePerio JM, Grace JT Jr, et al: The role of splenectomy in malignant lymphoma and leukemia. Surg Clin North Am 47:1163–1171, 1967

Mittelman A, Elias EG, Wieckowska W, et al: Splenectomy in patients with malignant lymphoma or chronic leukemia. Cancer Bull 22:10–13, 1970

Molander DW, Pack GT: Lymphosarcoma: Choice of treatment and end-results in 567 patients. Role of surgical treatment for cure and palliation. Rev Surg 20:3–31, 1963

Moore RM, Singleton AO, Pickett WH: Splenic artery ligation in palliation of ascites. Ann Surg 131:774–780, 1950

Morris PJ, Forbes JF: HL-A in follicular lymphoma, reticulum cell sarcoma, lymphosarcoma, and infectious mononucleosis. Trans Proc 3:1315–1316, 1971

Munnell ER: Current concepts of thoracic surgery in the management of lymphoma. Ann Thorac Surg 11:151–159, 1971

Nies BA, Creger WP: Tolerance of chemotherapy following splenectomy for leukopenia or thrombocytopenia in patients with malignant lymphomas. Cancer 20:558–562, 1967

Nuland SB, Cornelius EA, Spencer RP: Scan evidence of organ involution and improvement of hypersplenism in Hodgkin's disease following splenic artery ligation. J Nucl Med 11:692–694, 1970

O'Brien PH, Hartz WH Jr, Derlacki D, et al: Splenectomy for hypersplenism in malignant lymphoma. Arch Surg 101:348–352, 1970

Pack GT, Molander DW: The surgical treatment of Hodgkin's disease. Cancer Res 26:1254–1263, 1966

Papp JP, Penner JA: Spontaneous splenic rupture in lymphoma: Report of 3 cases. South Med J 64:631–632, 1971

Rambo WM, Richardson SN: Indications for splenectomy in hematologic disease. Am Surg 34:579–584, 1968

Rappaport H, Crosby WH: Auto-immune hemolytic anemia. II. Morphologic observations and clinicopathologic correlations. Am J Pathol 33:429–458, 1957

Rege V, Patel R, Briggs WA: Leucocyte antigens and disease. II. Association of HL-A5 and lymphomas. Am J Clin Pathol 58:14–16, 1972

Rigby PG, Rosenlof RC, Pratt P: Rural leukemia and lymphoma. Proc Am Assoc Cancer Res 6:54, 1965 (Abstr)

Rodd JJ van, Leeuwen A van: HL-A and the group five system in Hodgkin's disease. Trans Proc 3:1283–1286, 1971

Rood JJ van, Leeuwen A van, Schippers A, et al: Human histocompatibility antigens in normal and neoplastic tissues. Cancer Res 28:1415–1422, 1968

Rosenberg SA, Diamond HD, Jaslowitz B, et al: Lymphosarcoma: A review of 1269 cases. Medicine 40:31–84, 1961

Rosenthal MC, Pisciotta AV, Komninos ZD, et al: The autoimmune hemolytic anemia of malignant lymphocytic disease. Blood 10:197–227, 1955

Rousselot LM, Rella AJ, Rottino A: Splenectomy for hypersplenism in Hodgkin's disease: A reappraisal. Am J Surg 103:769–774, 1962

Rudders RA, Aisenberg AC, Schiller AL: Hodgkin's disease presenting as "idiopathic" thrombocytopenic purpura. Cancer 30:220–230, 1972

Sandusky WR, Leavell BS, Benjamin BI: Splenectomy: Indications and results in hematologic disorders. Ann Surg 159:695–710, 1964

Schultz JC, Denny WF, Ross SW: Splenectomy in leukemia and lymphoma: Report of 24 cases. Am J Med Sci 247:30–35, 1964

Schwartz SI, Adams JT, Bauman AW: Splenectomy for hematologic disorders. Curr Probl Surg 1–57, May 1971

Schwartz SI, Bernard RP, Adams JT, et al: Splenectomy for hematologic disorders. Arch Surg 101:338–347, 1970

Scott RB: The surgical aspects of the lymphomata. Ann R Coll Surg Engl 22:178–196, 1958

Sedgwick CE, Hume AH: Elective splenectomy: An analysis of 220 operations. Ann Surg 151:163–168, 1960

Sherwood LM, O'Riordan JL, Aurbach GD, et al: Production of parathyroid hormone by nonparathyroid tumors. J Clin Endocrinol 27:140–146, 1967

Slaughter DP, Economou SG, Southwick HW: Surgical management of Hodgkin's disease. Ann Surg 148:705–710, 1958

Sloane GL, Averbook BD, Kaplan MR: Splenectomy in hematologic disorders. Am J Surg 104:94–103, 1962

Spratt JS Jr, Hoag MG: Incidence of multiple primary cancers per man-year of followup: 20-year review from the Ellis Fisckel State Cancer Hospital. Ann Surg 164:775–784, 1966

Strawitz JG, Sokal JE, Grace JT Jr, et al: Surgical aspects of hypersplenism in lymphoma and leukemia. Surg Gynecol Obstet 112:89–95, 1961

Strum SB, Rappaport H: The persistence of Hodgkin's disease in long-term survivors. Am J Med 51:222–240, 1971

Strumia MM, Strumia PV, Bassert D: Splenectomy in leukemia: Hematologic and clinical effects of 34 patients and review of 299 published cases. Cancer Res 26:519–528, 1966

Sybesma JP, Borst-Eilers E, Holtzer JD: HL-A antigens in Hodgkin's disease and other lymphomas. Vox Sang 22:319–324, 1972

Sykes MP, Karnofsky DA, McNeer GP, et al: Splenectomy in far-advanced Hodgkin's disease: Report of five cases. Blood 9:824–36, 1954

Thorsby E, Falk J, Engeseth A, et al: HL-A antigens in Hodgkin's disease. Trans Proc 3:1279–1281, 1971

Tillman HH: Malignant lymphomas involving the oral cavity and surrounding structures: Report of twelve cases. Oral Surg 19:60–72, 1965

Tubiana M, Attie E, Flamant R, et al: Prognostic factors in 454 cases of Hodgkin's disease. Cancer Res 31:1801–1810, 1971

Welch CS, Dameshek W: Splenectomy in blood dyscrasias. N Engl J Med 242:601–606, 1950

Williams RD, Andrews NC, Zanes RP: Major surgery in Hodgkin's disease. Surg Gynecol Obstet 93:636–640, 1951

Wiseman BK, Doan CA: A newly recognized granulopenic syndrome caused by excessive splenic leukolysis successfully treated by splenectomy. J Clin Invest 18:473, 1939 (Abstr.)

Zervas JD, Delamore IW, Israëls MC: Leucocyte phenotypes in Hodgkin's disease. Lancet 2:634–635, 1970

Zollinger RM, Martin MM, Williams RD: Surgical aspects of hypersplenism. JAMA 149:24–29, 1952

Zollinger RM, Williams RD: Surgery of the spleen. Minn Med 42:881–887, 1959

Zubrod CG: Summary of informal discussion on radiation therapy for Hodgkin's disease. Cancer Res 26:1264–1267, 1966

Index

3 a
4 b
5 c
6 d
7 e
8 f
9 g
0 h
1 i
8 2 j